Penelope Quest is a qualified teacher with 15 years' experience as a lecturer and senior manager in further and higher education, where she taught mainly marketing, management, communication and personal development. Her academic qualifications include a Masters Degree in Health and Healing Science, and a BA in Psychology and Education.

She first became interested in Reiki in 1990, taking the first and second levels of training in 1991 and 1992, and then worked part-time as a Reiki Practitioner for several years before becoming a Reiki Master/Teacher of both the Usui Shiki Ryoho and Usui/Tibetan traditions in 1994, and a Karuna Reiki Master in 1996. Since then, she has taught Reiki to thousands of students, and in 2000 and 2003 she gained further experience and qualifications in the original Reiki techniques and training methods from the Japanese traditions and lineage. In addition she has extended her knowledge by studying a wide range of other subjects, including meditation; neurolinguistic programming (NLP); Emotional Freedom Technique (EFT); sound healing; Shamanism; dowsing; feng shui; kinesiology and other topics that promote understanding, personal growth and a holistic view of the person.

Her books – *The Basics of Reiki*; *Self-Healing with Reiki*; *Living the Reiki Way*; and *The Reiki Manual*, as well as *Reiki for Life* – have become bestsellers in the UK and internationally. She is a former Vice-chairman and Education Co-ordinator for the UK Reiki Federation, and was involved with the RRWG (Reiki Regulatory Working Group, now called the Reiki Council) during the initial process of formulating the new guidelines for professional Reiki practice. She has also been a consultant on Reiki for both the Open University and the NHS, and now teaches Reiki and leads occasional shamanic retreats and workshops on personal and spiritual development, energy psychology, earth energies and abundance theory.

Also by Penelope Quest

The Basics of Reiki
Living the Reiki Way
Self-healing with Reiki
The Reiki Manual
(with Kathy Roberts)

REIKI
FOR LIFE

The Complete Guide to Reiki Practice for
Levels 1, 2 and 3

PENELOPE QUEST

piatkus

PIATKUS

First published in Great Britain in 2002 by Piatkus Books
Reprinted 2002, 2003 (twice), 2004 (twice), 2005, 2006 (three times),
2007 (three times), 2009, 2010, 2011
This fully updated and expanded edition 2012
Reprinted 2013, 2014

A CIP catalogue record for this book
is available from the British Library.

ISBN 978-0-7499-5658-5

Illustrations by Rodney Paull

Typeset in Baskerville by Phoenix Photosetting, Chatham, Kent
Printed and bound in Great Britain by
Clays Ltd, St Ives plc

Papers used by Piatkus are from well-managed forests
and other responsible sources.

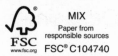

MIX
Paper from
responsible sources
FSC® C104740

Piatkus
An imprint of
Little, Brown Book Group
100 Victoria Embankment
London EC4Y 0DY

An Hachette UK Company
www.hachette.co.uk

www.piatkus.co.uk

Dedication

This book is dedicated to Mikao Usui, without whom the world would not have received the wonderful gift of Reiki.

Disclaimer

This book gives non-specific, general advice and should not be relied on as a substitute for proper medical consultation. Reiki does not replace normal allopathic medical treatment; it helps to enhance the process of harmony of the mind, body, emotions and spirit, and is a means of supporting and complementing medical treatment. If you have any acute or chronic disease you should consult a qualified medical practitioner.

While all suggested treatments are offered in good faith, the author and publisher accept no liability for damage of any nature resulting directly or indirectly from the application or use of information in this book, or from the failure to seek medical advice from a doctor.

Contents

Part 4: Your Continuing Steps Along the Reiki Path

Part 5: The Japanese Tradition

Acknowledgements

I would like to express my heartfelt gratitude to the many people who have helped, directly or indirectly, with this book:

To Kristin Bonney, who started me on my Reiki journey and set me a good example to follow; to William Lee Rand, who initiated me as a Master in Usui Reiki, Usui/Tibetan Reiki and Karuna Reiki®, and who encouraged me to always be myself in Reiki; to Sensei Hiroshi Doi, and his students Andrew Bowling and Richard Rivard, for helping me to gain knowledge and experience of the original Japanese techniques; to Frank Arjava Petter and Chetna Kobayashi, for bringing the first translations of Mikao Usui's and Chujiro Hayashi's original Reiki manuals to the West; to the UK Reiki Federation and The Reiki Council (formerly the RRWG) for the information on Practitioner training issues; to the many spiritual teachers who have guided and inspired me, especially Gill Edwards, Esther and Jerry Hicks, Neale Donald Walsch, Caroline Myss, Donna Eden and Dr David R. Hamilton; to my friend and fellow Reiki Master Helen Galpin, for allowing me to use some of her meditations; to the many Reiki Masters I have known, who have unselfishly shared their knowledge and experience with me; to all my Reiki students, for the love and learning they have brought me; and to my son, Chris, and daughter, Kathy, for their loving support.

Introduction

When I wrote the first edition of this book in 2001, I had by then been using Reiki for ten years, and it was an exciting time for the Reiki community in the West, because a few years earlier some new information had finally come out of Japan, mostly due to the German Reiki Master, Frank Arjava Petter, who was living in Japan at that time, and to a Japanese Reiki Master who had also trained in Western Reiki techniques, Hiroshi Doi. We learned much more about the origins of Reiki and its founder, Mikao Usui, as well as many methods for using Reiki that had not, until then, been known by Western Reiki Masters (teachers). I had attended the very first Japanese Reiki Techniques workshop in the UK in May 2000, taught by one of Hiroshi Doi's students, so I was able to include what I had learned in that first edition.

Ten years later, as I write this updated and expanded edition of *Reiki for Life*, it is perhaps an even more exciting time for the Reiki community, because we now have access to even more details about the way Reiki is practised and taught in Japan, and I feel very privileged to have had the opportunity to do further training to qualify as a *Shihan*, the term used for a teacher of the Japanese Reiki traditions. In addition, in recent years I have successfully studied for a Master of Science degree in Health and Healing Science, and have been fortunate enough to meet and learn from some of the leading scientific and spiritual teachers in the field of mind–body connection and holistic health–healing, such as Gill Edwards, Esther and Jerry Hicks, Byron Katie, Brandon Bays, Jan de Vries, Dr Rosy Daniel, Leo Rutherford, Tim Wheater and Dr David Hamilton, among others. Another advantageous experience was the time I spent in 2005 and 2006 on the Reiki Regulatory Working Group's Education and Accreditation Committee, helping to produce an acceptable Core Curriculum for Reiki Practitioner training in the UK.

One of my core beliefs is that information is empowering, which is why I was keen to share some of my increased knowledge and experience with the readers of one of my most successful books, *Reiki for Life*. This has become an internationally acclaimed classic text on Reiki, hence this new revised edition, which also includes many more illustrations, which I hope you'll find helpful.

I originally chose the title for this book because it reflects my understanding of Reiki:

1   Once you have acquired the ability to access Reiki healing energy, you retain that ability for the rest of your life.

2   Because Reiki promotes healing and well-being for the whole person, it is definitely a practice that is 'for' an improved life.

3   The title also reflects the fact that Reiki can potentially transform your life, as it stimulates personal and spiritual growth, encourages healthy changes in lifestyle, increases inspiration and intuition, and brings about realisations of our deeper, spiritual nature, which can be powerful and life-changing.

This new revised edition of *Reiki for Life* is therefore aimed at anyone interested in healing and self-healing with Reiki at any level, from absolute beginners to Practitioners and Masters. Unlike other books on Reiki, it uniquely explores the true depth, power and promise of this wonderful healing system, but I hope it also demystifies it, presenting it in an understandable and easy-to-read way. The book is divided into five parts:

Part 1 begins by explaining what Reiki is, how it was discovered and how it links with other energies in humans, animals, plants and the rest of the environment. It outlines some of the latest fascinating research into energy, healing and the mind–body connection, discusses the processes of healing from both conventional and non-traditional viewpoints, and provides comprehensive information about Reiki training, including what to expect on courses at each of the three levels – First Degree, Second Degree and Third Degree/ Master.

Part 2 covers everything you need to know at Reiki First Degree, including methods for self-healing and all the hand positions for treatments on yourself and on other people, how to use Reiki with animals, plants and even inanimate objects, as well as some creative ways of using Reiki, such as working on personal problems or world situations.

In Part 3 there is a thorough explanation of the real impact and creative power of Second Degree, and I have included much more information about the three Reiki Second Degree symbols, including how to use them for self-healing, for 'hands-on' treatments on others, and how to carry out distant healing, including ways of 'sending' a Reiki treatment to anyone, anywhere, at any time, with the same effectiveness as a 'hands-on' treatment. A wide range of other advanced techniques are included, too, such as using Reiki to empower goals, heal emotional problems, create sacred space, and to protect yourself and those you care about.

Part 4 looks at methods for cleansing and clearing your personal and environmental energies and the increasing importance of spiritual development as you progress along your path with Reiki. It also discusses what is needed to set up as a professional Practitioner, including an outline of the recently introduced National Occupational Standards for Reiki in the UK, as well as the role and responsibilities of a Reiki Master and how to train at that level.

Part 5 introduces the latest and most comprehensive information about the Japanese way of training in Reiki, including the spiritual practices and techniques taught at each of the three Japanese levels, *Shoden*, *Okuden* and *Shinpiden*, roughly equivalent to the Western Reiki 1, 2 and Master. These include meditations, special methods for self-cleansing and removing toxins from the mind and body, as well as alternative ways of using Reiki, such as patting or stroking with the hands, or using the breath or the eyes to deliver Reiki during treatments. I've also included a list of different styles of Reiki in the Appendix.

This book provides an essential resource for Reiki practice in the 21st century, and its aim is to help anyone at any level to reach their full potential as a healing channel for Reiki. The emphasis throughout *Reiki for Life* is therefore on enjoying the healing and self-healing benefits of Reiki, and having fun being creative with it, while still treating it with the respect it deserves as one of the world's most precious gifts for healing and spiritual growth.

Whether you're only just exploring the idea of Reiki for the first time by reading this book, or whether you've already done one or more Reiki courses, I hope Reiki brings you as much healing and joyful satisfaction as it has brought me.

With Reiki blessings,
Penelope Quest

Part I

Simplicity and Power: Reiki Healing Energy

Chapter 1

The Discovery of Reiki

WHAT IS REIKI?

Reiki is a safe, gentle, non-intrusive hands-on healing technique for use on yourself or with others, which uses spiritual energy to treat physical ailments without using pressure, manipulation or massage; however, it is much more than a physical therapy. It is a holistic system for balancing, healing and harmonising all aspects of the person – body, mind, emotions and spirit – and it can also be used to encourage personal and spiritual awareness and growth. In this chapter we deal with the meaning of the word Reiki, how, when and where Reiki was discovered, and how it has developed as a healing system both in the West and in Japan where it originated.

THE WORD REIKI

The Japanese word *Reiki* (pronounced 'Ray Kee') is often translated as 'universal life-force energy', but a more accurate version is 'spiritual energy'. The word is divided into two parts:

Rei is translated as 'sacred', 'soul' or 'spirit', the 'wisdom and knowledge of all the Universe' or 'atmosphere of the Divine'. It means the Higher Intelligence that guides the creation and functioning of the universe; the wisdom that comes from God (or the Source, the Creator, the Universe or All That Is), that is, all-knowing, and which understands the need for, and the cause of all, problems and difficulties, and how to heal them.

Ki is the life-force energy which flows through every living thing – plants, animals and people – and which is present in some form in everything around us, even in rocks and inanimate objects.

Reiki is represented in the Japanese *kanji* calligraphy in two slightly different ways. The image on the left is the more modern form, while that on the right is an older and more traditional way of writing the word Reiki.

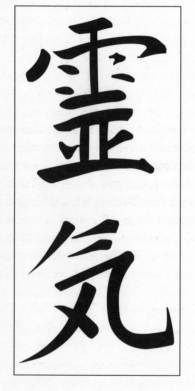 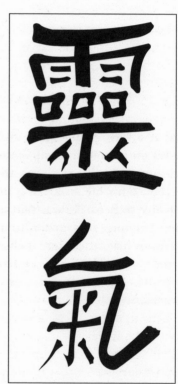

Modern kanji *for* Rei Ki   *Older* kanji *for* Rei Ki

In Japan, the word Reiki can be used to describe any form of healing using spiritual energy, but in the West when we talk about Reiki we are usually referring to the form of healing practice developed by a Japanese Buddhist priest, Dr Mikao Usui (1865–1926), who, after many years of study, discovered a way of accessing and using this healing energy, and of passing this ability on to other people. During the last few years of his life he founded a healing system called Usui Reiki Ryoho, which means the Usui Spiritual Energy

Healing Method, and this has become widely known throughout the world simply as 'Reiki'.

HOW REIKI CAME TO THE WEST

Reiki as a healing system has been used and taught in the West since the late 1930s and until the early 1990s the story of how Reiki was discovered was an oral history, handed down from teacher to student in a very traditional way. There is more accurate information about the Japanese origins of Reiki in a later section, but the story originally told to Reiki students in the West was that Dr Mikao Usui was a learned scholar who taught in a Christian seminary. One day he was challenged by one of his students, who asked him if he believed in the Bible stories of Jesus' healing, and, if so, when were they going to be taught how to heal? It was said that, as an honourable Japanese gentleman, upon realising that he could not teach his students any healing techniques, he dedicated the rest of his life to finding out how Jesus and the Buddha had been able to heal. He was said to have travelled widely and learned other languages in order to research both Christian scriptures and Buddhist teachings, including Japanese and Sanskrit Sutras (sacred texts). He finally ended up in a Zen Buddhist monastery where the Abbot advised him to meditate to find the answers he was seeking.

Then, at the end of a 21-day fasting retreat Mikao Usui was apparently struck by a great light. He saw the sacred symbols he had earlier found during his research, and he acquired a deep understanding of them, receiving a spiritual empowerment (empower means 'to give to' or 'to enable', and a spiritual empowerment means to transfer wisdom, insight and ability by means of an inpouring of spiritual energy) and achieving enlightenment, a state of spiritual insight brought on by joining with and becoming one with the Light. When it was over, despite weakness after his long fast, he was able to rush down the mountain, but he injured his foot in his haste. When he bent down to hold his toe he found that the bleeding stopped and the pain went away and he was healed. Later he healed a young girl's toothache and his friend the Abbot's arthritis, so he came to a realisation that he had finally discovered the healing power for which he had been searching.

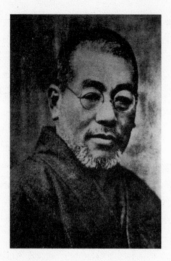

Mikao Usui

The story then told that he spent many years healing people in Japan before passing his knowledge and teachings on to Dr Chujiro Hayashi (1879–1940), a naval commander. After Usui's death, Hayashi was said to have opened a Reiki clinic, the Hayashi Reiki Kenkyu Kai (Hayashi Spiritual Energy Society). One day in 1935, a young woman from Hawaii, called Hawayo Takata (1900–80), who was visiting relatives in Japan, came to the clinic to be healed of a serious illness. She was so impressed with the success of her treatment that she begged to be able to learn Reiki, and Hayashi eventually agreed to teach her. She lived with his family and worked without pay in his clinic in exchange for the privilege of being able to learn the first and second levels of this healing system. She returned to Hawaii in 1937 and opened the first Reiki clinic in the West, where Hayashi and his family visited her. He passed on the final level of the Reiki teachings in 1938 before he returned to Japan, so that she would be able to teach this healing art to others.

The story Mrs Takata told was that during World War II Hayashi and all of his Reiki students in Japan were killed, and she was therefore the only Reiki teacher alive. Mrs Takata continued to teach Reiki and run her clinic in Hawaii, but also travelled extensively throughout the US and Canada, treating people with Reiki and training them in how to use Reiki for themselves. She held classes in two levels of Reiki training, which she called First Degree and Second Degree; however, it was the 1970s before she began to impart the final level of teachings, the Third Degree, which she called Reiki Master (a rough translation of *Sensei*, meaning respected teacher in Japanese) so that others would be able to pass on the teachings when she had gone. By the time of her death in December 1980, after 42 years of teaching Reiki, she had trained 22 Masters, and it is through them that Reiki has spread so widely throughout the Western world:

George Araki
Dorothy Baba
Ursula Baylow
Rick Bockner
Patricia Bowling
Barbara Brown
Fran Brown
Phyllis Furumoto
Beth Gray
John Gray
Iris Ishikuro

Harru Kuboi
Ethel Lombardi
Barbara McCullough
Mary McFadyen
Paul Mitchell
Bethel Phaigh
Shinobu Saito
Virginia Samdahl
Wanja Twan
Barbara Weber Ray
Kay Yamashita

THE TRADITIONAL WESTERN SYSTEM OF REIKI

Mrs Takata established a system of teaching Reiki that survives to this day, although since the early 1990s there have been a number of changes made by various Masters, which will be outlined in later chapters. She taught the system in three levels, as taught by Hayashi; however, she adapted the teaching to suit Western students; for example, teaching First Degree or Second Degree as workshops held over just a few days, rather than expecting students to work in her clinic for months. Master level was usually taught as a form of apprenticeship, working alongside Takata for at least a year. She used the ceremonial spiritual empowerment, which Hayashi had taught her, which she called an initiation or attunement, to transfer the healing ability to her students. She also taught the four Reiki symbols. These are sacred shapes that alter the way Reiki can be used and which also increase its strength. Reiki treatments were carried out using a series of 12 basic hand positions, each held for five minutes, and she encouraged her students to treat themselves with Reiki every day. In addition, realising that in the West her students related money to importance, and wanting people to value the incredible gift of Reiki, she charged high course fees – US $150 for Reiki First Degree, $500 for Reiki Second Degree and $10,000 for Reiki Master. To put this into context, in the early 1970s when Takata began to teach Reiki Masters, $10,000 would have bought a house in the US.

THE DEVELOPMENT OF REIKI IN THE WEST

After Hawayo Takata's death, a group of her Masters met in Hawaii in 1982 to discuss how Reiki should progress, and who should become the next leader, or 'Grand Master'. It appears there were two 'favourites' for the post – Phyllis Lei Furumoto, Mrs Takata's granddaughter, and Dr Barbara Weber Ray. Phyllis agreed to follow in her grandmother's footsteps and was therefore elected by the majority of the Masters. Soon afterwards, Dr Barbara Weber Ray broke away to found her own system of Reiki called The Radiance Technique, which she later renamed Real Reiki.

That historic first meeting in 1982 allowed Western Reiki Masters to share their experiences for the first time, and they discovered differences in the way they had been taught – perhaps because Mrs Takata had taught the system as an oral tradition, not even allowing her student Masters to take notes. They made some decisions to standardise the system and these have had a major influence on the development of Reiki in the West, establishing what we now call the Western tradition of Usui Reiki. The Masters agreed on how the system should be taught and the exact form of each of the four Reiki symbols. They also adopted the same pricing structure Mrs Takata had inaugurated. At a further meeting in British Columbia in 1983, The Reiki Alliance was formed. This is an organisation of Reiki Masters who recognise Phyllis Lei Furumoto as the 'Grand Master', and whose purpose is to support each member as teachers of the Usui System of Reiki.

Until 1988, following the tradition which her grandmother started, only Phyllis Furumoto, as Grand Master, was entitled to train other Masters, but in a gathering at Friedricksburg that year she announced that any suitably experienced Master could teach other Masters. This significant decision is what opened up Reiki in the West to the inevitable changes that result from expansion.

By the early 1990s the number of Masters and Practitioners had grown extensively, and an increasing number of Masters moved away from the system agreed by the Reiki Alliance to work independently, changing the way they taught Reiki. Written manuals and books about Reiki began to appear, additional hand positions were used, extra symbols were added, and the time between levels was shortened, so that sometimes Reiki First Degree and Reiki Second Degree (nowadays more frequently called Reiki 1 and Reiki 2) were taught on two consecutive days. The way the Master level was taught also changed considerably. Instead of an apprenticeship system, where one or two trainee Masters would work alongside an established Master for a year or more, the Reiki Third Degree began to be taught in large groups on courses lasting just a few days. Also, students were allowed to progress through the three levels very quickly – often within one year, and sometimes within only a few months or even weeks. This resulted in a massive expansion in the number of Masters, with a consequent growth in the number of people learning First and Second Degree Reiki, so that Reiki rapidly spread all over the world.

REIKI AT THE END OF THE 20TH CENTURY

In the late 1990s, new information began to come to the West from Japan, which showed that Usui had been a Buddhist priest, not a Christian priest, and that he had passed his complete teachings on to about 20 people, not only to Chujiro Hayashi. It turned out that not all the Reiki Masters in Japan had been killed during World War II, and it became apparent that Reiki had continued to be taught there continuously since Mikao Usui's death. Indeed, an organisation existed which was dedicated to preserving the original teachings of Dr Usui – the Usui Reiki Ryoho Gakkai. This fuller and more accurate picture of Reiki's discovery and development came particularly from two men – Frank Arjava Petter, a European Reiki Master living and working in Japan with his Japanese wife, Chetna Kobayashi, and Hiroshi Doi, a Japanese Reiki Master who has trained in both Japanese and Western Reiki traditions. Others who have contributed to our current knowledge of Japanese Reiki include Dave King, Melissa Riggall, Chris Marsh, Andrew Bowling,

Frans Stiene and Robert Jefford, all of whom have spent time researching in Japan.

THE NEWLY FOUND HISTORY OF REIKI IN JAPAN

Despite the amount of research that has been done, it is unlikely that we will ever have a totally accurate account of Mikao Usui's life or his system of healing. Even though contact has been made in recent years with some of Usui's original students, all well over 100 years old, they were unwilling to reveal the whole story, because the prevailing culture in Japan is to keep information they consider to be sacred away from Western eyes. We do now know, however, that Usui was born into a Samurai family in Taniai-mura (now Miyama-cho) in Japan on 15 August 1865, and that he began his study of Buddhism at the age of four, when he was sent to the local monastery school run by Tendai Buddhist monks. He studied martial arts from the age of 12 – including *aiki jutsu* and *yagyu ryu*, reaching Menkyo Kaiden, the highest level of proficiency, by his mid-twenties – and of other ancient Japanese systems as he got older, including *ki-kou*, an ancient healing technique that is a combination of mindful targeted breathing, simple flowing movements and restful poses – the Japanese form of the Chinese martial art and energy balancing system known as qigong. He also learned meditation and healing. During his adult life he held many different jobs, including a position as a government officer, a businessman, and a journalist, and for a time he was secretary to the Mayor of Tokyo. For a while he is also said to have worked as a missionary, although where and to what purpose is unclear, but this may simply be a reference to his charitable work in prisons. Although he is referred to as a Buddhist priest, in effect he was a lay Tendai priest called a *zaike*, so he lived a relatively normal life with a wife and children. He is known to have studied other forms of Buddhism, including Shingon, Mahayana (Mikkyo) and Zen, as well as Shinto, an ancient faith common in Japan – many Japanese follow both Buddhism and Shintoism.

Usui was undoubtedly influenced as he grew up by the expansiveness that was characteristic of the reign of Emperor Mutsuhito (known as the Meiji Emperor) who came to the throne when Usui was nearly three years old. During his reign, known as the Meiji Restoration period (1868–1912) a new wave of openness began, as

Japan's previously closed borders were opened for the first time in many centuries. The country went from an agrarian economy to an industrial one, and this resulted in an eagerness to explore the benefits of Western influences, with a consequent freedom for Japanese nationals to travel outside their own country. Many Japanese scholars were sent abroad to study Western languages and sciences, and Usui is known to have travelled widely, and to have pursued a life of study. It states on his memorial, situated in the graveyard of the Pure Land Buddhist Saihoji temple in Tokyo, that he visited China, the US and Europe, and that he was fond of reading, acquiring knowledge of medicine, history, psychology and world religions. Although he is often referred to as Dr Usui, there is no evidence currently available that he had qualified as a medical doctor, so the reference may just be a mark of respect.

As part of his lifelong study of Buddhism, he would have been working towards achieving *Satori*, the state of Spiritual Enlightenment, and his memorial confirms that he had an experience of mystical enlightenment on Mount Kurama (Kurama-yama), near Kyoto. The date is uncertain, as some sources suggest 1922, although 1914 is quoted in some Japanese books and seems to be quite possible, as he appears to have begun teaching some aspects of his healing system in 1915 and to have become widely known as a healer perhaps as early as 1917.

Apparently, after advice from one of his Buddhist teachers, he decided to undergo *shyu gyo*, a strict spiritual discipline involving meditation and fasting for 21 days, until he either died or became enlightened. On the last morning of his fast he experienced 'a great Reiki over his head' (a quote from Usui's memorial), which enabled him to become enlightened, and to acquire the ability to access healing energy (Reiki) and to pass that ability on to others. Usui then spent the few years before his death on 9 March 1926 practising and teaching his healing system – Usui Reiki Ryoho, or Usui Spiritual Energy Healing Method – during which time he passed on his knowledge to others so that the teachings could continue. His memorial states: 'If Reiki can be spread throughout the world it will touch the human heart and the morals of society. It will be helpful for many people, not only healing disease, but the Earth as a whole.' His wishes have come true, perhaps even beyond what he could have envisaged, and there are now millions of people around the world using Reiki.

THE DEVELOPMENT OF REIKI IN JAPAN

As I have mentioned, it is a facet of Japanese culture that knowledge or important information is normally kept secret (or sacred, as the words are synonymous in the Japanese language) within family groups, which is the main reason why it has taken so long for information to come to the West about Reiki's development. Initially Usui is believed to have used Reiki only on himself and his family, and it is reported that Reiki cured his wife of a serious illness at that time. So important did he realise his discovery to be, that he decided to begin teaching people how to access this healing energy, and he made *Shoden* (meaning 'the entrance', the first level of Reiki training) 'freely available to all of the people' – a direct quote from one of his teaching manuals, the *Usui Reiki Hikkei*.

There is reliable information that about 2,000 people learned Reiki from Usui (which he also called *Teate*, meaning hands-on or palm healing), but most of these would only have achieved the first level, *Shoden*. It appears that between 30 and 50 people may have learned the second level, *Okuden* (meaning 'the deep inside'), equivalent to the Western Second Degree, but only approximately 20 acquired the third level, *Shinpiden* (meaning 'the mystery/secret teachings'), which is what we call Third Degree, or Reiki Master. It is believed that these included five Buddhist nuns, four naval officers and at least eight other men, but little else is known about them, despite the fact that all of Usui's students who achieved *Okuden* and *Shinpiden* were recorded with the education departments in Japan. Some of these records may have been lost in the earthquake which affected Tokyo in 1923; nevertheless, the following ten are listed:

Juzaburo Ushida (rear admiral)
Kan'ichi Takatomi (rear admiral)
Tetsutaro Imaizumi (rear admiral)
Chujiro Hayashi (admiral)
Haru Nagao (occupation unknown)
Toshihiro Eguchi (schoolteacher)
Yoshiharu Watanabe (philosopher)
Sono'o Tsuboi (tea ceremony master)
Imae Mine (musician)
Masayuki Okada (author of the inscription on Usui's memorial)

In April 1922 Dr Usui opened his first clinic in Harajuku, Tokyo, where he practised and taught Reiki. His healing skills must have been extraordinary, as he was renowned all over Japan, and admired as 'the pioneer of restarting hands-on healing from past generations', and the number of people helped by Reiki is reported to have been several hundred thousand, including many of those injured in the Tokyo earthquake in September 1923 – although this number must have included people helped by Usui's students, as well as those helped by him personally.

The emphasis of Usui's teaching was really more about a spiritual awakening than on purely physical healing. The importance of self-healing was therefore imparted, as well as the benefits of living a 'proper' life, using the Reiki Principles as a foundation. Below is a version of these Principles, which comes from an original document thought to be written in Dr Usui's own handwriting (in Japanese *kanji*), which has now been translated and appears in Frank Arjava Petter's book *The Legacy of Dr Usui*; however the latest information is that this was written by Ushida Sensei, the second President of the Usui Reiki Ryoho Gakkai, and a copy of this document can be found on page 328:

Shoufuku no hihoo	The secret method of inviting happiness
Manbyo no ley-yaku	The wonderful medicine for all diseases (of the body and the soul)
Kyo dake wa	Just today
1 *Okoru-na*	1 Do not get angry
2 *Shinpai suna*	2 Do not worry
3 *Kansha shite*	3 Show appreciation
4 *Goo hage me*	4 Work hard (on yourself)
5 *Hito ni shinsetsu ni*	5 Be kind to others
Asa yuu Gassho shite, koko-ro ni nenji, kuchi ni tonaeyo	Mornings and evenings, sit in the *Gassho* position and repeat these words out loud and in your heart. (*Gassho* means to sit quietly with your hands together in the prayer position, with your thumbs pointing to the centre of your chest – see illustration on page 327.)
Shin shin kaizen	(For the) improvement of body and soul,

Usui Reiki Ryoho Usui   Spiritual Energy Healing Method
Chosso Usui Mikao   The founder, Mikao Usui

In addition, Dr Usui used 125 inspirational poems (*Gyosei*) from the Meiji Emperor as a guide to his students in their personal and spiritual development. Here is one example of the stylised *waka* (also called *tanka*) poetry written by Emperor Mutsuhito, which Dr Usui taught to his students:

Sky
The spacious sky
Spans serene and clear
So blue above
Oh, that our souls could grow
And become so open.

All 125 *waka* poems are given in *Spirit of Reiki*, by Walter Lubeck, Frank Arjava Petter and William Lee Rand.

Dr Usui incorporated other aspects of his many years of Buddhist and martial arts training into his Reiki teaching, including meditation, self-cleansing and a simple but powerful method of spiritual empowerment called *Reiju* (see Chapter 22), as well as some Shinto and *ki-kou* energy practices. It seems that he worked intuitively on people, placing one or both hands wherever he detected energy imbalances that seemed in need of healing. Once he began to teach others to do Reiki, however, he found that instructions were needed, and he wrote the *Usui Reiki Hikkei*, which was a manual to be given to his students. Frank Arjava Petter and his wife Chetna Kobayashi have translated a copy of Usui's manual (*The Original Reiki Handbook of Dr Mikao Usui* by Frank Arjava Petter), and it gives instructions for the treatment of particular illnesses and parts of the body using specific combinations from the total list of almost 70 hand positions. The latest opinion is that this manual may have been produced in collaboration with (or even authored by) Chujiro Hayashi, who was a medical doctor; he, and some other naval colleagues, wished to learn palm healing to help with their treatment of patients.

THE FOUNDING OF THE USUI REIKI RYOHO GAKKAI

Mikao Usui is also credited with founding the Usui Reiki Ryoho Gakkai (meaning the Usui Reiki Healing Method Learning Society), an organisation dedicated to keeping the Reiki teachings alive, although it is possible that his followers started it after his death, naming Usui as the founder as a mark of respect. This society has continued to practise and teach Reiki in an unbroken line since 1926, the first few leaders being *Shinpiden* students taught by Usui. They do not take the title of Grand Master, but are simply referred to as Presidents of the society, and they are listed as:

1 Mikao Usui (1922–6)   5 Hoichi Wanami (?–1975)
2 Jusaburo Ushida (1926–35)   6 Mrs Kimiko Koyama (1975–99)
3 Kan'ichi Taketomi (1935–60) 7 Masayoshi Kondo (1999–2010)
4 Yoshiharu Watanabe (1960–?) 8 Ichita Takahashi (from 2010)

(The dates for the fourth and fifth Presidents are unconfirmed – but it is believed that each President served until the date of his or her death.)

The Gakkai members follow Usui's teachings very closely, and they have in their possession the two manuals produced by Usui (the *Usui Reiki Hikkei*), one of which is an explanation of his energy healing method, the Usui Reiki Ryoho, and the other gives details of the various healing techniques, including specific hand positions for different diseases and physical problems, as mentioned above. The Gakkai hold regular meetings in Tokyo and elsewhere in Japan for their members, where the students sing *waka* poetry, chant the Reiki Principles, do *Hatsurei-ho* (a combined meditation and cleansing practice – see Chapter 21), and each time they attend they receive a *Reiju* empowerment from one of the *Shihan* – teaching *Shinpiden* members – for cleansing, purification and to strengthen their ability to access Reiki.

ISSUES RAISED WITHIN THE REIKI COMMUNITY

For a number of years, questions have been asked about why the story Mrs Takata told about the rediscovery of Reiki became

Christianised, but this may well have been because both during and after World War II she was training people in America in a Japanese technique based on Buddhist teachings. Perhaps without introducing the idea that Usui was a Christian priest, things might have become very awkward for her, especially after the bombing of Pearl Harbor. We now realise that it would have been almost impossible for Usui to train as a Christian priest, because Christianity was banned in Japan until 1877, well after Usui began his Buddhist training, and no record can be found of Usui attending or teaching at any of the colleges or universities in either Japan or the US that Mrs Takata included in her story. (One of my Reiki Masters, William Lee Rand, has letters from each of the institutions confirming that no record of Mikao Usui can be found as either a student or tutor).

When, in the late 1990s, information came out of Japan about a range of techniques which did not seem to have been taught in the West through the Takata lineage – for example the *Hatsurei-ho*, and alternative ways of using the hands during treatments, such as *Oshi-te Chiryo-ho* – tapping with the fingertips (see Chapter 21) – there was confusion, even indignation, in the Reiki community. Some people wanted to reject the new information, and stick to what they already knew, while others wanted to throw out all they had learned in the West, and use only the techniques from the Japanese traditions. Others were angry that we had been denied the chance of learning these valuable methods, and were critical of the Western lineage.

The spirit of Reiki training in the West was probably originally very similar to that in Japan. It seems possible, though, that Mrs Takata did teach many of what we now know were Usui's original methods, although she did not use their Japanese names, and some were seemingly only taught to Masters. Perhaps because the Masters she trained were not allowed to make notes, they simply forgot, or they didn't realise the importance of some of the techniques because they did not come from a Buddhist background where the spiritual and energetic significance of each method would have been more obvious.

EXPLORING THE DIFFERENCES

In Part 5, the Japanese Reiki training and techniques are covered more comprehensively, but I'd like to briefly introduce some of the differences. We know that in Japan the numbering of the levels is reversed, so what we would refer to as the first level, *Shoden*, equivalent to our First Degree, is actually their sixth degree. This is itself divided into four parts: *Roku-To* (Sixth Degree), *Go-To* (Fifth), *Yon-To* (Fourth) and *San-To* (Third), and this is probably why we have four attunements in the traditional Western system of teaching Reiki. *Shoden* can be learned by anyone, but the second level, *Okuden*, which is divided into two parts, *Okuden-Zenki* when the student would be taught a range of techniques such as using the eyes and breath to deliver Reiki, and *Okuden-Koki* when the symbols and mantras are taught, is only given when a student can demonstrate that they are accessing an appropriate amount of Reiki healing energy, and are proficient at the techniques, which may take many years. They are expected to practise Reiki daily, to obey the five Principles and to make an effort to live those principles in their daily lives, encouraging mental and emotional growth and development. They are also expected to practise a number of meditations daily, including *Hatsurei-ho* at *Okuden* or *Shinpiden* level, for self-cleansing and spiritual enhancement, and to continue their spiritual development, partly by attending regular training seminars where they receive *Reiju* empowerments. Receiving regular *Reiju* helps them to develop their intuitive skills so that they become better able to detect and treat physical illnesses, a process which is called *Byosen* – being able to feel energy from a source of illness, and being able to judge a symptom and the number of days of healing that will be required; or *Reiji-ho* where the hands go intuitively to affected areas automatically and start sending Reiki (see Chapter 20). Very few people in Japan ever reach the advanced level of *Shinpiden*, the equivalent of a Western Reiki Master, even after many, many years of practice.

Reiki has developed differently in the West, perhaps because we have not had the same spiritual background or the cultural understanding of energies resulting in the need for a self-cleansing tradition. Although some Masters did bring their students together regularly to practise Reiki, no *Reiju* empowerments were given, because these were unknown to us until 1999 when they were demonstrated by Sensei Hiroshi Doi at a training session to Western Reiki Masters in Canada that year. There has also been less emphasis on developing sensitivity in the hands with Reiki, which probably accounts for the system we have of 12 or more hand positions being held for five minutes each. This enables the Reiki to flow everywhere in the body, so that each person can receive the Reiki wherever they need it.

Since Mrs Takata's death, many Masters have chosen to change the way Reiki is taught so that there are now more than 30 different types of Reiki being practised in the West (see the Appendix), some based very closely on Takata's system, and some that have introduced many new 'channelled' (receiving insight from spiritual sources) symbols, different attunement procedures and other 'New Age' practices, and no doubt more will appear in the future. Now that we have discovered Usui's original techniques, however, these can be integrated into Reiki practice, so we have even more tools available to us. The aim of this book is to show the enormous potential of integrating these two healing systems whose roots are firmly based in Eastern philosophy and wisdom but whose body is expanding with the collected wisdom of many Western and Japanese Masters and Practitioners. In the next chapter we look in more depth at Reiki as a healing energy, and at its relationship to other energies such as those that comprise the human energy body.

Chapter 2

Reiki and Energy

ENERGY IS ALL THERE IS

Reiki is an energy – as explained in the last chapter, the word means 'spiritual energy' – and when we use it in healing, it acts holistically, affecting all of the energies that comprise the human body, or animals or anything else in the natural world. To make later sections easier to understand, I want first to introduce energy in a wider and more scientific context, especially electromagnetic energy, because this is what makes up our physical body, as well as the energy field that surrounds and interpenetrates it.

We talk about 'energy' in different ways, perhaps referring to energy sources such as coal, gas, wind-power or electricity, or the calorific value of food, but the definition of energy is much broader than that. Einstein and later quantum physicists have explained that at the quantum level – which is incredibly tiny, between 10,000 and 100,000 times smaller than an atom – every-thing that exists in the universe is energy, which is vibrating and oscillating at different rates. What this basically means is that phys-ical matter – that is, the 'stuff' that we're familiar with, from the planet itself to the smallest insect – and energy, are just two forms of the same thing.

What this new branch of physics has established is that the whole universe is really a dynamic web made up of these energies, and that everything in it can be described as part of what is called the Zero Point Field. The concept of zero-point energy was developed in Germany by Albert Einstein and Otto Stern in 1913, so the term originates from the German *Nullpunktenergie*, which means 'an ocean of microscopic vibrations that exists in the space between things'. This explanation has a knock-on effect to our understanding of other words; for example, when we think of 'vacuum' or 'outer space' we may think they are totally empty, but because every atom in everything that exists is 99.999 per cent empty space, it means that there is therefore 0.001 per cent of 'something'! This means that there is no true 'emptiness' anywhere, because it is still 'full' of microscopic zero-point energy. Therefore, what we think of as being totally empty is still a part of this ever-moving, ever-changing Zero Point Field.

Max Planck, known as the father of quantum theory, coined the phrase 'the Divine Matrix', which can be used to describe the Zero Point Field, way back in 1944, saying that this was the origin of everything, from the birth of the stars to the DNA of living things, but it has taken until recently for the bulk of the scientific world to catch up with him.

Now, I realise that at this point you may be wondering why I'm including complicated quantum physics in a book about Reiki. Don't worry, what I've said above is about as scientific as I'm going to get, but it *is* relevant because this 'new' science actually now explains that when we experience 'good health' it means that we are achieving a state of perfect subatomic communication between every part of the body; 'ill health' is a state where that communication breaks down, so basically, we become ill when our energy waves are out of synch.

This 'communication' is both at the subatomic level (the biophotons that make up our physical bodies), and at the subconscious level (our thoughts and emotions). Let's look at the physical process first.

Biophotons are tiny emissions of light that are produced and used by all living things. When we eat a vegetable, for example, we absorb the biophotons created with the sun's energy, which have been used and stored by the plant as it grew. We, in turn, store these biophotons in the DNA of our cells, to be used to organise the 100,000 chemical reactions that take place in each of our 60 trillion cells every second. In other words, biophotons produce changes in our physical body chemistry. They communicate with all the cells in our bodies instantaneously, at the speed of light, in a synchronous wave of energy that creates a perfect harmony – or potentially perfect health.

If we then consider the subconscious process, you may be surprised to read that at the subconscious level every thought, and
the emotion it carries, also produces changes in our physical body
chemistry, and even our DNA, and these both have an impact on
our health. Perhaps we shouldn't be too surprised by this; after all,
when we feel sad, our body produces tears, and when we're embarrassed blood flows to our cheeks to produce a blush, so it's not too
much of a stretch for the imagination to realise that there are other
effects taking place internally.

As an example, a neuropeptide called oxytocin is released into
the bloodstream when we are feeling loving or compassionate – it
is even sometimes known as the 'love hormone'– and this has wide-
ranging health benefits, from helping our digestion to reducing
inflammation, as well as protecting our cardiovascular system (see
Why Kindness is Good For You, by Dr David R. Hamilton for more on
this).

Experiments carried out by both the US army and the Institute
of HeartMath have graphically demonstrated that everything is
connected, and that our thoughts and emotions – which are forms
of energy too – have a greater impact than we might have believed.
(The Institute of HeartMath is an internationally recognised non-
profit research and education organisation that was set up in
California in 1991. It is dedicated to helping people reduce stress,
self-regulate emotions and build energy and resilience for happy
and healthy lives.)

Both sets of experiments involved taking samples of DNA and
moving those samples to a different location from the DNA donor,
and then getting the donor to experience various emotions (for
example, by watching a series of video images). What was then
observed were both the responses of the donor and also the
responses of the samples of DNA when the video images were displayed. The donors' responses were measured electrically, and the
DNA samples were observed under microscopes at exactly the same
time, even though they were in another room in the same building,
and even in some cases up to 350 miles apart. The reactions of the
DNA samples coincided with those of the donors: the double helix
spiral of the DNA tightened and shortened when negative emotions
such as fear, anger or frustration were experienced by the donor,
and some DNA codes even switched off; when the emotions were
positive, such as when the donor was looking at something that

made them feel happy, loving or grateful, the DNA strands relaxed and lengthened.

Not only does this show that everything is connected (part of the Divine Matrix of energy) but it also validates another theory of quantum physics: the Heisenberg principle, that once something is joined (for example, our body and our DNA scrapings, such as small samples of skin tissue) it remains connected, whether it is physically linked or not. (For very readable information on this topic, see books by Lynne McTaggart, Gregg Braden and Bruce Lipton listed in Further Reading.)

THE HUMAN ENERGY PERSPECTIVE

Energy is all there is. Some energetic vibrations we are familiar with, such as sound, light, radio waves or X-rays. These are all part of the electromagnetic spectrum, and from a scientific perspective the only difference between these various forms of energy is that each oscillates at a different frequency or rate of vibration.

Human beings are also comprised of electromagnetic energy, and every cell, atom and subatomic particle that makes up the human body is vibrating at different rates depending upon their biochemical make-up; for example, the specific electrical output of the human heart can be measured on an ECG machine (electro-cardiogram). Also, the electromagnetic output of the whole body can be measured using an electro-myograph, and the normal biological frequency for the human body is around 250cps (cycles per second); however, some pioneering research that is very relevant to our understanding of human energy (bio-energy) was carried out by Valerie V. Hunt, a scientist and Professor Emeritus of Physiological Science at the University of California. She was the first to develop the protocols and instruments necessary to detect and record the body's high-frequency energy fields, and her groundbreaking research has led to the first truly scientific understanding of the relationship between energy field disturbances, consciousness and disease. In 1985 Dr Hunt became the Executive Director of the BioEnergy Fields Foundation—a non-profit research and educational organisation dedicated to the continued study of human bio-energy and the application of that research within the fields of medicine, education and self-development, including the evaluation of alternative treatments such as sound and hands-on healing.

In experiments they carried out on a variety of people, recording the output at sites on the body traditionally associated with high energy spots known as chakras (*chakra* is a Sanskrit word meaning wheel or vortex), some very interesting results were obtained. Most people in the study recorded the normal range for the human body, which is around 250cps, but when the tests were carried out on people who used or were receiving healing energies (such as Reiki), and others who had considerable psychic ability, it was found that their energy frequencies registered in a band between 400 and 800cps. Even higher frequencies – more than 900cps – were found in people who were described as 'mystical personalities': people who were not only psychics and healers but who also followed a very spiritual path and were able to meditate deeply. As you will see in later chapters, when I talk about Reiki 'raising your energetic vibrations', Valerie V. Hunt's pioneering research has now provided scientific evidence to prove that this is true. (See her book in Further Reading for more information.)

Science, therefore, has finally confirmed something that has been part of the spiritual wisdom of many cultures for thousands of years: that an unseen energy flows through and connects all living things. In one of the world's oldest scriptures from India, the Rig Veda, which is thought to date back 7,000 years, there is a description of a force that underlies creation from which all things are formed. This energy has various names, depending upon the culture or spiritual tradition, and probably the most commonly known is *Ki* (Japanese) and *Chi* or *Qi* (Chinese), but it can also be referred to as *Prana* (Indian), Light or Spirit or the Holy Ghost (Christian), or as Vitality or Life-force.

As this book is about Reiki, I will refer to it by its Japanese name *Ki*, or as life-force, but before we examine Reiki's connection to this life-force energy in more detail, I want to explain the human energy body in greater depth. The theories I shall be discussing about the aura and chakras come from India and other areas of the Far East rather than from the Japanese Reiki traditions, as you will see in Part 5, but they are often included in Reiki training, and because of the 'New Age' adoption of these ideas they provide a reasonably familiar and understandable way of looking at human energies.

The Human Energy Body

The physical body is something we all know about – we can see it and feel it – yet every cell in it is still energy or light, vibrating at a slow enough rate to make it into visible physical matter. Surrounding and interpenetrating our physical body is another body of energy, this time made up of much faster, finer and lighter vibrations, and this is most commonly called the aura, the auric field, the biofield or the human energy body. This auric field is as much a part of you as your physical body – indeed your physical body is really just the densest inner layer of this flowing energy field. The higher frequencies of the energies that make up the aura mean it is harder to see with the naked eye, although it can be detected by some scientific equipment, and can also be photographed using a specially developed Kirlian camera. (Named after its Russian inventors, the Kirlian camera uses a process that records on photographic film the field radiation of electro-magnetic energy emitted by an object.) Each person's energy field has its own distinctive energy signature; its energetic vibrational frequencies are unique, just as fingerprints are unique to each individual.

In addition to the aura, our energy body contains chakras – the energy centres – and a range of energy channels flowing through the body, called meridians. Perhaps the easiest way of understanding this is to think of the energy body in similar terms to your physical body. The aura is the energy equivalent of your whole physical body, the chakras are the energetic equivalent to your brain and major organs, and the meridians are similar to your veins and arteries, but instead of blood, they carry energy – *Ki* – all over the body.

The Aura

The aura is a field of energy or light that completely surrounds the physical body above, below and on all sides. It is made up of seven layers, with the inner layers closest to the physical body being comprised of the densest energy, and each succeeding layer being of finer and higher vibrations. Most people have an oval (elliptical) aura, which is slightly larger at the back than at the front, and fairly narrow at the sides, and it also stretches above the head and below the feet. A person's aura is not always the same size; it can expand or contract depending upon a variety of factors such as how healthy you are, how you are feeling emotionally or psychologically at any given moment, or how comfortable you feel with the people who are in your immediate surroundings.

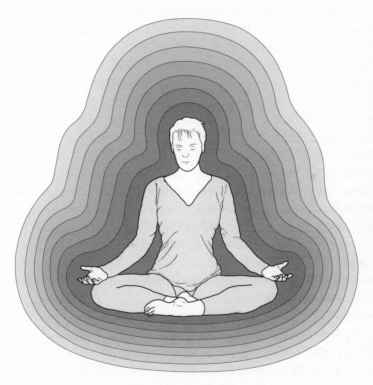

The layers of the aura surrounding the body

This aura is spiritual energy, which is present from birth (and probably before) until death. After physical death, no aura can be detected, because the life-force no longer exists. In a living person, however, the outer edges and the individual layers of the aura can be detected using dowsing rods or a pendulum, and they can also be sensed with the hands. The densest layers, nearest the body, can also be seen with the naked eye by most people with a little practice, and some psychic people can see the whole energy body quite clearly. Painters over the centuries have depicted the aura around the heads of angels, saints and prophets as a bright golden halo, indicating their pure and spiritual energy.

Detecting auras is the first thing I teach in my Reiki classes, because apart from being great fun it also allows people to gain a real understanding of the concept of energy and life-force, before they learn to use the higher vibrations of Reiki healing energy to permeate, clear, balance and energise the whole energy body. For the majority of people, the layers of the aura seem to be alternately positive and negative energy; this does not mean they are good or bad, but it simply indicates a different set of vibrations, similar to positive and negative polarities in magnetism. Some people's auric layers are all the same – all positive, or all negative – and others have the first three layers positive, and the next four negative, and so on. Each person is individual, so there is no right or wrong in this – just as there is no right or wrong about having dark hair instead of blond. That's just the way it is.

The biggest shock for most people is finding out how large the aura can be. Of course, it varies from person to person, and it changes from day to day anyway, but the outer layer of the aura can be anywhere from about 2m (6½ft) to 20m (66ft) or even further away from the person's physical body. This means that whenever we are with other people, our auras are intermingling, and whether or not we are mindful of it we are 'picking up' signals from other people's auras all the time.

Although we may not be consciously aware of the fact, we all use our auras as sensing devices – what you might call 'the eyes in the back of your head'. Have you ever felt particularly drawn to sit next to someone, or felt a sense of discomfort when sitting next to someone else, even though you don't know them? This could be because your aura has already 'picked up' either complementary or discordant energies within the other person's aura. (This doesn't mean that that person is 'bad'; it's just that their energies are very different from yours!) Or have you ever experienced a strange prickling sensation at the back of your neck, and you've realised that someone has been looking at you from behind? Perhaps you've even been able to sense the atmosphere within a room before you have opened the door? It's not surprising, really, when you consider that your aura may extend 10m (33ft) or more ahead of you, so it will already be in the room picking up the vibrations of other people's auric fields; this is because the finer and lighter vibrations of auric energy can pass easily through the denser energy of physical matter.

DETECTING THE AURA

Sensing the aura with your hands

Something you might like to try is sensing your own aura between the palms of your hands. Hold your hands out in front of you with the palms facing each other, about 60cm (2ft) apart, and *intend* to detect your auric energy (it is your intention that switches on this ability, just as it is your intention that switches on the flow of Reiki once you have been attuned to it). Close your eyes so that you can concentrate on any sensations in your hands and fingers, and then slowly bring your hands closer together. You may find that your palms get warm, or your fingers begin to tingle, and as your hands get quite close together you may feel a resistance between them, almost as though you have a balloon between your hands. That's your auric energy!

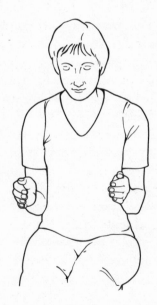

THE CHAKRAS

Chakra is a Sanskrit word, meaning wheel or vortex, and there are seven major chakras in the human energy body located at (1) the perineum/base of the spine; (2) near the navel/sacral; (3) at the solar plexus; (4) in the middle of the chest/the heart; (5) in the throat; (6) at the centre of the brow; and (7) the crown of the head. In addition, there are more than 20 minor chakras, such as in the palms of the hands, on the knees and on the soles of the feet. A healthy chakra can be seen psychically, vibrating evenly in a circular motion, resembling a funnel which is fairly narrow close to the body, but which becomes wider as it gets further away.

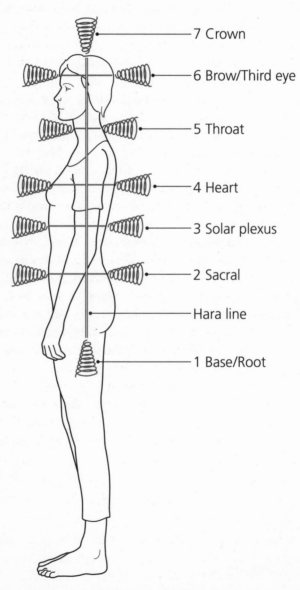

7 Crown

6 Brow/Third eye

5 Throat

4 Heart

3 Solar plexus

2 Sacral

Hara line

1 Base/Root

The seven major chakras

Chakras are an essential part of our body's energy system, because they are intimately connected to our physical health, as each is linked with specific parts of the body and to systems within the body. You will see in later chapters that when carrying out a Reiki treatment, either on yourself or on another person, your hands are placed near to the major chakras, as this is where life-force energy – and Reiki – can be most easily absorbed, transformed and distributed throughout the physical and energy bodies. It is also possible to become sensitive enough to 'read' or 'sense' your own or others' energy bodies so that the Reiki healing energy can be directed into those areas that need it.

When a particular chakra is healthy, balanced and fully open, so are its connected body parts, but if a chakra is blocked, damaged or partially closed, then the health of the connected body parts and systems will begin to reflect this. Our chakras, like our aura, are affected by everything that happens to us – good things as well as bad. For example, falling in love has an amazingly beneficial effect on our whole energy body, making it sparkle and zing with colour, whereas emotional or mental traumas, and even negative words, can have detrimental effects on our energy levels. When we use the term 'broken heart' to describe the feeling of devastation after the loss of a loved one, this is actually reflected in the energy body, as the heart chakra appears to have breaks or tears in it. Feeling 'choked' with emotion appears as imbalances in both the throat and the heart chakras; the sacral chakra, near our navel, is the seat of our creativity, so writer's block might show as a dark mist or spots indicating obstruction in the natural flow of energy there.

In the chart overleaf, I have shown not only each chakra's number, name and location but also the colour vibration, body parts and systems linked with it, and the aspects of our lives associated with it, as well as a phrase that indicates its major influence.

Chakra number	Chakra	Location	Colour	Body parts/ systems	Associated life aspects
7	Crown (*sahasrara*)	Top of head	Violet, purple or white	Pineal/pituitary, nervous system, mind and whole body	Enlightenment, knowledge, spirituality, understanding, self-realisation, unity, connection, fulfilment, completion, mysticism, universal consciousness 'I have'
6	Brow or third eye (*ajna*)	Centre of forehead	Indigo	Pituitary/ pineal, brain, hypothalamus, endocrine system, head, eyes, face	Clairvoyance, intuition, insight, imagination, spiritual awareness, vision, individual consciousness 'I see'
5	Throat (*vishuddha*)	Throat	Blue	Thyroid, parathyroid, metabolism, ears, nose, mouth, teeth, neck, throat	Communication, creativity, self-expression, abundance, sound, vibration, receiving 'I speak'
4	Heart (*anahata*)	Centre of chest (sternum)	Green or pink	Thymus, respiration, circulation, immune system, heart, lungs, upper back, arms, hands	Unconditional love, balance, unity, compassion, kindness, affinity, giving, limitless, infinite 'I love'
3	Solar plexus (*manipura*)	Solar plexus	Yellow	Pancreas, muscles, digestive system, liver, spleen, small intestine, gall bladder, middle back	Personal power, autonomy, will, purpose, control, self-determination, self-empowerment, energy, self-esteem, intellect, destiny 'I can'

Chakra number	Chakra	Location	Colour	Body parts/ systems	Associated life aspects
2	Sacral (*svadhisthara*)	Abdomen (navel)	Orange	Ovaries/testes, reproductive system, uterus, lower digestive organs, kidneys, prostate, urinary tract, lower back	Relationships, emotions, intimacy, sharing, sexuality, sensations, food, appetite, pleasure, movement, imagination, the unconscious 'I feel'
1	Root or base (*muladhara*)	Perineum/ base of spine	Red	Adrenals, skeleton, skin, blood, large intestine, pelvis, hips, legs, feet, elimination system	Survival, security, trust, grounding, physical body, money, home, job, sense of belonging, nature, biology, earth 'I have'

THE MERIDIANS

Meridians are the final component of the human energy body. Meridians are the channels that carry our life-force, or *Ki*, around our body, and the major meridians route the energy longitudinally through the body, connecting with all of the body's major organs, but there are other smaller meridians which criss-cross throughout the body connecting all the parts together so that *Ki* can flow every-where. It is on these meridians that the various points exist that are used in a range of complementary therapies such as acupuncture or acupressure, or that connect all parts of the body with the areas on the feet and hands used in reflexology.

THE HUMAN ENERGY BODY AND HEALTH

The state of the energy body is a very important element in the health of any individual, because if blockages and damage in the aura are not cleared and healed, they can eventually manifest them-selves as physical illness or disease. Everything that happens to us affects the aura, whether those are negative or positive experiences, although of course it is the negative experiences that create the blockages and eventual damage.

Every negative thought you have ever had, every negative word you have spoken, and every negative action you have performed will have had an effect on your aura and whole energy body – including effects on your physical body, such as the effects emotions had on the DNA in the HeartMath experiments described earlier – although these effects would normally only be lasting if the negative thoughts, words or actions were consistently repeated. Similarly, any negative words spoken to you, or negative actions performed against you, can potentially form damaging energy patterns in your aura, particularly if they evoke your emotions. Even reading the newspapers, which are usually filled with negative news, or watching violent or horror movies or television programmes, has a dampening effect on your energy field. All of these things will lower your energy body's vibrations, or life-force, but fortunately we are able to take in more life-force, or *Ki*, every day, and thankfully our lives are not normally filled with only negative experiences. The positive experiences we have – the love and affection we receive from our family and friends, the pleasure we feel from watching children at play or viewing a beautiful sunset, the satisfaction of a creative project or success at work – all contribute to raising our vibrations, or *Ki*, so the effects balance out for much of the time. It is therefore usually only major traumas and significant negative experiences that have the opportunity to damage our energy field beyond our normal ability to replenish and repair it.

THE ROLE OF *KI* – LIFE-FORCE ENERGY

Knowledge that our bodies are filled with life-force energy – *Ki* – and that this is directly connected to the quality of our health, has been part of the wisdom of many cultures for thousands of years, and has resulted in the development of many different forms of 'energy medicine'. Some of these require direct physical contact with the body, such as acupuncture, shiatsu and reflexology; some require beneficial body movements, like ta'i chi or qigong, whereas others are taken into the body in various forms, such as herbal, homeopathic and flower remedies. Of course, it is not only people who have energy fields within and around their bodies. All animals, birds, fish, insects and plants have detectable auras and, indeed, so do what we might term 'inanimate' objects, such as rocks, crystals, minerals, metals and water.

The amount of *Ki* or life-force within you varies from day to day – there is a natural rhythmic ebb and flow in the energies within our bodies – but we absorb *Ki* in various ways in order to 'top up' our supply of life-force, as we naturally use some each day. We absorb some in the form of food and drink – remember all animal and plant life, and even water, is filled with *Ki* too – and we also take in *Ki* from the air we breathe and absorb it through our auric fields. *Ki* energy is everywhere; it is the connective force of the universe, so there is a limitless supply.

The levels of life-force in our bodies have an impact on our inherent healing ability, as *Ki* helps to nourish the structure, organs and systems of the body, supporting them in their vital functions and contributing to the healthy growth and renewal of cells; however, the amount we absorb is not constant, and it can depend on many factors, so we don't always sufficiently replenish our supply of *Ki*. If this happens over some time, our energy body can become too depleted, and this is when we become weaker and more susceptible to illness, the ageing process and even physical death, because our *Ki* is what defines us as living beings. Without it we would not be alive. This means that when our *Ki* is high and flowing freely around our whole energy body, we feel healthy, strong, fit and full of energy. We also feel confident, ready to enjoy life and take on its challenges, and are much less likely to become ill. If our *Ki* is low, on the other hand, or there is a restriction or blockage in its flow, we feel weak, tired, listless and lethargic, and can become much more vulnerable to illness or 'dis-ease'.

REIKI AS AN ENERGY

To bring all of the above information into context, the difference between *Ki* (life-force energy) and Reiki (spiritual energy) is:

Ki is the term we use to describe the energy that surrounds and permeates everything.

Reiki is a specific band or frequency of energy for healing and self-healing that works synergistically with *Ki*, but at a higher vibration. Reiki comes directly from the Source (or God, the Creator, All That Is) and is directed by that Higher Intelligence through your Higher Self/Soul for healing or wholing (to make whole) anything, whether animate or inanimate.

Because Reiki energy is vibrating at a very high rate, it is not normally visible to the human eye, but its use by a practitioner can be detected around the healer's hands by a Kirlian camera, and some people do see it, usually as a white/gold stream of energy, similar to the spiral shape of the DNA double helix. Unlike *Ki*, however, which is present everywhere and in everything, Reiki does not flow automatically through everyone from birth. It flows only through people who have been 'attuned' to its vibrational frequency. This attunement, or spiritual empowerment, is the way in which the healing ability of Reiki is passed energetically from a Reiki Master to a student during a sacred ceremony, which is a vital part of a Reiki course or workshop.

CONNECTING WITH REIKI ENERGY – THE SPIRITUAL EMPOWERMENT

In Buddhism, a spiritual empowerment is a familiar but very special element in spiritual practice, and it is where wisdom, existential knowledge, insight and ability is passed from the Master, by thought and intention, deep into the student's mind, body and spirit. You may remember from Chapter 1 that Dr Usui received a spiritual empowerment on Mount Kurama, where he achieved a deep knowledge and understanding of the Reiki symbols, and acquired the ability to heal. The spiritual empowerment that is carried out by a Reiki Master is similar in nature, but less powerful, since Dr Usui received the whole understanding and the full strength of Reiki in one single empowerment from the Highest Source, which also allowed him to become enlightened. As he had been involved in spiritual practice for about 50 years by that time, he was no doubt energetically far better prepared for such a tremendous experience and vast amount of healing energy than any of us would be.

In Usui Reiki there are a number of spiritual empowerments spread out between the various levels, so that the student has time to 'acclimatise' to the levels of energy involved. We usually call these sacred ceremonies initiations or attunements, as they 'initiate' the student into a new life with Reiki (initiate means to begin) and 'attune' the student to the unique vibrations of the Reiki spiritual healing energy (attune means to bring into harmony with). The attunement (more about this in Chapter 4) sets up an energetic channel in the student, through which the Reiki energy can flow from the Source, through the student's energy body – the crown, brow, throat and heart chakras – and out through the hands.

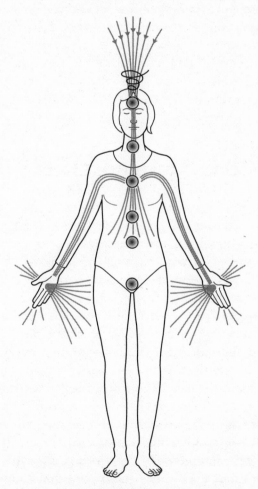

The flow of Reiki after attunement

In effect, this attunement is really 'reopening' an existing channel within our energy body to our enlightened selves – our Soul/Spirit/Higher Self; that part of us which is always and completely connected to the Source/God/All That Is. Although the Reiki may appear to come from outside ourselves, entering through the crown chakra, this only seems that way because we have a limited awareness of our whole existence, and cannot 'see' the full extent and potential of our being, our Soul/Spirit/Higher Self, extending way beyond the confines of our physical bodies. The 'spiritual empowerment', which takes place during the attunement, is just that: it empowers a part of our spirit, Reiki, which we did not consciously know how to access before, so that we become aware of it for the first time.

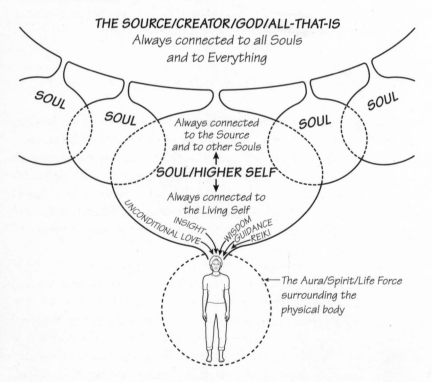

As soon as students have received this attunement they are able to access and use Reiki healing energy for themselves or to treat others, and will continue to be able to do so for the rest of their lives, as this healing energy comes through their Soul/Higher Self, channelled from an inexhaustible source – God/Creator/All That Is/ the Universe – whenever they want it to.

This 'instant' acquisition of healing ability is one of the things that makes Reiki unique, but it is probably also the most puzzling aspect of the practice to Western minds. We are not accustomed to anything so valuable being achieved so effortlessly, yet in the East, spiritual empowerments are a well-known and accepted way of acquiring energy, knowledge, wisdom or insight. Although Reiki may have its roots in Eastern spiritual practices, it is not a religion, so it can be made available to anyone, regardless of their personal beliefs. Also, Reiki does not depend on a person's intellectual capacity or level of spiritual development, so people of all ages and from all backgrounds can acquire the ability to channel Reiki healing energy simply and easily by attending a Reiki First Degree course and receiving the attunement(s). No specialised knowledge or skills are required, so Reiki is a very accessible way of learning how to help yourself and others.

OTHER HEALING ENERGIES

Perhaps I should make it clear that Reiki is not the only healing energy that exists; indeed, a 5,000-year-old book called the Neijing, published as *The Yellow Emperor's Classic of Medicine* by Huang Di (the Yellow Emperor), cites the possibility that there may be 32 different strands of healing energy. I have only experienced a few of these – for example, traditional Usui Reiki, Usui/Tibetan Reiki and Karuna Reiki, but I would certainly agree that they seem to feel and act differently.

Also, there are some people who are described as 'born healers', because they naturally develop the ability to draw spiritual energy into themselves for healing purposes, sometimes even as children, and it is also possible to attend courses from the National Federation of Spiritual Healers (now called The Healing Trust) to learn how to do this. In addition, we *all* have the ability to use our own life-force energy (*Ki*) to help with healing; for example, it feels natural to place a hand on some part of us that is hurting or to put our arms comfortably around a child who has fallen, or to spend time empathising with a friend who is upset. But none of these is Reiki. The healing energy you use can only be called Reiki if you have received an attunement as part of the system of Reiki originated by Mikao Usui.

Reiki Energy as a Healing Treatment

After an attunement, a student can use Reiki on themselves or on other people, and many people who train in Reiki go on to become Practitioners or therapists, offering Reiki treatments in their own home or natural health centres, and even in some hospitals and clinics. The process of a Reiki healing treatment is very simple, and the person receiving it will usually either lie on a massage couch or sit in a chair, and they remain fully clothed, although they are usually asked to remove their coat and shoes.

When a person who has been attuned wishes to use Reiki, they don't need to go through any complicated ritual – simply *intending* to use Reiki starts it flowing into their energy body, as shown in the diagram on page 35, and out through the palms of their hands. The Practitioner then places their hands very gently on specific places on the head and body of the person who wishes to receive a Reiki treatment (more information on hand placements in Chapters 6 and 7), and either holds them still, or occasionally taps gently with the fingertips or pats lightly with the flat of the palm (see Chapter 21), so there is no need for manipulation, massage or pressure of any kind.

Because Reiki is a very high vibrational energy, it can flow into, over and through anything, including solid matter. This enables it to work holistically on the whole person – chakras and aura, body and mind – consciousness, emotions and spirit. As Reiki flows into our aura and physical body, it helps to break down energetic disruptions or blockages, clearing and balancing the chakras and straightening the energy pathways (meridians) to allow the life-force to flow in a healthy and natural way around the whole body.

This influx of high-frequency healing energy stimulates and accelerates the body's own natural healing ability, so that pain relief and physical healing can take place quickly and easily – sometimes at quite extraordinary speed. Also, because Reiki is guided by your Soul/Higher Self, it can make its way to those areas of the physical body and energy body that are most in need of healing, without any conscious direction from either the healer or the recipient. In addition, Reiki automatically adjusts to suit the recipient, so that each person receives as much or as little as they need at that time, at an appropriate rate of flow. It acts to heal, harmonise and balance the whole self, and as it is guided by a higher wisdom and always works for the highest good of the person receiving it, it cannot be harmful in any way. The potential for healing with Reiki is unlimited, so anything can be treated, but it is important to rid yourself of specific expectations of what it will do, and how fast it will perform.

Many physical symptoms can be eased very quickly, while others may need lots of Reiki before starting to respond, but it is essential to remember that it is a person's own body – either your own, if you are self-treating, or a client's if you are treating someone else – that is actually doing the healing, as you will see in the next chapter.

Occasionally, people report amazing, even miraculous, effects from Reiki treatments, while some gain partial or complete relief from symptoms for a time, and others experience little obvious effect. Reiki is not a guaranteed 'cure-all', because 'healing' is not always the same as 'curing'. Healing doesn't always occur on the physical level first. Because Reiki works holistically and is guided by a Higher Intelligence (your Soul/Higher Self, connected to God/the Source), it may be that healing needs to happen first at the emotional level, with the releasing of anger, guilt or hatred, or it may be required first at the mental level, releasing negative thoughts, concepts or attitudes, before the physical symptoms can be addressed. Also, healing is a very personal issue, and if ten people displaying identical physical symptoms were given Reiki by the same Practitioner, there would be ten potentially different outcomes, because their mental, emotional and spiritual states would not be the same.

Ultimately, if the healing is to be permanent you have to take responsibility for healing the cause. This may mean changing how you think or the way you relate to other people, or even altering your whole lifestyle, from your diet and home environment to your close relationships, your job or career; however, when Reiki flows through you it can help with these adjustments too, allowing you to approach the changes in a calm, relaxed and accepting state of mind.

In the next chapter we take a broad look at healing, and at why people become ill, as well as the role Reiki can play in achieving health and well-being.

Chapter 3

Healing and Wholing

Healing is described in the dictionary as 'to be restored to health; to repair by natural processes, as by scar formation; to cure', but the origin of the word itself is 'making whole'. To make whole means healing on all levels – mind, emotions and spirit, as well as the body. As we saw in the last chapter, the use of Reiki helps to clear blockages in a person's energy field, and it works holistically – healing, harmonising and balancing the whole person – to promote better health and greater well-being. Before we look in more depth at the ways in which Reiki can be used for healing, I want to introduce the topic of healing in a more general sense, from the way your physical body repairs itself, to conventional and metaphysical approaches to healing, including looking at illness as a message from your body. You will then be able to see in later chapters how Reiki fits into the whole healing process.

THE PHYSICAL HEALING PROCESS

On a purely physical level, our bodies have an amazingly sophisticated and intelligent set of healing processes to repair and maintain themselves, from our vital organs to our bones, muscles and skin. Inside our bodies, cells are continuously lost through wear and tear, and replaced by cell growth and division. At one time it was believed that a few parts of our bodies, notably the brain and the nervous system, were unable to be repaired or replaced in this way once we reached adulthood; however, new research has shown that even these cells can replicate, given certain conditions. During each year, approximately 98 per cent of the cells in your body are replaced, so in effect you have virtually a new body each birthday. Your bone cells take about three months to regenerate your skeleton, although the calcium in the bone takes longer, about a year; your liver gradually replaces itself roughly every six weeks; your skin is renewed monthly and your stomach lining every four days.

This constant replication and repair is what enables all physical healing to take place; without it, we would all probably bleed to death from our first childhood cut! Of course, many things can impact on your body's natural healing ability: whether you eat a healthy balanced diet; whether you drink plenty of water so that you are not dehydrated; whether you are too tired or under a great deal of stress; your age and general state of health; and so on. For example, poor nutrition reduces healing rates and increases susceptibility to infection which further delays healing, and studies such as those on wound healing by Janice Kiecolt-Glaser (1995) and on HIV by Steve W. Cole (1998) in the US have also proved that psychological stress has a similar delaying effect on the body's healing processes.

HEALING AS A HOLISTIC ISSUE

So from the above information you can see that healing is not something that happens 'out there', something which someone else 'does' to you. There is really only one 'healer' of your body, and that is *you*, because *all* healing is self-healing. Your body possesses the mechanisms to heal itself, so all anyone else can do – whether that person is a doctor, a nurse, a complementary therapist or a Reiki 'healer' – is to kick-start that natural process in some way, whether by conventional or alternative means.

Of course, your body copes every day with lots of other potential hazards; for example, if it is invaded by a virus, such as the common cold, your immune system is mobilised, and all those rather unpleasant symptoms you experience, such as a high temperature and a runny nose, are actually the effects of your body fighting off the infection, rather than effects from the virus itself. Indeed, taking medication to lower your temperature when you have a simple cold could be undoing much of your body's good work, because the virus is being killed off by the rise in temperature.

(Although of course there are some circumstances where it is essential to bring a temperature down if it gets dangerously high, such as with small children.)

If your body is so good at healing itself, why are there times when it isn't completely well? Why do people continue to suffer from chronic or incurable illnesses? The reason is because healing – and health – are holistic issues, not simply physical ones.

As an example, your body produces pre-cancerous (altered) cells every day, but almost all the time your immune system detects and destroys them. If your immune system is not operating as effectively as usual, however, it is possible that not all of them will be destroyed. There are a number of possible reasons for this: perhaps your body is already struggling to fight off another major infection, or your immune system has been seriously affected by some stressful event such as a close bereavement (or even a happy but nevertheless stressful event like a wedding), or perhaps it's because your body doesn't have the right nutritional balance to work at optimum strength. Any of these causes, and there are a number of other possibilities, can be at the root of the growth of cancerous cells in an otherwise healthy body.

In many cases, even if this happens, providing the immune system can return to normal working capacity fairly quickly it will tackle any early cancerous growth and destroy it, and you will be none the wiser. If the cancer develops, of course, there are various conventional medical interventions that can help: surgery, chemotherapy, radiation treatment. But you have probably also heard of people who have gone on to develop mature cancerous growths, yet who have managed to mobilise their own body to destroy the cancer, sometimes with astonishing speed, even without medical intervention. These people always have a very positive attitude and an overwhelming determination to 'get better', as well as having supportive people around them to help them to release emotional blockages and to gain insight into the reasons for their illness. Also, they have usually used a variety of techniques such as Reiki or spiritual healing, or other complementary therapies to help them to activate their own healing ability, because the causes of any serious illness are likely to be complex and multi-levelled. Remember though, that you should always consult your doctor if you feel ill and be guided by them.

THE HEALING–CURING DICHOTOMY

This brings us to the relationship between healing and curing. Let's start by unravelling some common misconceptions. Many people use the words 'healing' and 'curing' interchangeably, yet they don't necessarily mean the same thing. *Curing* means to completely eradicate an illness or disease, whereas *healing* can occur on many different levels.

1 **Healing on the physical level:** This might mean eradicating an illness completely, or it could simply mean limiting or alleviating the symptoms for a time.

2 **Healing on the emotional level:** This could allow you to calm any fears and to reach an acceptance of the effects of the illness.

3 **Healing on the mental (psychological) level:** This could enable you to think differently about your illness, perhaps bringing to your attention the lessons your illness is trying to teach you, and promoting understanding of the causative issues.

4 **Healing on the spiritual level:** This could enable you to develop a more loving and forgiving relationship with yourself, or perhaps even to make a peaceful transition into death.

Let's take one graphic example to demonstrate the difference between healing and curing. In the case of someone who develops gangrene in the lower part of their leg, it may be necessary to amputate the leg below the knee in order to *cure* the illness. Hopefully, if the disease has been caught in time, the gangrene will indeed be eradicated, and in practical terms the body's normal repair and replication processes will heal the wound caused by the operation.

However, an amputation certainly does not *heal* the person, because such an operation has an enormous psychological, emotional, and even spiritual, impact upon the person. It can have a broad range of effects, from the way the person views themselves and how easy or how difficult it is for them to accept their new body image; to the person's relationships with other people – whether they still feel loved, or attractive, or whether they expect (or receive) rejection from others because of their disabling condition. It impacts also on the way they live their lives on an everyday level, coping with the challenges to mobility or dexterity which the loss of a limb can cause; their beliefs about their future aims, ambitions and potential, and possibly even whether they believe life is worth living any more.

Healing is therefore a very personal thing, but many people still seem to think of it as being healing at a physical level, whereas the reality is much wider. Even medical science is at last coming round to an understanding that healing is not simply a collection of physical processes; it involves the whole person – body, mind, emotions and spirit. In a later section (page 48), I talk about the research on the placebo effect (for example, the effectiveness of a 'sugar pill' when compared to actual medicine) as a result of the mind–body connection; placebos can only work because our minds have influence on the workings of our bodies.

A HOLISTIC AND METAPHYSICAL VIEW OF HEALING

There are three possible ways of thinking about health and healing:

1 The bio-medical model

Looking at health and healing from a purely physical perspective has been the predominant Western view for several hundred years: the bio-medical model of health and healthcare. This is sometimes referred to as allopathic or conventional medicine, and it regards the physical body as a machine or a complex set of systems and chemicals. Illnesses or diseases are therefore simply malfunctions, evidence of a physical breakdown which needs to be 'fixed' by an 'expert'. The methods used for this are of course physical: chemicals in the form of pills, injections or sprays; minor or major surgery; radiation treatment; physical manipulation; and other similar treatments that concentrate solely on the physical symptoms, and give little or no credence to anything other than physical causes. In this way, the person who is ill is often viewed not as a person, but as a diagnosis, so they are described as an 'asthmatic' or a 'diabetic', for example. From this viewpoint, people are seen as helpless victims – of bacteria or viruses, of faulty genes, or simply as victims of bad luck or adverse circumstances – and a person is not treated as a whole because the body is seen as a separate entity, not connected to or influenced by the mind and emotions.

2 The holistic model

Holistic is really 'wholistic', meaning that the whole person is treated, so the physical body is not viewed or treated separately but is seen as a *part* of the whole person, with the other aspects – mind, emotions, spirit, and even environment and lifestyle – being equally important. The holistic model doesn't just concentrate on the symptoms of an illness or disease, it begins to look for causes. It assumes that although some physical causation is obviously a factor in illness, such as a virus or being genetically predisposed to a disease, there are other issues to consider. A person's state of mind, level of emotional stability, living conditions or stress at work could all be a part of his or her health crisis. It is now accepted, for example, that high stress levels, such as facing redundancy at work or going through a divorce, deplete the immune system, leaving people more vulnerable to viruses or infections.

From the holistic viewpoint, unless the underlying causes of illness or disease are healed, the person will soon become ill again. The symptoms may go away temporarily, but then they will re-emerge, often as something even more serious. This is the general viewpoint of complementary and alternative medicine, and more people, including many doctors and nurses, are becoming sym-pathetic towards this view of health. Patients are encouraged to look at their lives and lifestyles to see where improvements can be made, and may be persuaded to look towards complementary and alternative therapies to help them with their health problems, either by encouraging relaxation and a greater sense of harmony and balance or to help to accelerate their healing processes. Some therapies, such as osteopathy, chiropractic, acupuncture and homeopathy, are already officially recognised as being effective – and cost effective – alternatives to conventional medical practices, and others are becoming well respected for their proven beneficial effects, such as aromatherapy, reflexology and healing (spiritual healing and Reiki).

3 The metaphysical model

Using the metaphysical approach, everything is seen as energy, and all energy is interconnected; as we have seen in the last chapter, science, in the form of quantum physics, upholds this view. The computer on which I'm writing this book, the chair I'm sitting on, the plant on the window ledge, my own physical body and even the air that surrounds me are all energy or light, vibrating at different rates. Some are vibrating relatively slowly, which makes them dense and heavy enough to be seen and felt as physical objects, and others are vibrating very quickly, which makes them finer and lighter, like the air, for example.

From this perspective, everything that we call physical or real is seen as the product of creative consciousness. Creative conscious-ness is described as God/dess, or the Source, The Creator, or All That Is, or even as the Universe, and as everything is connected that means that each of us, every individual, is also a part of that consciousness. This viewpoint is very empowering but also very challenging, because it sees each of us as co-creators with God/dess, actively creating our own reality, using our consciousness or thought processes to attract events, situations or people into our lives. The metaphysical view is that everything that happens to us, everything we experience, has meaning and purpose, so there is no such thing as luck (good or bad) or coincidence, and we are not helpless victims of random events but powerful creators of our lives, using the circumstances we create to help us to develop and grow as people – and as souls.

> We are spirit having a human experience,
> not humans having a spiritual experience.

The world we collectively create – this planet Earth – reflects the mass consciousness, the overriding beliefs, concepts, attitudes, fears and desires of the majority of people. The world we individually create – what we think, say, do and experience, who we meet and relate to, where we live, and so on – reflects our *personal* beliefs, concepts, attitudes, fears and desires. From this perspective there are two phrases that probably sum things up: 'what you resist, per-sists' and 'you get out what you put in'. What these both mean in slightly different ways is that whatever you put your attention to, that is what you will get. Therefore, if you are constantly thinking and talking negatively about something you don't want or don't like, such as an illness or money problems, you will constantly be re-creating it because you are still putting your conscious energy into it (that is, resisting it) – so of course it won't go away. Nothing will change until you 'change your mind'. Similarly, if you put out lots of positive thoughts, words and actions, your consciousness, or conscious energy, will start to create whatever you focus on, so more and more good things will begin to happen. Clearly, this means that your thoughts, speech and actions are very important, because negative conscious energy attracts and manifests negative things, while positive conscious energy attracts and manifests positive things.

I know these are quite mind-blowing concepts, and some people find them very frightening, because it turns the responsibility for our lives well and truly over to us. No one else is responsible. No one else is to blame. And equally no one else deserves the credit. Not even God/dess. Pretty scary stuff! But once you get used to the idea, this viewpoint is incredibly empowering, because it puts you in the driving seat of your life, it gives you the power to change and to become who you really want to be and to live the life you really want to live.

A LITTLE MORE SCIENCE!

I described in the last chapter the experiments that showed that a person's DNA, even when not directly connected to the person, is affected by that person's emotions. In that research, each person was asked to think of experiences that had made them sad or fearful, and their DNA double helix was observed tightening, whereas when the person thought of loving or happy experiences, the DNA strands relaxed. In other experiments Professor Emeritus William A. Tiller of Stanford University's Department of Materials Science found that the pH level of water changed when someone focused their attention and emotions on it, and this happened even if the person was just in the vicinity of the water. Japanese doctor and scientist, Masaru Emoto, has found that expressing negative emotions into water (such as despair) created distorted water crystals, whereas expressing loving emotions created beautiful symmetrical crystals. Since our bodies are composed of about 70 per cent water and contain thousands of miles of DNA, this research suggests that both might be affected by what we think about and how we feel.

A former pharmaceutical research scientist, Dr David Hamilton, became fascinated when, time after time, patients receiving placebo pills reported the same level of improvement as people receiving an actual drug. This fascination led him to research the mind–body connection, and the effect our beliefs, thoughts and emotions can have. Basically, the reason placebos work is because the person receiving the placebo *believes* they have been given a drug which will help their condition, so their body replicates the effects they believe will happen. This even occurs in experiments where one group had a real surgical operation and others received a sham operation, where cuts were made to the skin, but no inner work was carried out. Probably the most quoted case was a randomised placebo-controlled trial involving 180 patients to evaluate the efficacy of arthroscopic surgery for osteoarthritis of the knee carried out by J.B. Moseley and his co-workers in Houston, Texas (2002). The placebo group received skin incisions but no actual surgical intervention. Despite this, the outcomes (pain and function) for both groups of patients over the following two years were practically identical. If just thinking that you have had an operation can have virtually the same effects as actually having one, surely there could be no better proof that our mind–body connection is central to our health! If we *believe* we can get better, then we probably will! As Dr Hamilton says, every part of your body is wired to the brain; nerves connect it to the skin, bone, muscles, tendons and internal organs. This is why thinking about raising your arm results in you raising your arm. This is also why your beliefs, thoughts and emotions impact on your health. Loving and compassionate thoughts have been shown to encourage the release of serotonin, dopamine and oxytocin, all of which help to increase happiness levels, and these changes in the neural structures of the brain stimulate the nervous system to combat inflammation and help damaged cells to regenerate faster, so helping the healing process.

Another study by the Institute of HeartMath in the 1980s showed that volunteers who were told to spend just five minutes every morning focusing on things that made them feel loving or compassionate experienced an increase in their IgA factor (an important aspect of the immune system) which lasted several hours; in contrast, volunteers who spent five minutes a day thinking about things that made them feel angry or frustrated experienced a decrease in the IgA factor, which again lasted several hours. So, even five minutes a day of choosing to think positively or negatively can have an impact on our capacity to maintain a healthy body.

As a very basic example, think of the effects of the adrenalin rush when we're in danger, getting us ready for 'fight or flight'. That protective instinct in the body was essential when we were faced with a sabre-toothed tiger, but the response was meant to reduce when the danger was over. Life for many people today, however, produces this state of high adrenalin almost all the time, as we deal with stress at work, at home, in our relationships and so on, and this is injurious to our health. Basically, where emotion goes, a chemical flows.

The relatively new field of psychoneuroimmunology (PNI), which studies the links between the mind, stress and our nervous and immune systems, has firmly established links between stress and almost every major disease, including allergies, arthritis, autoimmune disorders, cancer, diabetes, heart disease, hypertension, infertility, irritable bowel syndrome, peptic ulcers and strokes.

These are just a few examples of what is now a sizeable and growing body of scientific research that shows that our beliefs, thoughts, attitudes, concepts, perceptions and emotions, or in other words our consciousness, has a direct effect on our physical bodies. I think this is really exciting. For very readable books that expand on this subject, try those by Dr David R. Hamilton, Gill Edwards, Candace B. Pert and Valerie V. Hunt, see Further Reading.

CONSCIOUSNESS

What exactly is 'consciousness'? The metaphysical approach assumes that each person's consciousness is made up of three parts:

1 **The Super-conscious, or Higher Self**, which is that part of us that we might call our soul or spirit; our true self which is fully connected to the God/dess Consciousness and that has full knowledge of our life purpose and the lessons and experiences we have chosen for this life. It is that very wise part of ourselves that is totally loving and supportive, and always working with us for our greatest and highest good by subtly guiding us and providing us with intuition and deep insight, whether we choose to acknowledge and act on this wisdom or ignore it.

2 **The Conscious Self**, sometimes referred to as the ego, is who we think we are, in other words our thinking, speaking, acting self, our personality, our beliefs, attitudes, concepts, likes, dislikes and so on – everything that makes us recognisable as ourselves. The Conscious Self is not necessarily aware of the helpful insights provided by either the Higher Self or the Subconscious Self, but can operate independently until such time as the person is ready to begin to discover more about themselves, developing and growing personally and spiritually so that they become more 'in tune' with the other aspects of their consciousness.

3 **The Subconscious**, which works with the Higher Self to provide intuition and insight to the Conscious Self through dreams, visualisations, instinctive 'feelings' or 'gut reactions' and other aspects of 'body wisdom'.

BODY WISDOM

Our physical body has its own conscious energy system, or body wisdom, which is always working for our greatest and highest good. Because of this it tries to tell us when something is going wrong, either with our thinking or in our lives generally. Its messages take the form of symptoms, illness or disease; so, when we have a headache, catch a cold or flu, have toothache or become more seriously ill, our body is trying to tell us something, trying to get us to understand the signal and do something about it. But that is the difficulty, because we don't always understand this kind of 'body language', and some people are completely unaware of it, so its significance is lost.

Most people react to illness or disease by trying to get rid of the symptoms as quickly as possible, usually by seeking medical advice or intervention. An advertisement on television a few years ago caught my attention, because it was extolling the virtues of a popular analgesic as something 'for people who don't have time to have headaches'. I found this quite alarming, because while there is nothing wrong in seeking relief for symptoms, if you really want your body to be healed, you also need to understand the illness at the causative level. If you have constant headaches, 'masking' them with medication and carrying on as if nothing was wrong is not a long-term solution. You are not listening to what your body is trying to tell you, so, although the symptoms might abate briefly, they will return because you are not taking your body's advice and acting upon it.

Your first priority is to ask yourself *'Why* am I ill?' Because, from the metaphysical perspective, illness or disease is created by the body – albeit as a helpful message. As the body is simply a part of our consciousness, this means that we actually create our own ill health. Again, this may be a very challenging concept, but as I pointed out earlier, the metaphysical viewpoint is really very empowering, because if we have the power to create ill health with negative beliefs, thoughts and emotions, then we also have the power to create good health with positivity.

This is definitely *not* a 'blame theory', however. Although you may ultimately be responsible at a deep spiritual level for having created an illness, this is not being done at a conscious level so there is no blame attached, and therefore you should not harshly judge yourself – or anyone else – for being ill. You don't suddenly wake up one morning and say, 'Oh, I think I'll break my leg/slip a disc/develop ME today, that'll stop me rushing around doing too much, and I can have a good rest and some time to think about my direction in life!' From a human perspective that would be utter madness! But from a Soul/Higher Self/Subconscious Self level the pain of the broken leg or slipped disc, or the problems associated with living with ME, are simply experiences on your journey through this physical life, and they do what they are supposed to do: they stop you in your tracks; that is, they stop you making further progress down the wrong path. If you heed the messages, all well and good, and you can heal and move on, but if you don't, then they will lead to different life experiences, although from the soul perspective even that is still OK. All experience – good, bad or indifferent – is good experience for the growth and development of the soul, but not necessarily pleasant as a human being living through it.

I appreciate that these metaphysical theories can be very difficult to come to terms with if you haven't heard them before, and they may well challenge your belief system or your concept of how the world works, and of course you are free to take them on board or ignore them, the choice is yours. But if reading about them has sparked at least an interest in finding out more, then there are some recommended books in the Further Reading section, which you might find useful. To summarise this metaphysical viewpoint:

- Every illness or disease, accident or injury has a message for you, and the more serious the illness or injury, the more serious and urgent the message.

- Nothing is accidental or coincidental.

- Every experience is useful and valid and contains some valuable information for you, even some of the minor things – such as cutting your finger with a knife while chopping vegetables. Why were you distracted? What were you thinking about at the time? What are you feeling 'sore' about?

UNDERSTANDING YOUR BODY'S 'LANGUAGE'

Your body sends you messages every day: to highlight that something is not right in your life; to nudge you into noticing that you are going in the wrong direction; or to bring to your attention that there are lessons to be learned which you are ignoring. The trouble is we are not speaking the same language, especially if we think every 'accident' is accidental, every pain is just something to be got rid of, and every illness is just an inconvenience and something to be suffered until it is over.

If you are frequently unwell, could the underlying reason (or 'dis-ease') be that you are unhappy or too stressed at work, but the only way you will give yourself permission to take time off is to be ill? Is being sick perhaps a way of getting more attention or affectionate responses from your family or partner? Do you 'need' an illness to slow you down because you have reached a stage in your spiritual life when you need lots of time by yourself for inner reflection? These are just a few examples of the possible messages offered by the body for you to examine, learn from and then take action, making the necessary changes in your life to bring about harmony and good health. Of course there isn't room in this book to give anything other than a very short outline of some suggested metaphysical causes of illness and disease, so I have recommended some books in the Further Reading section that deal with this issue if you want to explore it further.

The list below shows just a few of the possible relationships between parts of the body or specific illnesses and facets of our inner selves, as a very rough guide. This list is only a brief example of a complex issue, and it is not intended to be regarded as the 'truth' in every case. See if they 'feel' right to you; they are generalisations and each case is individual, so you may need to explore the issue in more depth. In the meantime, however, it may sound simplistic to say that if you have a sore throat you may be experiencing problems expressing yourself, but just be prepared to look at that, honestly, to see if it has any relevance for you. If not, that's fine, but please remember that most of us are very good at hiding our motivations from ourselves, so probing our deeper reasoning can be an uncomfortable and disturbing experience. Therefore, even if at first you want to deny it outright, it could be worth having another look.

Causative issues linked with body parts

Left side of body	Represents our feminine side and our inner journey, as well as creativity, imagination, spiritual and psychic issues
Right side of body	Represents our masculine side and our outer journey, as well as money or job issues, or other practical, physical and material concerns
Head	Who or what is being a 'headache' to you? Are you living too much 'in your head' and not paying enough attention to your feelings?
Eyes	How do you 'see' the world? What are you not prepared to see? Are you looking at things from an unhelpful perspective?
Ears	What is it that you are unwilling to hear? Are you avoiding listening to your inner guidance?
Mouth	Have you 'bitten off more than you can chew'? Has something or someone 'left a nasty taste in your mouth'? Are you desperate to 'get your teeth into something'?
Throat	Have you swallowed your anger and hurt? Are you expressing your feelings? Are you telling the truth? Are you feeling guilty about something you've said?
Shoulders	Are you carrying too many burdens and responsibilities? Do you always put yourself last in your list of priorities? Is your life too stressful?

Arms	Who or what are you holding on to? Are you afraid to let go? Who or what would you like to embrace? Are you doing what you want to do?
Hands	Associated with giving (right hand) and receiving (left hand). What issues or situation can't you 'handle'?
Fingers	What can't you 'grasp'? What opportunities are 'slipping through your fingers'? Do you ignore the little details to concentrate only on the 'bigger picture'?
Upper back	Associated with stored anger and resentment, feeling unsupported, and trying to be perfect. Are you 'pushing back' your feelings?
Chest (heart/ lungs)	Relationship issues, self-esteem and feelings of worth or worthlessness, suppressed emotions, feeling smothered or controlled by others, your public image, and deeply buried issues about deserving (or not wanting) to be alive
Stomach	Who or what can't you 'stomach'? What are you finding difficult to digest? What are you worrying about? Who or what would you like to eliminate from your life?
Lower back	Survival, security and self-support; job, home and money issues; responsibility issues. Do you feel the people around you are giving you enough support? Do you often feel worried about inconsequential things that might be masking bigger issues?
Legs	Associated with progress through life, fear of change, fear of the future, and family or parental issues. Who or what is holding you back? Why can't you move forward?
Knees	Linked with stubbornness, inflexibility and indecision. What decision are you afraid to make? Are you being obstinate over something?
Ankles	Do you need to change direction? Is your life unbalanced?
Feet	Associated with security and survival, reaching our goals or completing tasks, fear of taking the next step, being 'ungrounded'. Who or what can't you 'stand' any more?
Skin	Touching and feeling issues; oversensitivity. Who or what is 'getting under your skin'?

USING ENERGY FOR HEALING

As mentioned in the last chapter, everyone is born with an ability
to heal, because we all have our own supply of life-force energy,
or *Ki*, and this can act as a healing energy if we wish. But if we
constantly give our life-force away to heal other people, our supply
can become too depleted, and then we can gradually find ourselves
becoming listless, depressed or ill.

This can also happen if we come into contact with people who
are, quite unconsciously, 'energy drains', sometimes called 'energy
vampires'. That may sound alarming, but you might have experienced something like that – always feeling exceptionally tired when
you are with a particular person, or perhaps always being very
irritated or anxious around someone, even though there doesn't
appear to be any cause. Fortunately, this type of energy draining is
usually quite a rare occurrence, and the person who is sucking your
energy is almost always unaware of it; however, they may be ill or
just have an energy field with an unnaturally low vibration which
automatically attracts higher vibrations.

SPIRITUAL HEALING

Hands-on healing has been used for thousands of years in virtually
every religion, culture and society. Some healers use their own life-
force energy to heal others, but they can easily become exhausted
if they use too much, because the body needs sufficient time to
replenish its energy supply. Other spiritual healers work by being a
focus for the energies supplied by 'unseen friends' or spirit guides
(people in the spiritual realm who have agreed to help humanity
in this way) and they place their hands to direct energy wherever
their guides tell them it is needed. Some spiritual healers, however,
are able to draw healing energy into themselves from the Source,
which then flows into the person they are healing. This method is
similar to using Reiki, but as I said in the last chapter, it isn't Reiki
unless they have received an attunement to that particular energy.
I have had many spiritual healers attending my Reiki workshops,
and they have all reported that the Reiki energy feels quite different to them, and it seems to flow instantaneously unlike the other

healing energies they work with that tend to build up more slowly. This would seem to confirm that Reiki is a unique strand of healing energy with its own vibrational frequency, although I personally believe all healing energies come from the same Source.

REIKI AS A TOOL FOR HEALING

It can therefore be a great advantage to work with Reiki as a healing tool, because you can channel it into your energy body and out through your hands, and then when you place your hands either on yourself or on another person who needs healing, the Reiki will flow without depleting your own personal reserves of life-force energy in any way. Also, because Reiki is guided by your Soul/ Higher Self, it works holistically, so its effects are not limited to the physical body but also affect the mind, emotions and spirit, healing, harmonising and balancing the whole, as in the following:

Physical: Reiki supports and accelerates the body's own natural ability to heal itself, helping to alleviate pain and relieve other symptoms while cleansing the body of poisons and toxins. Reiki balances and harmonises the whole energy body, promoting a sense of wholeness, a state of positive wellness and an overall feeling of well-being. It also works with a person's physical consciousness, or body wisdom, to help them develop a greater awareness of the body's real needs; for example, the right nutrition, exercise and sleep pattern.

Mental: Reiki flows into all levels of a person's thinking processes, allowing them to let go of negative thoughts, concepts and attitudes, and replacing them with positivity, peace and serenity. This leads to a state of deep relaxation, with the consequent release of stress and tension. Reiki works with the energy field, especially the brow chakra (third eye) to enhance intuitive abilities, and it also works with all levels of a person's consciousness to encourage them to pursue their personal potential through greater insight and self-awareness.

Emotional: Reiki flows into all levels of a person's emotional energy – those of which they are aware, and those they keep hidden – to encourage them to examine their emotional responses to people and situations, allowing them to let go of negative emotions such as anger or jealousy, and promoting the qualities of loving, caring, sharing, trusting and goodwill. It can also help people to channel emotional energy into creativity.

Spiritual: Reiki flows into a person's whole energy body, soul and spirit, to help them to accept and love their whole self, and fosters a non-judgemental approach to humankind, allowing them to accept every person as a soul energy on its own spiritual path, not just as a human being with all its attendant failings and frailties. It promotes the qualities of love, compassion, understanding and acceptance, and encourages a person on their personal path towards spiritual development and connectedness with the Divine.

THE NEED FOR A CHANGE IN CONSCIOUSNESS

Whether we take a conventional or a metaphysical view, any illness, pain or disease is a signal from the body to indicate that something is wrong. From the conventional viewpoint, the indications are fairly basic. If we have a pain in the stomach area then a doctor will look for physical reasons, such as an ulcer, a viral infection or maybe even a grumbling appendix, and will prescribe appropriate treatment, which could range from antibiotics to surgery.

From the metaphysical point of view, the message is seen at the causative level, so a stomach pain might indicate that there is something happening in your life which you are, literally, finding 'hard to stomach'. Reiki usually alleviates such physical symptoms quite quickly, but because it also works at the causative level, it will help to raise to the surface the issues that are at the root of the physical problem. Perhaps what you cannot 'stomach' is the way you are being treated by your boss or colleagues at work, but once the stomach ache goes away you go back to work and carry on as normal. In this case, the *cause* has not been removed, even though the symptom has been relieved. Soon the tension returns, and the stomach ache comes back, or is replaced by some other, often more serious, symptom of stress. What is needed is a *change of consciousness*: a realisation that something must be done about the situation at work.

The problem needs to be tackled in a proactive way. This might mean being assertive and telling your work colleagues that you don't find their attitude acceptable, or talking to your boss about your dissatisfaction. It may even mean you really need to look for another job that you would find more enjoyable and perhaps better suited to your skills and talents, because sometimes illness can be a 'wake up' call to show us that we are not on the right track.

The main theme here is being involved in your own healing and taking responsibility for your own health and well-being. One of the best and easiest ways of helping you to do this is by learning how to use Reiki, so that you can be an active participant in your own self-healing, and that's what we deal with in the next chapter.

Chapter 4

Training in Reiki

People have lots of different reasons for attending their first Reiki course, but for many it is the desire to help others that finally motivates them to sign up for a workshop. Most of us know someone – a family member or a friend – who could do with a little help with an illness or other aspects of their health, and it is natural to want to do something positive for the people we care about. Others have a wish to help themselves to get over a health problem, and have heard that you can use Reiki to treat yourself. Some people, however, simply want Reiki to help them to relax, or cope with frenetic, stressful lives, while others want to add it to the range of therapies they already offer to clients.

Whatever the motivation, the most frequently quoted reason seems to be that 'it just felt right'. People progress, personally and spiritually, through all the experiences life gives them, and it seems that when the time is right Reiki finds you, rather than you finding Reiki. It will begin to turn up in your life in some way – you will read an article in a magazine, overhear a conversation in a café, find your best friend has recently completed a course, or a book just catches your eye in your local bookstore (perhaps even this one!). You may never have heard of it before, or you might have been thinking about it for some time, but there it is – Reiki.

As I explained in Chapter 2, all energy is connected, and when your Soul/Higher Self feels that Reiki is an appropriate next step for you, to help you grow both personally and spiritually, it sends out a signal, and Reiki, being guided by a Higher Intelligence, picks up the signal and finds you. From then on, it is likely to keep turning up until you get the message!

HOW DO PEOPLE ACQUIRE THE ABILITY TO USE REIKI?

Reiki is the simplest and easiest holistic healing method available to us, so anyone can learn to use it, whatever their age or gender, religion or origin. No specific prior knowledge or experience is required; you need only a desire to learn, a willingness to let this healing energy flow through you, and some spare time to attend a short course.

However, Reiki cannot be 'learned' in any of the ways with which we in the West are familiar. You cannot acquire the ability to channel Reiki by reading a book, or attending a lecture, or watching a television programme or DVD; although you can learn how to *use* Reiki in those ways – for example, where to place your hands when carrying out a Reiki treatment.

Reiki doesn't actually require any learning, in the traditional sense, because it is not knowledge-based. It is experience-based. You have to take part in a special ceremony of spiritual empowerment, usually called an attunement or initiation, where you become connected to the Reiki energy by a qualified Reiki Master who has been taught how to carry out that process, so that you become a Reiki channel, able to draw Reiki into yourself whenever and wherever you wish to.

Becoming a Reiki channel

The spiritual empowerment 'attunes' your energy body to the particular vibrational frequencies of the Reiki energy, meaning it brings your energies and the Reiki energies into harmony with one another, so that the Reiki can flow easily into and around your energy field. This process also creates or, more accurately, reactivates a permanent spiritual channel (a type of conduit in the energy body to carry spiritual energy) within your energy field, through which Reiki (and only Reiki) can flow into your crown chakra, and through your brow, throat and heart chakras to your arms and then down to the centre of each palm, and out (see the illustration on page 35). This channel is not visible (except perhaps to people with exceptional psychic gifts), but I usually describe it as an energy equivalent of a fibre-optic tube. Just as light can flow down a fibre-optic tube and be seen shining out of the other end, so Reiki flows down this channel in your energy body until it flows out of your hands.

'Channelling' healing energy is similar to 'channelling' other forms of spiritual energy, which is something that has been a part of many spiritual traditions throughout history. It is a word that can also encompass forms of mediumship, communicating with spirit guides (human spirits who have lived before, and whose work is now to help humans to follow their own spiritual path), 'speaking in tongues' and other mystical experiences. Some Reiki Masters claim to have 'channelled' additional symbols, or new methods of attunement, or specific hand positions to enhance their healing, and other people speak of 'channelling' information from highly evolved spiritual guides. What this means in real terms is that they have received insight and inspiration they believe to be from a source outside of themselves, or possibly from their Souls/Higher Selves, which may take place during meditation or visualisation, during a creative activity or simply when walking in natural surroundings. For some of these people this can produce a very profound spiritual experience of a psychic nature, while for others it seems more like a perfectly normal part of everyday life, like waking up from a powerful and enlightening dream. Channelling Reiki, on the other hand, is simple, easy and automatic once you have been attuned to its energetic vibration; it isn't 'spooky', it requires no rituals or complicated processes, and it feels perfectly natural.

THE LEVELS OF TRAINING

There are normally three levels of training, although sometimes you may encounter Reiki Masters who split the training into four, five or even seven parts. The levels are usually described as Reiki 1, 2 and 3 or Reiki I, II and III or often as Reiki First, Second and Third Degrees – but this does not refer to (or confer) any academic level or qualification. (The Third Degree is usually referred to as Reiki Master.) In the Japanese tradition, these levels are called *Shoden*, *Okuden* and *Shinpiden*, and you will find a full explanation about those levels and what they include in Part 5.

The Attunement/Initiation Process

The word 'attune' means to bring into harmony, and the process of being 'attuned' to the energetic frequency of Reiki is how you are 'initiated' into Reiki – how you become a 'channel' for Reiki. The attunement process makes Reiki unique, and is the reason why the ability to heal can be developed so quickly, yet so permanently. It is a sacred ceremony of spiritual empowerment, and the actual process is kept secret until someone becomes a Reiki Master, when the Reiki 3 student is taught the Master Symbol and the attunement procedure for each of the three levels of Reiki.

As I have described earlier, the attunement carried out in a Reiki class is a version of the spiritual empowerment that Dr Usui received on Mount Kurama, but gentler and less powerful than he experienced. Its purpose is to form a connection between the Reiki energy and the Reiki Master, which is then transferred to the student. When the Reiki Master 'brings in' the energy in order to commence the attunement, this has the effect of altering the space around the Master and student(s), filling it with Reiki to provide a protective environment. When I am carrying out an attunement I can always feel this difference, and some students also remark upon it afterwards, but on some occasions I have actually seen this take place, and the whole room seems to be bathed in violet light.

Another effect is that the Reiki Master becomes filled with lots of Reiki in a very tangible way and, again, I always see and feel this. On several occasions I have taught Reiki in a dance studio, which had mirrors down one side, and as I carried out the attunements I looked up and saw my reflection, and was amazed to see myself surrounded by a very visible bright golden aura, spreading out to at least 2m (6½ft) around and above me, and I could also see the stream of Reiki coming down into my crown chakra. Also, every time I carry out attunements, I notice an incredible increase in my body heat as the Reiki fills me, and this is one reason why I limit the number of students I teach in a class, as the more students I have, the greater the amount of energy I have to carry, so the hotter I get!

What happens in an attunement?

Although each attunement has the same elements, each Reiki Master decides exactly how they should be carried out, and sometimes this will depend on the way the Master prefers to teach. Some Masters like to teach on a one-to-one basis, so they will obviously carry out the attunement process on that individual. Other Masters teach groups of students, so they will often gather all the students together, usually seated on chairs set out in a straight line, a circle, or a horseshoe shape. Sometimes, however, even if the Master teaches a group, they may prefer to perform the whole attunement on one student at a time, so any other students in the class are asked to wait in another room, and take turns to receive the attunement.

Whichever way the Master prefers to operate, they will usually set out the room according to their own preferences, and often this will include having candles and incense burning, and possibly a small altar with crystals and other sacred objects on it, including perhaps a photograph of Dr Usui. Although none of these additions is essential, they help to highlight the special and sacred nature of the attunement. The room will then be cleansed with Reiki, to help to create a 'sacred space', and the students will be invited to take their seats. Before the attunement begins, the Master will normally explain to the student(s) what to expect, and will then ask them to hold their hands in the prayer position (called *Gassho* in Japanese) with their thumbs pointing to the middle of the chest. They will then be asked to close their eyes, and to keep them closed throughout the whole procedure. The attunement is normally carried out in silence, although appropriate soft background music may be played.

When the students have settled, the Master will then begin by quietly 'tuning in' to the Reiki vibrations before connecting with and channelling into themselves sufficient Reiki energy to carry out the spiritual empowerment. The process is usually carried out with the Master standing initially behind the student, then in front, and ending behind the student again. At various stages during the process there may be some gentle touching on the student's head and hands, and the student may be asked to raise their hands above their head for a few moments, but everything is gentle, supportive and restful. At the end of each attunement, the Master 'seals' the channel open, so from then on you have your own direct and permanent connection with Reiki.

The attunement is a very special, meditative experience, and the silent contemplation with eyes closed is for two reasons. The first is obviously because, as a sacred and spiritual ceremony, the procedures are intended to be kept secret until such time as any individual student trains to be a Reiki Master. The second, less obvious, reason is that when someone has their eyes closed this reduces any external distractions around them, stilling the mind so that they are more easily able to stay in an appropriate meditative state, which leaves them more receptive to, and aware of, any potential mystical experience.

Being initiated into Reiki is a powerful spiritual experience, although how it is experienced will vary from person to person, as the *Rei*, or God-consciousness, guides the whole process, adjusting it according to the needs of each individual. After the attunements are over, students often describe the beautiful spiritual or mystical experiences they have enjoyed, such as 'seeing' wonderful colours, or visions of beautiful healing places. Others report receiving personal insights or profound healing, sensing the presence of spirit guides or angelic beings or simply having a feeling of complete peace. Some students don't experience anything unusual, however, and can feel disappointed and think that the attunement hasn't worked on them. If this happens to you, please don't worry, it does *not* mean the attunement hasn't worked – it *always* works, provided it is being carried out by a qualified Reiki Master!

THE EFFECTS OF ATTUNEMENT TO REIKI

The attunement is only the start of your connection to Reiki, and over the ensuing weeks and months as you practise using it, the flow of Reiki gains strength so that within six to eight weeks after being initiated into Reiki you are experiencing the full flow of energy. Basically, the more you use it, the better it flows, and once you have received a Reiki attunement you will be able to use Reiki for the rest of your life. It doesn't wear off or wear out, the supply of Reiki is inexhaustible, and you can never lose the ability to channel it.

If for some reason you don't use Reiki for a long time, you may think it isn't flowing because you don't have any sensation of it in your hands. Some people ask to be reattuned if this happens, but there really is no need, because it is still there – you just need to carry out some self-cleansing (which I will describe later) and some self-treatments to bring back the full flow. If you choose to undertake a reattunement, however, it won't do any harm; it can be another pleasant experience and will also increase the amount of Reiki you can channel (see the later section on Multiple Attunements).

At each level of attunement (Reiki 1, 2 or 3) you become able to tap into a higher, wider channel of Reiki healing energy, and the vibrationary rate of your energy body is increased. After an attunement some people go through a shift in their awareness immediately, describing the sensation as almost like being reborn, so that they experience everything around them more intensely: colours are brighter, their sense of smell is enhanced and sounds are sharper. Others feel a buzzing or heightened sensitivity in the crown chakra for a short while, or describe a sense of floating or light-headedness. All of these reactions are absolutely normal. Nevertheless, experiencing very little is quite common too, and while it may be a little disappointing for some students, as I have already mentioned, it definitely doesn't mean the attunement has not worked.

Because Reiki is guided by a Higher Intelligence, it therefore adjusts to suit each person, so everyone's experience of a Reiki attunement is slightly different, even though the process is identical for everyone. If someone has already been doing energy work for some time – perhaps t'ai chi, qigong or martial arts, or they already do some form of spiritual healing – then their bodies are already tuned in to higher energetic vibrations, so they are able to absorb and channel more Reiki right from the moment they are attuned. The same is often true of people who have done a lot of spiritual work, including deep meditation. If a person has never done anything in terms of energy or spiritual work they will still be able to channel Reiki, but the flow of energy they experience may initially be a bit less. After a few weeks of practice, however, there is very little difference between the amount of Reiki flowing through the energetically or spiritually experienced or inexperienced person.

It is this unique attunement process which is one of the major differences between Reiki and other 'hands-on healing' methods. It is possible to learn how to channel other forms of spiritual healing, and there are various organisations that teach it, such as The Healing Trust (formerly the National Federation of Spiritual Healers) in the UK, and there are similar establishments in other countries. Do bear in mind, though, that it can take many months to learn and, as I explained earlier, the energy channelled by spiritual healers is not Reiki but energy of a different vibration.

THE FLOW OF ENERGY

The channel which is created during the Reiki spiritual empowerment becomes active immediately, so within minutes you can begin
to draw Reiki through yourself, which can then be used either for
your own healing or to heal others. From then on, whenever you
intend to use Reiki, simply thinking about it, or holding your hands
out in readiness to use it, will activate it – there are no complicated
rituals to follow.

Reiki does not flow through you all the time, however. You can
put out your hand to pick up a cup of tea, for instance, but that
won't switch the Reiki on! What starts the Reiki flowing is your
intention to use it. Later on, however, when you have been using
Reiki for some time, you may find that the Reiki does occasionally
'switch on' without you actively *intending* it to happen, but if you
have been practising Reiki quite a lot on yourself and on others
your unspoken intention is to use Reiki whenever it is needed. As
it is Divinely guided, if there is a person (or an animal) nearby who
is really in need of it, then their Higher Self (and animals have a
form of higher consciousness too) will know that you are a Reiki
channel, and will request it. The Reiki will just respond, because on
a subconscious level you have given permission – you have chosen
to become a Reiki channel.

This process can only happen, however, because Reiki is *pulled*
by the recipient, not *pushed* by the Practitioner. Healing cannot be
forced on to anyone; however, this doesn't have to be a conscious
process, either for the Practitioner or the recipient, because it is
controlled by the recipient's Higher Self, not by their thought processes. Therefore, the person receiving the Reiki doesn't need to do
anything or think about anything in particular. It is helpful if the
recipient is consciously willing to receive the energy, but even this
is not strictly necessary. Reiki will flow into animals, and they don't
know what it is! If a person's Soul/Higher Self knows they need
healing, it will draw Reiki into the person's energy body, overriding
any conscious objections. When I do public demonstrations of Reiki,
I often come across people who are very sceptical, and who patently
do not believe Reiki can work. If they can be persuaded to allow me
to place my hands on their shoulders to see if the Reiki will flow,
they are almost without exception astonished at the results, and
often they are then the first to sign up to take a Reiki course.

SENSATIONS OF REIKI FLOWING THROUGH YOUR HANDS

Another effect following a Reiki attunement is that whenever you *intend* it to, Reiki begins to flow out of the palms of your hands. The way in which students experience this is very varied. As I explained earlier, Reiki adjusts to suit each recipient, so some people are fairly clear channels to start with, and in those instances more Reiki can flow through them; the more Reiki flows through, the more sensation you are likely to get. But people sense energy in different ways. Some experience the world in a very *visual way*, so they might see the energy as colours, getting very little physical sensation in their hands. Others experience the world *kinaesthetically*, being much more aware of physical sensations caused by the flow of energy – they may even experience the energy as a taste or a smell, although this is less usual. When they place their hands on themselves, or on others, to do Reiki, some people have immediate feelings in their hands of heat or gentle warmth, a cool sensation as though a breeze was blowing on them, or they sense tingling, prickling, tickling or buzzing in their hands and fingers. A few even experience these sensations going up their arms as well, and occasionally these sensations are experienced in the crown chakra, too. But you will not necessarily feel anything, at least at first, and it is important to realise that this is OK – sensations are not essential, the Reiki will still flow and will still have beneficial effects whether you feel anything or not.

If there are several blockages in your energy body it might take a little longer to establish a full flow, so you may gradually begin to experience some sensations after a few weeks or months – provided you use Reiki, that is. If you just give up straight away you are unlikely to clear the blockages sufficiently to get the Reiki flowing fully. You have still retained the ability to channel Reiki, you are just not using it.

Rid yourself of the idea that there are people who are 'no good at Reiki'; everyone who has been attuned has roughly the same potential to be a good Reiki channel, and the Reiki which flows through a brand new Reiki First Degree student is exactly the same as the Reiki that flows through their initiating Reiki Master. It may not flow as much or as fast, but it is the quality not the quantity that counts. True, a few people do turn out to be outstanding at channelling Reiki – and being treated by them is fabulous – like being under a waterfall of pure healing. But that ability is rare, and I have no plausible explanation for it.

Apart from the experiences I have already described, some people find they are very hungry during and after a Reiki course or they need much more sleep than usual. This is probably because they are not used to the higher vibrational energy flowing through them, so it is rather like getting your physical body going when you first start taking exercise – it is just tiring. Others, conversely, seem to have lots of extra energy – but that just demonstrates that each person has an individual experience of Reiki.

Most people do feel on a 'high' – buzzing with excitement and enthusiasm – when they have finished the course because, for many, an attunement is definitely a peak experience, so I recommend that when you have attended a Reiki workshop you try to slip back into normal life as gently as possible afterwards. This might not be easy, as often the courses are held at the weekend and you may have to get back to work on the Monday. If you do have the chance to take an extra day off, however, just allow yourself to 'come down' slowly, perhaps sleeping longer and then spending the day doing gentle things like walking, reading, meditating or listening to relaxing music – and giving yourself Reiki.

After each level of attunement the vibrationary rate at which you operate is raised, and in order for this to happen there has to be a clearing of old physical, mental, emotional and spiritual patterns and thoughts which inhibit the growth of consciousness. One of the major effects of an attunement, therefore, is what is called the 21-day clearing cycle, where your whole energy body is cleansed and cleared by the Reiki. This is not a permanent effect, however, so you will need to use Reiki to cleanse your energy system quite regularly, but there are details of that in a later chapter.

THE 21-DAY CLEARING CYCLE

This clearing cycle usually takes about three weeks, hence the title, but can sometimes be accomplished more quickly, or take a little longer. During the first few weeks after each Reiki attunement, at whatever level, the Reiki that flowed into your physical and energy bodies so powerfully during the attunement begins to work on clearing specific parts of your auric field associated with the physical, emotional, mental and spiritual aspects of the self. It does this through the chakras, seeming to clear, harmonise and balance one chakra each day for the first week, and then the cycle repeats itself as often as necessary until the clearing work is completed, which is why it may take less than three weeks, or as long as five, six or seven weeks, depending upon how much clearing and balancing work is required.

The clearing begins gradually, starting at the root or base chakra on day one, then the sacral chakra on day two, and the solar plexus chakra on day three, and so on, right up to the crown chakra on day seven. During the clearing process, you may find that facets of your life associated with each of the chakras are highlighted, perhaps through dreams or memories, or people coming back into your life to trigger certain thoughts and feelings to help you let go of them. The following points might help you to identify these areas, and they also describe what some people call the four etheric bodies – physical, emotional, mental and spiritual – within your energy field.

Physical: There are two chakras most closely associated with your physical energies. The root chakra, which is related to your basic survival instinct and feelings of security, can trigger issues about money, your home and job, or your physical body. The sacral chakra relates to physical sensations and sexuality, so issues of intimacy and sex, as well as those associated with food, appetite and other sensual pleasures can come up.

Emotional: The two chakras associated with emotional energies are the solar plexus and the heart. With the solar plexus chakra, issues to do with your feelings and beliefs about yourself might come up, such as autonomy, life purpose, willpower and self-esteem, while the heart chakra's issues link to your ability to love unconditionally and include giving and receiving, compassion for others and loving acceptance of yourself.

Mental: The throat and brow chakras are associated with your mental energies. The throat chakra throws up issues about communication, self-expression and your sense of deservingness. With the brow chakra, also called the third eye, issues raised might include psychic and spiritual awareness, your ability to respond to intuition or insight, and your recognition of yourself as a unique individual consciousness.

Spiritual: The crown chakra is linked with your spiritual energies, and issues about knowledge and intellect, as well as your capacity to understand on a deeper, more spiritual level, may be raised, including a desire to explore aspects of mystical union with the Divine and connectedness with all life.

During the second and third weeks this clearing cycle is repeated in the same way – root chakra on day one, sacral chakra on day two, and so on. I usually describe this to my students as a sort of energetic 'spring cleaning' where the Reiki gently flows through and breaks down the blockages in your whole energy system.

HEALING CRISIS

As the blocks that are preventing your progress are brought forward, the trapped and blocked energies need to be released by your energy body. Sometimes this is achieved quite easily and you may feel colder than usual, as energy, while being released, often has an icy feel. The intensity of the clearing and the way it is experienced depends upon each person, as everyone is unique, with their own personal life experiences, thought patterns, emotional baggage and so on. The effects of the release of any blockages can vary from feeling more emotional or irritable than usual, or having the urge to laugh or cry frequently, to a sense of detachment and the need to spend more time alone. Other blocked energy may need to be released through your physical body, however, and you may experience a temporary 'healing crisis', such as having a cold or sweating a lot, or even occasionally being sick or having diarrhoea for a while. These are simply ways to release toxins out of the body and they are perfectly natural (if a little uncomfortable), so please don't be alarmed. These effects do not always happen, however, so don't turn them into a 'self-fulfilling prophecy'.

The reason some people occasionally experience more severe physical reactions is usually because there are deeper blockages to release – for example, perhaps they are harbouring very deep resentment or hatred against someone, either consciously or sub-consciously. These intense emotional feelings have to be cleared from the energy body, and as they can be represented by almost tangible, dense energy, they need to flow into the physical body in order to be released. The easiest route is through the body's excretory system, but if the body is in any way dehydrated, other more extreme routes may need to be chosen (like vomiting), because it is in the body's best interests to be rid of this toxic energy as quickly as possible. Another reason this can happen is if the person is spiritually ready to release and clear issues on a deeper level, but this may be more likely to happen after a Second Degree or Master-level attunement.

It is important to remember, however, that Reiki is Divinely guided, and therefore always works for the highest good, so you can trust Reiki to know what is best for you and to do it – even if that sometimes results in some temporary discomfort.

HELPING THE CLEARING PROCESS

You can make the whole process as easy as possible for yourself by following these suggestions:

- Do lots of Reiki on yourself, especially a full Reiki self-treatment (see Chapter 6) for at least 30 minutes every day during this clearing cycle.

- Drink lots of water – at least six to eight glasses (approximately 2 litres (3½ pints) a day). This needs to be pure water (other drinks like tea, coffee, cordials, beer, wine, fizzy drinks, and so on, don't count because they either contain toxins, or act as a diuretic), but it can be either bottled or filtered tap water. Sparkling water is OK very occasionally, but as the carbon dioxide, which makes it fizzy, is actually one of your body's waste products, you are potentially accumulating more toxins. It is best to drink the water plain, rather than adding any flavours, although herbal teas are acceptable. **Note:** If you have any health problems, particularly any related to water retention, please seek medical advice before drinking extra water.

- Try to reduce your intake of obvious toxins such as alcohol, cigarettes or other drugs (but do *not* reduce the dosage of any drugs or medicines prescribed by your doctor).

- It is also helpful to eat very healthily at this time, concentrating on fresh foods, particularly organic vegetables and fruit, rather than pre-packaged ready meals and other processed foods, which often contain lots of additives and preservatives.

Over the 21 days, and for a number of weeks afterwards, you will probably notice a gradual strengthening of the Reiki as you use it, and may notice other changes in yourself, too. For this purpose I often suggest to my students that they keep a journal of their 'Reiki journey' for the first few weeks, where they can record what they experience during self-treatment, or during treatments of friends, family, pets or plants. They also find it a good idea to write down any vivid dreams, emotional episodes, feelings or meditations they experience, or changes they feel are taking place in themselves – and perhaps link them to the particular chakra which is being 'cleared' on that day.

MULTIPLE ATTUNEMENTS

Some students enjoy attunements so much that they want to repeat the experience as often as possible, which is one of the reasons why some people choose to progress very quickly through Reiki 1, 2 and 3. Other people choose instead to attend several Reiki courses at the same level, but with different Masters, sometimes because they are under the (mistaken) impression that they have not been attuned 'properly', or that because they have not used their Reiki for months – or years – it will not work any more, which is another mistaken belief. Some Reiki Masters are very much against this, but although I would not wish to encourage people to become 'attunement junkies', there is nothing intrinsically wrong with having a number of attunements at the same level, as each attunement helps to widen the Reiki channel, enabling even more Reiki to flow through.

Indeed, you may remember that in Japan it is usual for Reiki students to gather together about once a month with their Master to share treatments, ask questions and receive a simple attunement/ empowerment called *Reiju*. This is not identical to the attunement process used to initiate a person during a Reiki course in the West, but it does increase the power and flow of the Reiki they can channel, and is beneficial for their spiritual development, too (there is more information about this in Part 5).

Waiting for a reasonable time between attunements is sensible, because it then allows your physical body to adjust to the new, higher vibrationary rate that results from the previous attunement. This is the case whether you intend to take several attunements at the same level with the same or different Masters, and is even more important if you want to progress from Reiki 1 to Reiki 2, or from Reiki 2 to Reiki 3, because at each level of Reiki training the attunement expands your Reiki channel and increases the amount of Reiki that can flow through you. I recommend a minimum of three months between Reiki First and Second Degree (and most of my students choose to wait between six months and a year), and then a minimum of two, or preferably three, years of active Reiki practice on yourself and others, at Second Degree level before being attuned at Third Degree/Master level. This gives you time to gather practical experience of treatments, and also time to carry out self-healing, which is vital for everyone, but especially for those who want to be professional Practitioners, or who wish eventually to become Reiki Masters.

DISTANT ATTUNEMENTS

In recent years there has been a growth in the number of distant attunements offered, especially on the internet, and some Masters only perform distant attunements, either because they don't offer Reiki courses, or because they attract many students to their websites from overseas. There is no reason why an attunement cannot be 'sent' to someone, just as Reiki treatments can be sent (see Chapter 12), but one of the major disadvantages to not being with your Reiki Master in person is that it is more likely that you could believe that 'nothing has happened', so you might not think you can use Reiki. (I discuss this further in the next chapter.)

Next, we move on to Part 2 about Reiki First Degree, including how to carry out self-treatments, and how to treat your family and friends, and animals too.

Part 2

Activating Your Healing Channel: Reiki First Degree

Chapter 5

Reiki First Degree Training

Once you have made the decision to take a Reiki course, you need to find the Reiki Master who is right for you. Actually 'find' is probably the wrong word, because Reiki is a Divinely guided energy and, when the time is right, Reiki finds you, rather than the other way round. Also, it always guides you to the Master who will give you exactly what you need – because Reiki always works for your highest and greatest good. Every Master is unique, and each one of them brings something of themselves to their teaching, so of course it is important that you should feel that they are someone you can like, trust and respect.

People find their Reiki Master in all sorts of ways: by seeing a poster in a complementary health clinic, reading an advertisement in a magazine, being recommended by a friend or finding their details on the internet. Unfortunately, there are currently no professional bodies or societies offering official registration processes for Reiki Masters, although some offer listings of the Masters who are members, so it really is best to let your intuition and your common sense guide you, and you won't go far wrong. Some people prefer to get to know their potential Master before making a final choice, and probably the best way is to make an appointment to have at least one Reiki treatment from them, because that will give you a chance to discover whether you feel at ease with them, and will also help you to know what Reiki really feels like. Some Masters offer an introductory evening session where they demonstrate and talk about Reiki, often held the evening before a course without putting you under any obligation to join the course the next day. You can then discuss the possibility of training with them and you are always free to go away and think about it.

To help you to make an informed decision, there are some questions you might like to ask, such as how the Master structures the courses, what is included, whether there is time on the course for supervised practice, and so on. You might also like to know how many years they have been teaching, and do they also operate as a Practitioner, so that they can give practical advice and have plenty of experience to use as examples, and whether they host regular Reiki-sharing sessions where students can get together to practise Reiki and give each other treatments. Also, you might want to know whether the Master has trained in additional Reiki techniques from the Japanese tradition, or if they also teach meditation or other spiritual workshops, because this could give an added depth and dimension to their teaching.

The location of the course would be another factor in your decision. It could be important to you to train with someone in your local area, so that you can meet up with them later to discuss any areas of concern, or you might be prepared to travel to another area to train with a particular Master, and keep in touch by phone or e-mail afterwards. Some Masters travel widely, running courses at many different venues, whereas others work only in their own area, perhaps teaching at a local holistic centre or in their own home. I usually like to teach my courses as weekend residentials in one or two attractive centrally located venues that include overnight accommodation and meals, so that students are able to travel there easily from all over the country. I find this also allows them to take the necessary 'time out' from their normal, busy lives, making the course an even more special experience.

Your choice of Reiki Master is important, as the initiation process at each level of Reiki creates a very profound connection between the Reiki Master and the student, and it is therefore vital that the attunement is given by someone who embodies the energy of Reiki. In the West, we tend to distrust what cannot be explained, and a sacred spiritual experience, which empowers you with Reiki for the rest of your life, would certainly fall into that category. You need to feel personally and energetically comfortable and at ease with them, and to feel inspired by their example. You need to have confidence that they have both the technical knowledge of how an attunement is performed and the spiritual knowledge and experience to carry out the process mindfully, because being attuned to Reiki can be likened to opening a door to the Divine. You presumably wouldn't open the door of your home to people you didn't like or trust, and the same should be true of your relationship with your Reiki Master, whom you are inviting to open a door into your very being.

At the end of the day, the Reiki Master you find will be the right one for you. If you like practical, no-nonsense people, then you will probably be attracted to train with someone similar; if you are a real go-getter who cannot bear to wait for things, then you will find a Master who is willing to let you progress quickly through the levels. If you love history and tradition, then you will probably choose a very traditional Reiki Master; and if you are very interested in spirituality, you will find a Master who teaches mainly from that perspective. The point is that nowadays the choices are out there. In 1991, when I took my first Reiki course, there were very few Reiki Masters around – probably not even a dozen in the whole of the UK – and all of them were very traditional in their approach; I am not complaining about that because it was absolutely the right experience for me at the time because it reflected my own values. Since then there has been a great shift in the way Reiki is taught, and this has allowed an explosion in numbers, so there are now thousands of Reiki Masters in the UK, and many hundreds of thousands elsewhere in the world. Now, there are as many different types of Reiki Master as there are different types of people, which just means that everyone can find someone who suits them, and Reiki can continue to grow and spread rapidly around the world.

PREPARING FOR A REIKI COURSE

When you have found the right Reiki Master, you are ready to book on to a workshop at a convenient time and place; however, there are some advantages to preparing yourself before taking a Reiki course. A Reiki attunement is a special, spiritual experience, and as such the experience can be enhanced if you bring all your energies – physical, emotional, mental and spiritual – into harmony and balance during the week before a course commences.

Some aspects of our lives make this more difficult, so you might like to follow the suggestions below, but of course they are optional.

There are no serious disadvantages to not preparing for a Reiki course, so don't worry if you are reading this the night before attending one, or if you did a course ages ago but didn't do any of this. They are just about getting the most out of the more spiritual aspects of the course, plus they help to reduce the toxins in your body, which makes the clearing process after the course a bit easier. Please note that some of them involve changing your diet, which for most people is beneficial, but if you have any health problems, or feel concerned in any way, please seek medical advice first.

- It can be helpful to do a gentle 'detox' for a few days before an attunement, eating mostly raw, fresh vegetables and fruit – preferably organic – and drinking plenty of water.

- If that sounds a bit too drastic, then if you are not a vegetarian you may find it helpful to cut out meat, poultry and fish for a few days before the course. They can all contain small quantities of drugs or other toxins, and their energetic vibrations could also contain negativity from the fear the animals experienced during the catching, transporting and slaughtering processes. Instead, substitute lots of fresh organic fruit and vegetables, and also cut down or eliminate processed foods, which contain preservatives or additives.

- Try to drink plenty of water – the body needs about 2 litres (3½ pints) a day to operate optimally, some of which it can extract from the foods and beverages you take in, but you make your body's work much easier if you give it what it needs. **Note:** Remember to check with your doctor if you have any reason to suspect that an increased water intake could be detrimental.

- It is best to eliminate alcohol for a few days before and during the Reiki course, and possibly for a few days afterwards. Also, try to minimise your consumption of caffeine drinks such as tea, coffee and cola, other fizzy drinks, sweet or fatty foods and chocolate.

- If you smoke, try to cut down for several days beforehand and smoke as little as possible during and immediately after the course. If you take any non-prescribed drugs, please try to limit or eliminate your consumption of them for as long as possible before, during and after the course. **Note:** Do not cut out or reduce the dosage of any drugs or medicines prescribed for you by your doctor.

- Try to reduce or eliminate altogether any time you spend in any activities or situations that carry negative energy, such as watching the TV news, or violent or fear-inducing programmes or films; reading the newspapers, or books containing violence or horror; listening to loud music; being with people who have very negative views, or being in places which make you feel uncomfortable.

- Take some time out for yourself to spend quietly in contemplation or meditation, or walking in a park or the countryside, or listening to classical or New Age music, as these are useful activities to de-stress you so that you will be more in tune with the nature of the course.

All of the above suggestions can contribute to a healthier long-term lifestyle too, and you may find that after the Reiki course you will want to live more healthily; for example, some people find it much easier to give up smoking after being attuned to Reiki, and even more find that healthy eating is an attractive option, as the Reiki makes them more aware of the toxic load they may have habitually taken into their bodies.

WHAT TO EXPECT ON A REIKI FIRST DEGREE COURSE

What I am describing in this chapter is the Reiki 1 training normally offered in the West; however, an increasing number of Western Reiki Masters are teaching this level in a similar way to training in Japan, and calling the course 'Shoden', and this is described in Chapter 20.

Reiki courses (sometimes called classes, workshops or seminars) are usually relaxed and informal, and are often held at weekends, or on consecutive evenings during the week, to allow more people an opportunity to attend. In the West, until the mid-1990s, the First Degree was traditionally taught over four sessions – over two or four days, or four evenings – especially when taught by members of The Reiki Alliance. This gave a minimum of 12 hours of teaching, and included four separate attunements, allowing the Reiki energy to build up slowly over the four sessions, plus a comprehensive explanation of the Usui Reiki Healing System, as Mrs Takata had taught it.

This consisted of the story of how Reiki was discovered by Dr Usui, plus full training in the hand positions on the head and body for treating yourself and other people, and advice on how to use Reiki in cases of injuries or accidents, as well as using it with animals and plants. Time would be allowed for practising treatments on yourself and with other students, and for asking questions and sharing experiences, but it was taught as an oral tradition, so no notes were taken or handouts given to students. Some Masters, myself included, still prefer to teach Reiki in this way, although most of us now provide a set of class notes or even a comprehensive manual, and include more up-to-date information about Dr Usui and his discovery of Reiki.

Here is an example of how a traditional Reiki First Degree course in the West is often organised. It includes the introductory session, which some Masters offer, so that anyone interested can find out more about Reiki. There may be minor variations, but it is fairly typical:

Friday

A standard evening introductory meeting covers what Reiki is, how it was discovered, what it can be used for and an explanation of the three levels of training. (If no introductory evening is offered, this would be covered at the beginning of the first day.) There is also a demonstration giving each person the opportunity to experience receiving Reiki for a few minutes, and a question-and-answer session. (I also include a practical look at the human energy body, including using dowsing rods to detect the layers of the aura, plus sensing with the hands and seeing the human aura, and how this relates to Reiki, but not all Masters do this.)

Saturday

The first day of the course usually starts with introductions, so that people can begin to feel comfortable with each other. The rest of the day includes more information about what Reiki is, how it works, and some of the ways in which it can be used. Students are told what an attunement is, and then the first of four attunements is given, usually towards the end of the morning, and a second in the afternoon. (Some Masters lead a short meditation before each attunement.) A discussion of the Reiki Principles follows and the importance of self-treatment with Reiki is also discussed, demonstrated and practised. Sometimes there is time for a further practical session where students begin using Reiki on each other.

Sunday

The second day includes the other two attunements, the third being given quite early in the morning session, and the fourth just after lunch. (It is preferable to have at least three or four hours between the attunements.) There is an explanation and demonstration of the hand positions to give a full Reiki treatment, and then students are split up into pairs to practise on each other. Afterwards there is a discussion of some creative ways of using Reiki, including dealing with emergencies and treating animals and plants, plus a question-and-answer session and presentation of Reiki First Degree certificates.

Over the past 20 years many independent Masters have chosen to reduce the teaching time to one day or two evenings, or even half a day or one evening. These shorter workshops usually entail a single, non-traditional integrated attunement which 'delivers' the energy all at once. These classes don't often include any practice time for treatments, although usually some notes are given to participating students. Occasionally a Master offers just an attunement to Reiki, without any teaching backup, or they offer a 'distant' attunement, where the attunement process is carried out by the Master and 'sent' to you in your home or other preferred location at an agreed time, using distant healing techniques. Very short courses, or just going through an attunement process, or having a 'distant' attunement where your Reiki Master is not with you in person can lead to some confusion, and students who have no knowledge or experience of how to use Reiki for treatments or other purposes, seem to have very little confidence in their ability to channel Reiki, and often abandon the idea, assuming that it does not work.

Sometimes, however, Reiki courses include lots of 'extras', some of which can be very beneficial, such as learning about energy, auras and chakras, being shown additional hand positions for

specific ailments, or relaxation techniques using Reiki with meditation and visualisation. Other extras can be a bit confusing, such as
using crystals or colour healing, because although they are interesting, they don't necessarily relate to Reiki.

Class Sizes

Another variation is in class size. Many Reiki Masters teach groups
of students at the same time, some preferring small groups of
between four and six people, others have groups of up to 12 or 14,
some have much larger gatherings of between 20 and 30, and a
few have as many as 80 students in a class. Other Masters prefer to
work on a one-to-one basis or with only two students at a time. You
need to work out for yourself what you would prefer, as there are
advantages and disadvantages to each.

Being taught individually gives you lots of time to ask questions,
but it can be quite intense, and there is no one else to practise on
other than the Reiki Master, which might make some students
nervous in case they make a 'mistake'. Being in a pair has similar
results, although you have each other to practise on, but it is quite
important that you like each other if you are going to work together
so closely. Small or medium-sized groups give you a chance to
practise on a number of people, rather than just one, and you have
the opportunity of meeting other like-minded people and making
friends, possibly getting together later to practise Reiki with each
other. These groups also provide the likelihood that someone else
might ask the questions you would like to have asked, but were too
shy. Very large groups of 30 or more people obviously allow for
less individual attention from the Reiki Master but they do give
you the advantage of anonymity, if you like to get lost in a crowd. I
personally prefer to work with groups of about ten students, as this
provides enough people to form a friendly, supportive group but
does not overwhelm anyone and gives me time to take a personal
interest in each person. It also usually guarantees a wide variety of
personalities and interests that leads to lively discussion and lots of
questions, which provides a healthy learning environment.

WHEN NOT TO TAKE A COURSE

There are very few times when it might be inadvisable to attend a Reiki course, but there are some counter-indications. If a person is suffering from depression or other psychological disorders, such as schizophrenia, whereas in the long term it would probably be beneficial for them to be able to do Reiki on themselves, in the short term, receiving a Reiki attunement could potentially intensify their symptoms. I would therefore advise them to consider having plenty of Reiki treatments first, preferably from a very experienced Reiki Practitioner, or even one who has medical or nursing qualifications, until their condition becomes more stable, and I would also recommend that they seek medical advice, suggesting that they give their doctor permission to telephone the Reiki Master for further information. (Few doctors know much about Reiki, so just asking them if it is OK isn't very helpful.) Some Reiki Masters are also qualified doctors, so this would seem to be the ideal compromise, as they would be able to deal with any medical complications that arose.

Some other medical conditions also require caution. People with very high blood pressure, epilepsy or those fitted with pacemakers are probably best obtaining medical advice in the same way, although I have never experienced any problems with such people in my classes; however, because there is a slight risk that their symptoms could be intensified, if only briefly, it is probably better to err on the side of caution. The same applies to people who have recently had major surgery or who are recovering from a serious illness. For all of these cases I would recommend Reiki treatments first, until they are confident that their health has improved. As I have said, the risks are very small, and because I am confident that Reiki always works for the highest and greatest good, perhaps there are no real risks at all. Still, being a Reiki Master is a big enough responsibility without having to deal with medical complications, so it is better to be safe than sorry.

Some people become concerned about whether an attunement will affect the high levels of medication they are on, because of the cleansing of toxins which the Reiki carries out immediately afterwards. Again, I have not encountered any problems in this area, and as Reiki works for the highest and greatest good, I don't believe it would ever rid the body of substances that were actually helping the person. After using Reiki on themselves for several weeks or months, some people do find that they are able to reduce their levels of medication, but please never do this without seeking medical advice and perhaps working with your doctor and increasing the frequency of medical checks you receive regularly, such as blood tests, to ensure that everything is proceeding smoothly.

PREGNANCY

Another condition I often get asked about is pregnancy. I have attuned a number of pregnant women, and there have never been any ill effects – other than some slight discomfort because the babies they were carrying became very lively during the attunement process. Actually there are very real benefits for an expectant mother to be able to use Reiki, because she can use it on herself and her baby prior to the birth, to help ease aches and pains and encourage restfulness, and to promote both pain relief and relaxation during the birth. After the birth, of course, Reiki can be used to accelerate the mother's healing, and to relax the baby and help both to sleep well. It is probably only on ethical grounds that I would advise caution here, because I cannot be sure whether when the mother becomes attuned to Reiki, the baby might also become attuned – although I suspect not – and the baby has no choice. One way in which this can be clarified is by the mother taking some time to 'tune in' to her own and her baby's Higher Selves, to ask permission; if it feels fine, then go ahead.

AFTER THE COURSE

It is a good idea to treat yourself gently for a day or two after the course, as you may find that you feel more emotional or vulnerable than usual, or that your temper gets frayed more easily, but these effects generally only last for a short time. If you have to go straight back to work afterwards, then try to give yourself some quiet time after work and maybe go to bed earlier than usual.

The 21-day clearing cycle, which occurs after attunements, was described fully in the last chapter, so please refer back to that as appropriate. Although you might be very keen to start trying Reiki out on your family and friends, I usually recommend to my students that they don't do too much, other than self-treatments, for the first three weeks while the cleansing is going on, but this is not a hard-and-fast rule. As you begin to use Reiki over the coming weeks and months, you will probably notice more sensations in your hands, or even a feeling of warmth over your whole body, as the Reiki reaches its full flow. Essentially, after your Reiki First Degree course you have a really valuable healing tool with which to help yourself, your family, friends and your pets – for life. Just enjoy it!

In the next chapter we explore how you can treat yourself with Reiki, and the benefits this can bring.

Chapter 6

Self-healing with Reiki

Using Reiki for self-healing involves taking responsibility for your own health and well-being. The word 'responsibility' really means 'being able to respond'. In this case it means responding to your body's messages, learning from them and moving forward with a better understanding of what your body needs – and what you, as a whole, need in your life. It also means treating your body and your whole self with love and respect. Giving yourself a Reiki self-treatment can be a very important part of being loving to yourself, and I will be describing how to do this later in this chapter.

Essentially, all healing is self-healing, because whatever interventions take place, whether conventional medical methods or complementary therapies, it is the body's own repair and replication capabilities that carry out the healing. Reiki can be tremendously valuable in helping you to achieve optimum health, but it is not a cure-all. It will usually help to alleviate symptoms and relieve pain and discomfort, but it still needs a change of consciousness, a willingness on the part of the person receiving the Reiki to allow changes in lifestyle, in attitude, in ways of being, so that the healing can be completed and fully integrated into that person's life.

Even if you use Reiki on yourself every day, but you continue with any harmful habits or behaviours which are taking a toll on your physical, mental or emotional well-being, whatever you are doing which is causing you harm will carry on harming you. Initially, you may well see a considerable improvement in your health, because Reiki is wonderful, and it can potentially do the most miraculous and amazing things. But Reiki is not an impenetrable shield, and it doesn't make you invincible. It involves you in your own healing, encouraging you to take responsibility for your own wholeness and health.

Being able to use Reiki on yourself for self-healing is one of the major advantages – and the main emphasis – of Reiki First Degree. As you start bringing Reiki into yourself regularly, it begins the process of dislodging blockages and obstacles within your energetic system, slowly and systematically affecting deeper and deeper layers of blocked and stagnant energy caused by suppressed or buried negative and damaging thoughts, emotions, attitudes and beliefs. When these blocks are dislodged and removed they come to the surface for review. This often means that memories of past events suddenly come into your mind, or you start to have very vivid dreams. Occasionally you may even find that previous situations recur, so you might begin to feel that all those old problems you thought you had sorted out long ago have come back to plague you. But if they do, it is only to make you face up to them, and when you do they will soon disappear.

This is a necessary part of the process of letting go, and the memories, dreams or situations have surfaced to give you an opportunity to heal them and learn from them. Naturally, this is an ongoing process, as you cannot rid yourself of years of blocked or stagnant energy overnight. But as the process continues, over weeks, months and even years, you will gradually find that you feel better than you have ever felt before – lighter, more vital and energetic, less concerned about other people's opinions, more in touch with your own feelings, and happier with yourself and your life.

INTENTION AND INVOCATION

Reiki doesn't need any complicated rituals before it will start to flow. All it takes is your *intention* to use it, which can, if you wish, be accompanied by a simple invocation such as 'Let Reiki flow now for the highest and greatest good.' Thoughts are a form of energy and can be very powerful, especially with the force of intention behind them, but actually Reiki will begin to flow from the moment you first think of using it. So, as you place your hands on whatever needs healing – yourself, another person or an animal – it is already flowing; however, where and how Reiki flows is not up to you – you are merely a channel for this healing energy – because it is Divinely guided, so it goes where it is needed, not necessarily where the person using it, or the person receiving it, wants it. Having the *intention* that it should flow for the highest and greatest good therefore helps to get rid of the ego, which might otherwise be involved.

For example, you might truly wish, with the best of intentions, to heal a friend's illness, but if it is for your friend's highest and greatest good for the physical symptoms to remain while they face up to the causative issues, then the Reiki will go to the causative levels – mental, emotional or spiritual. It may also bring some temporary relief of symptoms, but you can never guarantee what Reiki will do, because it is never under your control. You therefore need to rid yourself of expectations as to outcome – which can be very hard, I know, because most of us in the Reiki community have a deep desire to help people. But please realise that by channelling Reiki you are helping people, even if that help doesn't turn out to be exactly the way you hoped it would.

Making a Fresh Start

A Reiki initiation is a fresh start in life, and your first priority really needs to be self-healing, before you begin to use Reiki on other people, because when your own energies have been cleared you will be in a better position to help others. Remember the adage 'healer, heal thyself'? Well, this is the major focus of Reiki at First Degree level, and that means putting yourself first, giving yourself the time to focus on your life, your thoughts, your emotions and your body. It is about giving yourself time to listen to your body's messages, and that inner voice which tells you when something feels 'right'. Of course, in today's busy lives, finding time for yourself can be a challenge, but unless you are living exactly the way you want to live, as healthily as it is possible to be, then you need to be willing to make some changes in your life – and giving yourself some time and space for the things you need could be the first one.

It makes sense to take a good look at your life to see if it is helping or hindering you in achieving optimum holistic health. Are you eating a really healthy diet or are you snatching fast food on the run to your next meeting? Are your major relationships – with partners, children, siblings, parents and close friends – healthy and loving or stressful and tense? Are you happy with whatever work you do, whether that's in external employment or in the home, or do you really long to do something else? Do you have time to indulge in hobbies and interests that add to your life, or are you always working or rushing around making everyone else's lives easier? Have you achieved some of your dreams and goals and expect to achieve even more, or have you given up the unequal struggle and settled for whatever you can get? Do you think life is wonderful, fun and a joy, or do you find it all too much of an effort, and you can't think why you bother?

Basically, the only person who has the power to change your life is YOU. Magazines and newspapers these days are full of articles on how to understand your motivations, make changes and improve your life, and there are several books recommended in the Further Reading section too, which should give you lots of ideas.

It also helps to clear out your life on a very practical level, so I would recommend a really good spring clean, regardless of the season. Go through all your cupboards and drawers, shelves and wardrobes, old suitcases and boxes, attics and basements. At home – or even in your workplace, if possible – throw away, give away or sell *everything* that you don't love or don't use.

It may all sound like a lot of hard work, but you will get a real sense of achievement when you have done some clutter clearing – and you will find benefits energetically, too. Things that should really have been discarded long ago, such as clothes you never wear, magazines you never read, or kitchen gadgets that you have never used, all hold 'old energy' – energy that reflects the time they were new. You may have moved on, but if you hold on to too many useless possessions, they can hold you back energetically. If you throw out the old it rids your environment of stagnant, blocked energy, and leaves room for new energy to enter your life, so that you really can make a fresh start.

THE IMPORTANCE OF DAILY SELF-TREATMENT

Being able to give yourself Reiki each day is a vital part of your own self-healing. Because Reiki works holistically, your use of it helps the whole of you – body, mind, emotions and spirit – to reach a state of harmony and balance. An essential part of this self-healing is giving yourself a daily self-treatment.

During your Reiki 1 course you should be shown the hand positions (usually about 12) for giving yourself a Reiki treatment, and your Reiki Master may also include some additional hand positions for certain conditions. I recommend that when self-treating, each hand position is held for between three and five minutes, so a full treatment would take somewhere between 36 minutes and an hour. This can obviously depend upon what time you have available, and if absolutely necessary the time for each hand position can be shortened to one or two minutes. A little Reiki is better than no Reiki at all, and you can perhaps give yourself an extra-long treatment another day.

In terms of timing, there are CDs and tapes available of gentle music in three- or five-minute slots, especially made for use when doing Reiki treatments, so those might be helpful. There are also special timers, which you can set to go off regularly after an interval of your choice, which could be anything between two and 20 minutes, after which a gentle gong sounds. I find it easiest to count the seconds silently – it turns the treatment into a type of meditation, and in any case, I prefer to keep my eyes closed, so I cannot see the clock, although I find its rhythmic ticking helps me to count the seconds at the right speed. The more practice you get in self-treatment, the easier it will be to just let the energy dictate the time you need in each hand position, and even exactly where your hands should be placed. If you are always rushing your self-treatment, however, allowing yourself less and less time, perhaps you should ask yourself why. Why can't you spare about half an hour for yourself? Don't you feel you deserve it? Or are you living life at too hectic a pace? Are you giving your needs too little priority, rushing around after everyone else instead? Giving Reiki to yourself is a loving act, and giving yourself some loving attention is not selfish; it is sensible. If you feel loved and cherished – even if it is only by yourself – then you will have more love to give to others, too.

Self-treatments can be carried out almost anywhere and at any time of the day, but they are more comfortable if you are lying in bed or sitting in a comfy chair, so that your body and arms are well supported. For me, the best time is just after I have woken up in the morning – although I do set my alarm clock to ring again about 40 minutes later in case I get so relaxed I drift back to sleep. It is also really pleasant to do a self-treatment last thing at night before you go to sleep, although if you are tired you probably won't get much past the fourth or fifth hand position before drifting off into a peaceful slumber. Doing a Reiki self-treatment is therefore excellent if you have trouble getting to sleep or if you wake up in the middle of the night and cannot get back to sleep again.

Of course, your self-treatment does not always have to be at the same time each day – you can choose a point which is convenient to you, because it should be something you enjoy doing for yourself, not something you feel forced to do. You could try it just after the children have left for school or in your lunch hour; it is even possible to do at least some of the less conspicuous hand positions while sitting on a bus or train if you commute. The benefits of giving yourself daily self-treatments are cumulative – the more Reiki you receive, the better Reiki is able to remove blockages and promote deep healing on all levels. Once it becomes a habit, you will probably find that you really miss it if, for some reason, you don't give yourself a treatment, because apart from its health benefits, it is also a very pleasant, meditative experience.

Energy sensations when self-treating

One thing I need to point out, however, is that when you are treating yourself you rarely get as much sensation in your hands as when you are treating other people. I have been self-treating since 1991, and unless I am treating particular areas of my body that are sore, aching or injured, I don't feel anything in my hands at all – and many of my students report the same thing. Don't worry, this doesn't mean the Reiki isn't flowing; you will probably get other indications, anyway, such as feeling very relaxed, or the part of your body you are treating might feel especially warm. If your hands do become hot, cold, or tingly when treating specific areas, however, or if the part of your body which you are treating is experiencing similar sensations, this would indicate that more Reiki is required, so do please leave your hands in place until the sensation diminishes. There is no need to time the hand positions to the exact second. The timings are a rough guide, and there is no reason why you cannot have your hands in the same position for half an hour or more, if you feel you need to.

WHAT IS INVOLVED IN A FULL SELF-TREATMENT

The Reiki hand positions for a self-treatment follow the major chakras down the body, first down the front and then down the back, so it is quite easy to remember them, and once you have practised them for a while it will become second nature. Most Reiki Masters teach 12 hand positions for both self-treatment and treatment of others – four on the head, four on the front of the body and four on the back of the body. Each hand position should feel comfortable; otherwise you won't get the full benefit in terms of relaxation. Your hands should be laid gently on your body in the order shown below, and it is usual to keep your fingers close together, with the thumbs also close to the hand. This seems to help focus the energy more efficiently than if the fingers and thumbs are wide apart, perhaps because the hand chakra is deep in the centre of the palm, although Reiki does come out of your fingertips too.

You will notice that each hand is placed on a different side of the body. Treating each side of the body equally helps to balance the energies, encouraging a good flow of *Ki* around the body's energy system, so it is more efficient, although using only one hand is not detrimental in any way. If you have any form of disability or injury that prevents you from using two hands, such as a broken arm or an amputation, or you have suffered with a stroke, you can place one hand on one side, and *intend*, or visualise, that the other hand is in a complementary position on the other side. Energy follows intentional thought, so the Reiki will flow through appropriate parts of your energy body – even if an arm or leg is amputated, its subtle energy counterparts are still there – and will then flow into wherever you intend it to go.

You will see that the treatment is started at the head. The first three hand positions focus the Reiki towards the crown and third-eye chakras, and it then works down the front of the body, over the throat, heart, solar plexus, sacral and root chakras. Energy can flow into and out of the body through any of the chakras, but when it flows into the crown chakra first and from then down through the rest of the energy body, it seems to enable the Reiki to move more easily into the other chakras, as well as having a gentler, more calming and relaxing effect. If the energy is taken in first through the root chakra or the feet, although it is in no way harmful to do Reiki that way, it tends to have a more vibrant and energising effect, which some people find slightly agitating, so I don't generally recommend this.

Preparing for self-treatment

Before you start your self-treatment, it is a good idea to spend a few moments just gently centring yourself by breathing deeply and evenly, and allowing your body to relax. If you wish, you can carry out some energetic cleansing too (see Chapters 15 and 20). Generally, I recommend that you close your eyes, and as you raise your hands to place them in the first position, over the eyes, think and *intend* that you are beginning a self-treatment, and think and *intend* that the Reiki flows into you for your highest and greatest good.

SELF-TREATMENT HAND POSITIONS

The head

The first hand positions, on the back of the head, over the eyes, ears and neck, work together to treat the head and the brain, including all of its functions and control mechanisms for the whole body, from memory to movement, including the nervous system and endocrine system.

1 The back of the head

1A *Either* place one hand so that it cradles the back of the skull, with the other hand just above it.

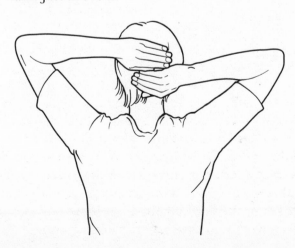

1B *Or* place one hand on the crown of the head and the other covering the back of the head.

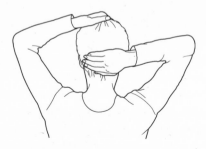

2 *The brow/eyes*

One hand held loosely over each eye, with the heel of each hand placed on your cheekbones, fingertips on your brow.

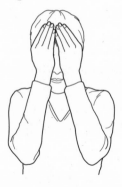

3 *The ears/temples*

One hand held loosely cupped over each ear, with the heel of each hand placed a fraction below the earlobe, and fingertips pointing upwards towards the temples.

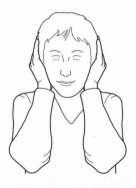

4 *The neck/throat*

4A *Either* one hand on top of the other, covering the throat.

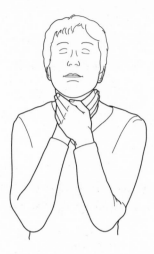

4B *Or* one hand on each side of the neck (it is OK to have the heels of the hands touching, or slightly apart).

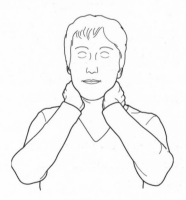

The front of the body

The hand positions on the front of the body treat the major organs and their associated body systems.

5 *The chest*

5A *Either* both hands crossed in the centre of the chest, over the heart chakra.

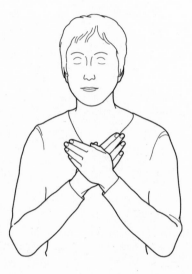

5B *Or* one hand on each side of the chest, very slightly above each breast. The fingertips can touch in the centre, or be slightly apart.

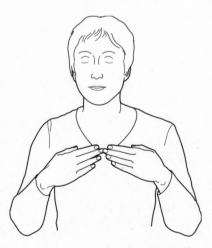

6 The solar plexus

One hand on each side of the body, covering the solar plexus (midriff). Again, the fingertips can touch in the centre, or be slightly apart.

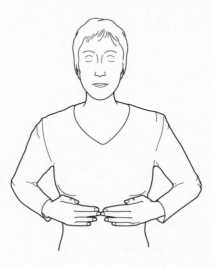

7 The waist/navel

One hand on each side of the body, fingers pointing towards each other, at about the same level as your navel, which can be either very slightly above or below your natural waistline.

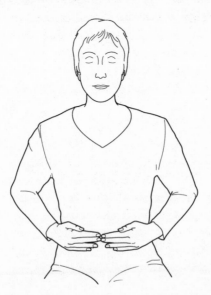

8 The pelvic area

One hand on each side of the body, fingers pointing downwards but slightly diagonally in a V-shape, sloping towards the pelvic area.

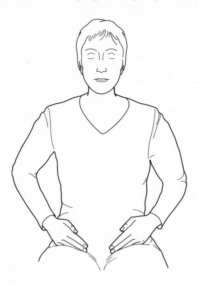

The back of the body

Although all the hand positions on the front of the body enable Reiki to flow around the whole body, and therefore into the back as well, treating the back separately allows Reiki to flow even more effectively into some particular parts of the body. The spine, for example, is a very important part of our skeleton and nervous system. The four hand positions on the back treat the whole of the spine from the base of the neck down to the coccyx, as well as treating other vital areas again, such as the heart, lungs, liver and kidneys.

When positioning the hands for the back of the body, some people find difficulty in having the palms of their hands flat against their body, particularly if they have any stiffness in their wrists or fingers, such as with arthritis. If this is the case, then you can place the *back* of your hand against your body instead and *intend* that Reiki flows out that way. The palm chakra, like all other chakras, spreads out of both sides of the hand, so the Reiki will flow out of the back of your hand just as well, if that is what it needs to do. For quite a lot of people this makes hand positions 10 and 11 much more comfortable.

9 The shoulders

9A *Either* place one hand on top of each shoulder.

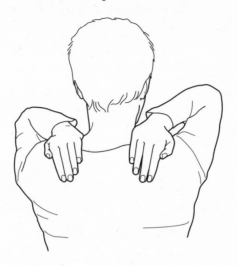

9B *Or* place one hand on top of each shoulder by crossing your arms in front of your chest.

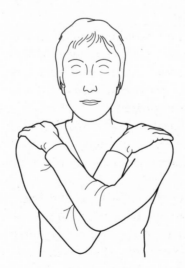

10 The middle back

10A *Either* place one hand on each side of the back, palms flat on the back, preferably mid-way between the shoulders and the waist, but if this is difficult, then as high above your waist as you can comfortably manage.

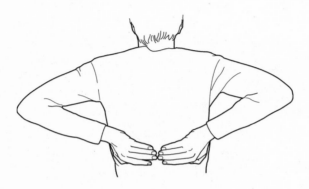

10B *Or,* if it is uncomfortable to place your palms flat on your back, then put the back of each hand against your back instead, as high above your waist as you can comfortably manage.

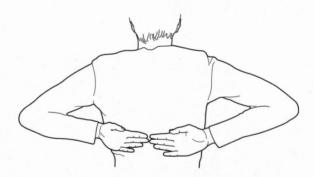

11 The waist

11A *Either* place one hand on each side of your body, with palms flat against your back, with your fingers pointing towards each other, and your thumbs tucked into your natural waistline.

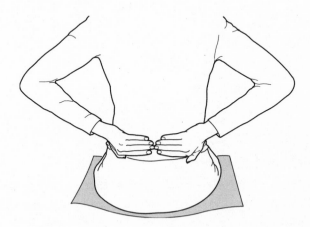

11B *Or*, if it is uncomfortable to place your palms flat on your back, then place the back of each hand against your back instead, with the fingertips pointing towards each other, this time with your little finger tucked into your natural waistline.

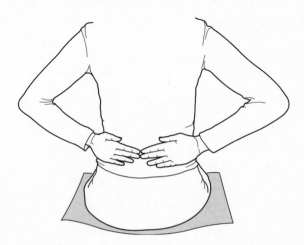

12 The buttocks

Place one hand on each buttock – it doesn't matter which way the hands are facing, as long as it is comfortable.

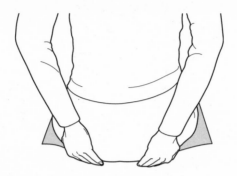

Additional hand positions

It is *optional* to give Reiki to the thighs, knees, calves, ankles and feet, or to the upper arms, elbows, forearms, wrists, hands or fingers. Naturally, if you have a health problem in any of those places, it makes sense to treat it. For any of the optional hand positions on the legs and feet you can either have one hand on each leg; for example, left hand on left knee, right hand on right knee, or alternatively you can place one hand under and one hand on top of each position, moving down the whole of one leg and foot, and then down the other leg and foot, moving from thigh to knee to calf to ankle to foot (see sample illustration below).

   Example: the knees

A *Either* place one hand on each knee.

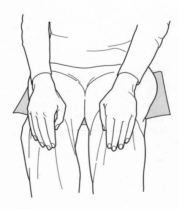

B *Or* place one hand underneath, and one hand on top of one knee at a time.

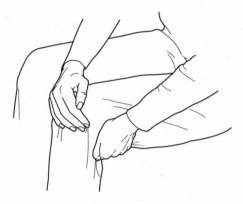

If you wish to treat your arms and hands, it is probably easier and more comfortable to do them one at a time, although it is just about possible to treat both arms together. Work downwards from the upper arm to the elbow, the forearm, the wrist and the hand.

Example: the elbows

A *Either* place one hand on each elbow.

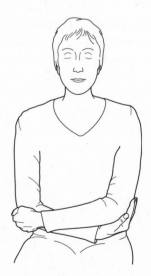

B *Or* place one hand on each elbow, one at a time.

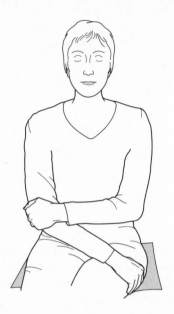

WHAT IS EACH HAND POSITION TREATING?

It is important to realise that each hand position, whether you are treating yourself or someone else, is in effect treating the whole of the body, because the Reiki flows into and around the whole subtle energy and physical bodies, through the meridians; however, the Reiki will always go where it is needed, and that is not under your control, or under the conscious control of the person you are treating. Also, because the Reiki can flow through the meridians of the energy body, which connect all parts, Reiki applied at the shoulder could equally well end up in the feet! As the Reiki flows into the body, each individual hand position allows the Reiki to move into particular areas with greater effect, and as Reiki flows into the physical parts of the body near to each hand position, it also flows into the psychological, emotional and spiritual aspects attributed to that area, healing or 'wholing' and bringing everything into harmony and balance. I have therefore included charts below to give you an overview of what each hand position could be treating. You will see that the metaphysical aspects – mind, emotions and spirit – have necessarily brief examples, and should not be seen as a full explanation, or as the only life aspects that Reiki will flow into at those points. For more information, I would recommend reading some of the books in the Further Reading section, especially *Your Body Speaks Your Mind* by Debbie Shapiro.

The head

Hand position	Body	Mind, emotions, spirit
1 Back of the head	From this position Reiki flows into the whole head and brain, nervous system, endocrine system, pituitary and pineal glands, as well as into the visual cortex	Your concepts, attitudes and ways of thinking and how these are affecting your life. Also your spiritual progress
2 Brow/ eyes	This position also treats the whole head and brain, nervous system, endocrine system, pituitary and pineal glands, as well as the eyes and face	Your perspective on the world and what you allow yourself to 'see' and what you 'face up to' or what you are avoiding
3 Ears/ temples	Once again, this position treats the head, brain, nervous system, endocrine system, pituitary and pineal glands, as well as the ears, sinuses, nose and face	What you are willing or unwilling to hear; whether you listen to your inner guidance
4 Neck/ throat	This position treats the neck, throat, tonsils, adenoids and vocal chords, as well as the jaw, mouth, teeth, gums, nose, sinuses and ears, plus the thyroid and parathyroid glands, which control metabolism and growth	Communication issues, such as unexpressed feelings, anger and hurt, being truthful to yourself and others; 'chewing things over' or finding things 'difficult to swallow'

The front of the body

Hand position	Body	Mind, emotions, spirit
5 Chest	This position treats the heart and the whole cardiovascular system, the lymphatic system, the immune system, the lungs and respiratory system, and the thymus gland, as well as allowing Reiki to flow into the arms and hands	Relationship issues, suppressed emotions, feeling smothered or controlled by others, trust issues, lack of independence, unexpressed grief
6 Solar plexus	From here Reiki flows into the liver, spleen, pancreas, gall bladder, stomach and the whole of the digestive system	Self-esteem, introvert/extrovert balance, feeling good about yourself or feeling worthless, putting others' needs before your own
7 Waist/navel	This position treats the kidneys and adrenal glands, the lower digestive organs, the prostate, bladder and urinary tract, and the female reproductive system – uterus and ovaries	Sexual and physical appetites, pleasure and creativity; enjoyment (or not) of life; taking pleasure in beauty, nature, sensations; procreation issues
8 Pelvic area	From here Reiki flows into the body's structure, including the whole skeleton, the muscles, tendons, and the body's largest organ, the skin, as well as the bladder, bowels and urinary/elimination system, the genitals and the male reproductive organs (testes), and the pelvis, hips, legs and feet	Survival, trust and security; money, housing or job issues; feeling unsupported; not letting go, feelings of fear or panic

The back of the body

Hand position	Body	Mind, emotions, spirit
9 Shoulders	Reiki flows into the shoulders, especially into the muscles which often hold a lot of tension, and also into the top of the spine at the base of the neck, and down into the arms and hands	Upper back: repressed anger or rage. Shoulders: too many burdens, too much stress. Arms: wanting to embrace, or being afraid to let go. Hands: giving and receiving, issues or situations you can't handle
10 Middle back	This position treats the upper part of the spine, as well as treating the heart and lungs again	Stored anger and resentment, feeling unsupported, trying to be perfect, as well as indefinable fears
11 Waist	From here Reiki flows into the middle part of the spine, as well as flowing again into the pancreas, digestive system, liver, kidneys, spleen and adrenal glands, and the female reproductive system	Ability (or inability) to 'let go and let flow'; holding on to negative feelings; being irritable and easily upset
12 Buttocks	This position treats the lower portion of the spine, including the lumbar region and the coccyx, and also allows Reiki to flow around the whole skeleton, as well as the skin, blood and urinary/elimination system, and again into the genitals, male reproductive system, hips, legs and feet	Lower spine: money and security issues, feelings of responsibility, inability to ask for help. Skin: someone or something getting 'under your skin'. Legs: progress through life, fear of change, fear of the future. Knees: stubbornness, inflexibility and indecision. Ankles: life imbalance, a need to change direction. Feet: fear of taking the next step, needing to be 'grounded'

(**Note:** In effect, each hand position treats parts of the skeleton and skin, but Reiki seems to flow into the whole of the skeleton and skin particularly when treating the pelvic area and buttocks.)

OTHER WAYS OF USING REIKI ON YOURSELF

Although doing a self-treatment every day is an excellent practice to promote self-healing, please don't feel that it is the only way to give yourself Reiki. Reiki can be as flexible as you are, so you can place your hands anywhere on your body and allow the energy to flow through you almost anywhere, at any time, throughout the day. You can add to your daily self-treatment as often as you like, giving yourself five or ten minutes of Reiki, or longer if you like, by just placing your hands on an appropriately convenient place – your chest, solar plexus, stomach or thighs are usually the easiest – and *intending* that Reiki should flow always for your highest and greatest good.

The point is, if you have some time to spare, give yourself Reiki. It doesn't require any conscious effort on your part. You don't even *have* to be sitting or lying down. Simply put your hands on any part of your body that you can comfortably reach and allow the Reiki to flow. You can then feel you are doing yourself some good, even when you are just being a couch potato!

GIVING YOURSELF 'FIRST AID' TREATMENT

There is no need to give yourself a full self-treatment every time you have a headache or cut your finger. Although a full self-treatment is always beneficial, it is not always essential, so if you have a stiff neck or aching shoulders, treat them. If you have a headache or sore eyes, treat them. If you fall and graze your knee, or trap your fingers in a door, treat them. All you need to do is *intend* that the Reiki should flow, and it will. If your injury is more serious, it makes sense to seek medical help or advice – but you can give yourself Reiki while you wait for professional attention (but see the cautions below).

As well as giving yourself Reiki for first aid, remember to give yourself lots of Reiki if you are ill. You cannot 'overdose' on Reiki, so if you are feeling ill, just place your hands on yourself any-where that is comfortable, and let the Reiki keep flowing for as many hours as you like. It will accelerate your body's own healing processes, and help it to fight off whatever 'bug' you have caught. Initially, it may exacerbate your symptoms – because many of the distressing symptoms we experience are actually the effects of the body's activities to fight off infection – but it will shorten the length of time you feel ill, which has to be a good thing.

TIMES FOR CAUTION

There are no known contraindications when using Reiki on its own, as it is intrinsically very safe, because it always works for the greatest and highest good; however, there are a few times when it might be sensible to exercise caution when giving Reiki to yourself – and also when treating other people, but those will be dealt with in the next chapter.

1 If you have the misfortune to chop off a toe or finger in an accident, for example, then the obvious thing is to pack the missing part carefully and get to a hospital as quickly as possible so that it can be reattached surgically. The slight caution here is that Reiki accelerates healing, so if you apply Reiki directly to the hand or foot, potentially the natural healing process of closing the wound will quickly begin to take place. One of my Reiki Masters reported the case of a student whose severed finger could not be reattached, even though the man in question went straight to hospital after the accident. The hospital staff couldn't understand why he had not gone there sooner, as the wound had healed so much it looked as though it had happened several days before. In a case like this, therefore, by all means give yourself Reiki, but not directly on the injured part. Instead, place a hand on your heart chakra or over your kidneys to help with the pain and shock, and although the Reiki will flow throughout the body, including to the injury, it will do so in a much gentler way, so the healing effect on the injury will not be so dramatic.

2 The same caution applies in the case of a bad break of an arm, leg, wrist or ankle etc. This will undoubtedly need professional setting and, again, if the healing process has already begun, this could potentially cause problems, because the bone(s) might not be aligned properly. Reiki your heart chakra or adrenal glands to deal with the pain and shock, rather than placing your hand directly on the break, until after the bone has been set and plastered. After that, give it as much as possible, and it should mend much more

quickly. I have known a number of people – all Reiki Masters – who have broken bones and managed to heal them completely within hours, using Reiki, so in the case of a straightforward break this is definitely possible – but it does take a great deal of belief in Reiki to trust its process, so I would always advise people to get profes- sional help.

3 Another reason for some caution is if you are taking medication intended to bring your body into balance, such as tablets or insulin injections for diabetes, or tablets for high or low blood pressure, or for thyroid problems. Treating yourself with Reiki is excellent, but because Reiki works to bring your body into better balance, it is sensible to keep a regular check on your state of health in case your medication needs some adjustment. Of course, you should never lower your dosage or stop taking your medication without medical advice, but most people with diabetes have kits to test their blood glucose levels, and people with high or low blood pressure often have their own testing equipment too, so if you notice any signifi- cant changes then do discuss these changes with your doctor. In the case of thyroid problems, if you notice any changes in the way you feel, then again, contact your doctor who may advise more regular appointments to assess your case.

QUICK ENERGY BOOSTS

Sometimes, when your energy is running low because you have been busy, or had a stressful day, you could do with a bit of a boost, so I came up with this technique, which seems to work well:

The ten-minute top-up

1   First, *intend* that the Reiki should flow for your highest and greatest good (just thinking that you want to use Reiki will activate it), and place one hand over your eyes, with the palm facing and touching your face, and the other hand at the back of your head, palm against the head. (It doesn't matter which hand is where – for example, left at the front or back.) Hold your hands in this position for two and a half minutes – count- ing to 150 is the way I keep a check on the time, but of course you can carry on for longer if you want to.

2 Next, place one hand on your throat, and the other hand on the centre of your chest, again for about two and a half minutes.

3 Then place one hand on your solar plexus, and the other one on your navel for another two and a half minutes.

4 Finally, place one hand on the top of your head, over your crown chakra, and the other one on your root chakra, either on your bottom (or underneath it, if you are sitting down), or with your hand between your legs for two and a half minutes.

Another useful tip is a hand position that works on hangovers. It is also good as a quick 'wake up', when you are feeling tired but you need to carry on with some tasks.

The 'wake up'

Place both hands, one hand crossed over the other, on the crown of your head. *Intend* that the Reiki should flow, and keep your hands in that position for at least five minutes.

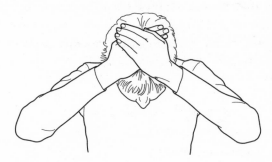

Those are the basics of self-healing with Reiki, but you will find other ideas in later chapters, and please do feel free to experiment. The classic self-treatment is a good structure to start with, but of course you can add to it; for example, at the end of the 12 hand positions I always treat each foot for a few minutes, holding it between both hands and then finishing with some gentle massage, which I find helps to 'ground' my energy, and helps me to become alert again after enjoying the deeply relaxed state during the treatment.

In the next chapter we look at methods for treating your friends and family with Reiki.

Chapter 7

Treating Family and Friends

Although the major emphasis of Reiki First Degree is self-healing, most people want to try out their Reiki on other people too. It would be inadvisable to set up as a professional Reiki Practitioner right from the word go, because obviously you will need plenty of practice in order to develop your knowledge and confidence, and there's more information about what is required in Chapter 17. I generally recommend that anyone wishing to practise professionally should take Reiki Second Degree to add to their capabilities, but to begin with let's explore what you can do with your Reiki First Degree skills.

THE LABEL OF 'HEALER'

Having the desire to help other people is very natural, and being able to treat people with Reiki is a very pleasurable experience. There can be a problem, however, and that is the label of 'healer', which some people will attach to you. The word implies a certain status and ability, and it is very easy to get caught up in the illusion of it all, and to enjoy the sense of esteem it can give you. But even if people do call us 'healers' it is not a factual description. The body does all its own healing, and because we are channels for Reiki that means we are able to act as catalysts, helping to get the healing process kick-started by delivering, through our hands, some healing energy. Actually, the more we push our own ego out of the way, the more we are able to go with the energy and let it direct us, and the stronger the flow of energy becomes. But it is important to remember that *we* don't do any healing; Reiki does – or at least, it is the Reiki that helps the person to heal him or herself.

WHAT IS A REIKI TREATMENT?

For many people, their first contact with Reiki is through receiving a Reiki treatment from a friend, a member of their family or a professional Reiki Practitioner. Normally a Reiki treatment takes about an hour, and is carried out with the client remaining fully clothed (except for coat and shoes) and tucked up comfortably with a blanket and pillows, usually on a therapy couch. (I am using the words 'client' and 'Practitioner' for simplification, but I mean anyone receiving and giving Reiki. Other terms like 'patient' and 'healer' are more emotive, and therefore I prefer not to use them.)

The treatment starts with the client lying on their back, and the Practitioner's hands are placed gently on the body in specific places and will normally be kept still for a few minutes – there is no pressure, massage or manipulation, unless the Reiki is being combined with another therapy. The responses during the treatment vary considerably. Some clients experience feelings of heat or tingling as the Reiki flows through them, or certain parts of their body might feel cold, especially after the Practitioner's hands have moved away. Usually the client feels very relaxed and peaceful as the energy flows through their body, and many clients drift off to sleep and have to be gently roused when it is time to turn over to lie on their front for the rest of the treatment.

Clients can sometimes become quite emotional as the Reiki begins to break down old patterns and blockages and bring them to the surface. They may laugh out loud or even shed some tears, or their legs or arms may suddenly jerk even while they are asleep. It is important to tell the client before the treatment that these reactions are possible, and to reassure them that they are perfectly normal – they are just caused by blocked or stagnant energy being released in different ways from the body.

Sometimes, after the treatment has ended, clients may experience a shift in consciousness, a realisation of the underlying causes of any problems they have been having, whether those problems are to do with their physical health, their relationships, or job, and so on. This is an important part of healing, and if the client wants to talk about it with you, that's fine, but this is where the boundaries can become blurred between being a friend or family member and being a complementary therapist or counsellor. Whatever issues are raised, it is important to remain non-judgemental, and to be as comforting and supportive as possible. If talking with clients in this way is something you don't feel very comfortable with, you might find it useful to take a short counselling course or read some books about the counselling process. If you believe the person needs much more support, then you could gently and tactfully suggest that they talk things over with a friend, a counsellor or a family therapist, for example.

Please remember, though, that if you are treating someone, even if it is a close friend or a member of your family, they may regard you differently – as a health professional – so your client is entitled to expect your complete confidentiality. It is vital *never* to talk to other people about any clients or their treatments, unless you need advice on how to handle a particular situation. In that case you could contact your Reiki Master and discuss the case, while preserving your client's anonymity by not revealing their name, or any personal details that might identify them.

Occasionally in the days immediately following a treatment some people experience something called a 'healing crisis', which is usually just a short period when they have temporary physical symptoms such as a sudden cold, as the Reiki energy works through the blockages and the body does its best to get rid of them. I always tell clients about this possibility, and encourage them to drink plenty of water during the next few days after a treatment, as this helps to flush any toxins out of the body in a natural way.

WHO CAN BE TREATED?

Receiving a Reiki treatment is great for anybody, whatever their age. Babies and small children usually love it, although they don't often want to stay still for long enough for a full treatment, and since they are so much smaller than an adult they don't need as much Reiki anyway. It is far easier to treat them casually, just allowing the Reiki to flow while you hold them or when they sit on your knee. Pregnant women usually find Reiki very soothing for themselves and their unborn child, and it can be really beneficial to both mother and baby to give Reiki during the birth process. Otherwise, adults of any age will find a Reiki treatment very helpful with any health or stress-related problems and, of course, people don't have to be ill to benefit from a Reiki treatment. It is lovely just to relax and be nurtured for a while.

EQUIPMENT

You don't really need any expensive equipment in order to give Reiki to someone – all you need is your hands; however, if you intend carrying out any Reiki treatments, it is sensible to have something suitable for people to lie on. The best option, if you can afford it, is a therapy couch, and there are several different types on the market. Costs vary depending upon which country you live in, but a search on the internet should reveal the range of prices for new portable couches, which are probably the most useful type to have, and some of these have adjustable leg heights, which can be beneficial. You may find one second-hand, which will be cheaper, but the best source of information about suitable therapy couches is to look on the internet, in the Yellow Pages, or in advertisements in a health magazine.

One thing to watch for, however, is that many therapy couches are made for the massage market, so they are designed to be low enough to allow the therapist to be able to bend over a client and exert some pressure. When practising Reiki you need a couch that allows you to stand beside your client with your hands held at a comfortable height, which is usually somewhere around the middle of your chest, but no lower than your waist. Of course, your hands will be supported on your client's body, but nevertheless it can be uncomfortable to hold your hands still for about five minutes if you have to bend your back to reach. You probably won't need to invest in an expensive couch unless you intend to become a Practitioner, so in the meantime there are other inexpensive alternatives.

First of all, you could use your dining table. These are usually about the right height. If it is sturdy and long enough, you could place some thick foam on top and cover it with a sheet. Another alternative could be a heavy-duty decorating table with foam on top. The heavy-duty models are made of stronger materials, and have wooden braces that can be screwed into place to make the whole thing solid.

If you are reasonably agile, you could do treatments with a person lying on a camp bed or a sun-lounger with you sitting on the floor with your legs under the bed. It is also possible to do treatments with people lying on the floor or on a conventional divan bed, but while these might be reasonably relaxing for the person you are treating, they can be very uncomfortable for you unless you are used to kneeling or sitting cross-legged on the floor for long periods. It is also possible to give someone a Reiki treatment while they are sitting in a chair, and I discuss that later in this chapter.

In each of the above cases, you will also need several pillows, pillowcases and fitted sheets (stretch towelling are best) to fit over the therapy couch or over the foam layer, if you are using that, and a soft blanket to cover the client.

PREPARATION

If you are going to give someone a full Reiki treatment, I would recommend that you wait until you have completed your own 21-day cleansing process, and have performed plenty of self-treatments. Once you are ready to begin, please remember that it is important that anyone you treat should come into a comfortable, safe and supportive environment, and they also need you to behave in a professional manner, even if they know you really well. Before you give anyone a Reiki treatment it is important that you should prepare yourself and the space in which the treatment is to take place.

There are two priorities for your self-preparation: energetic protection and cleansing. When I was originally taught Reiki in 1991, no mention was made of either, other than ensuring that we washed our hands before starting a treatment, which seemed sensible since we would be touching people, albeit they would be fully clothed. Over the years, however, I have come to realise that some further preparation *is* necessary, and certainly since 2000 when I learned Dr Usui's original techniques, I have recognised that there was considerable emphasis on self-cleansing in the Japanese tradition.

Self-cleansing

The first priority for your own sake, and especially for the comfort of your client, is to pay particular attention to personal hygiene. So, in addition to washing your hands (and probably brushing your teeth) before treating anybody, you need to ensure that you – and your clothes – are clean and fresh. There is nothing worse than having someone leaning over you with garlic breath or smelling of sweat or stale tobacco. You should also remove your watch and any metal jewellery (except for a wedding ring), or anything else that might catch on a client's clothing, or jangle distractingly.

Energetic protection

It is just as important to be energetically cleansed, and there are various methods detailed in Chapters 20 and 21, which I would recommend that you try, such as the *Hatsurei-ho* technique, or the Reiki Shower. As you become more sensitive and intuitive, which often happens after taking a Reiki attunement, it can be a good idea to start protecting yourself energetically and psychically. Psychic protection and other cleansing techniques are dealt with more fully in Chapters 14 and 15, but the simplest method is to create an energetic barrier by imagining your aura filled with Reiki, and if you wish, you can see its outer edge like a translucent eggshell made of energy. Imagine the Reiki flowing out of your hands, filling the eggshell with healing white light, and *intend* that the Reiki protects you from any negativity or harm, so that any negative or harmful energies within your aura will be cleansed and released by the Reiki, and the outer edge of your aura will only permit love, light and Reiki to enter.

During a treatment, your client will be inside your auric field, so doing this will mean that both you and your client will be surrounded by protective Reiki, and any negative energies released by the client during the treatment will not stick to your energy field, but will be healed and transformed by the Reiki. Of course, you can set up a protective energy field around yourself at any time, not just when doing a Reiki treatment: before going shopping in a city centre, or if you are visiting a hospital, or anywhere else that could hold negative energies.

Preparing the space

Whatever kind of space you use should be clean and tidy, and you can further prepare it by cleansing it with Reiki. Just sit quietly for a few moments, resting your hands on your thighs, palms facing upwards, and then allow Reiki to flow through your hands and out into the room, *intending* that the Reiki should cleanse it of any negative energies. If you wish, you can visualise the Reiki flowing like a soft white mist all over the room, especially into all the corners.

Set up the therapy couch if you have one, with a clean sheet on it – or over the foam if you are using some alternative equipment, and place clean pillows and a soft blanket ready, perhaps burning some incense or essential oils to fill the room with a pleasant smell. (Some people are sensitive to certain smells, so don't do this until you have checked with the client, and be aware that some essential oils may have contraindications, so it is best to stick to something fairly safe, such as lavender.) If you plan to play some relaxing music, get the CD or tape ready in the machine, and test it for volume before you start. Also, ensure that the room is at an appropriate temperature and that there will be no interruptions from telephones, children, pets or other distractions.

Preparing your client

Lots of people are a bit nervous before having their first Reiki treatment (and you might be equally nervous at first), so always spend a little time beforehand talking to them about what Reiki is, and what to expect during the treatment, including where you will be placing your hands. Explain to them that you will not be touching any 'personal' areas, such as genitals or women's breasts. They usually find it reassuring when they realise they can remain fully clothed, except for taking off their coat and shoes, as people are often self-conscious about revealing their bodies.

Also tell them what sorts of experience they may have, such as feeling sensations of warmth, heat or tingling where your hands are placed, or sensing energy flowing around their body, or hearing their tummy rumble or noticing their limbs jerking slightly. Explain that they will probably become very relaxed, but might feel a bit emotional, so reassure them that if they need to laugh or cry that it is quite normal and is also absolutely OK with you, and they don't need to feel embarrassed. Talk to them about the reason they have come for a treatment, and give them a chance to ask questions. If you are treating family or friends, you don't usually have to take a medical history or keep written records of treatments, but if you think you might like to be a professional Practitioner some time in the future, then these would be good habits to get into right from the start – see Chapter 17 for more information. Also, reassure them that they don't need to do anything consciously in order for the Reiki to flow into them, other than being willing to let it happen.

The person receiving Reiki should take off their coat, shoes, watch, spectacles and any metal jewellery (but there is no need to ask anyone to remove a wedding ring), but should otherwise remain fully clothed. When the person is lying on their back at the beginning of the treatment a pillow should be placed under their head and another one under their knees. When they turn over to lie on their front, move the pillow from under their knees and place it under the ankles, to take the pressure off their back. Sometimes putting a soft blanket over the client helps to make them feel nurtured and more relaxed, and it also prevents them from feeling cold, as their body cools down when they are lying still or when negative energy is being released during the treatment.

It is important that both you and your client should enjoy the treatment, so before you start, make sure that both of you are comfortable, that the therapy couch is at a comfortable height for you, and that the client is warm enough.

I usually explain that it is preferable for them to close their eyes, so they can fully relax, and I discourage talking or asking questions during the treatment; although if a client is initially nervous I will, of course, continue to answer in as gentle and supportive a manner as I can. I find that by the time I have reached the third hand position (or even earlier) their speech becomes slurred as they enter a state of deep relaxation, after which they generally go quiet, often drifting off to sleep. I find that playing soft, relaxing music – classical or 'New Age' – often helps people to feel at ease, although you should check if this is acceptable to your client.

WHEN YOU ARE READY TO BEGIN THE TREATMENT

There are explanations later in this chapter about how to treat someone who cannot lie on their front, or who needs to be treated in a chair, but the following description covers the classic 'hands-on' treatment on a therapy couch (or suitable alternative). Also, there are details about what each hand position is treating (for body, mind, emotions and spirit) in the last chapter – they are the same whether for self-treatment or treatment of others.

When you have made sure your client is comfortable, it is time to make your own preparations. Spend a few minutes centring yourself by breathing deeply and evenly, and allowing your body to relax, after which you are ready to 'tune in' to the Reiki by *intending* that it should flow. You might like to silently invoke the Reiki by saying to yourself, 'I am now starting a full Reiki treatment on [name of person] and wish Reiki to flow into him/her for his/her highest and greatest good.' This is not strictly necessary, as when you raise your hands to start the treatment, your thoughts have already been acted upon, and the Reiki will have started to flow, but it reaffirms your intentions.

HAND POSITIONS FOR THE TREATMENT OF OTHERS

When doing a treatment, your hands are always used with the fingers closed, and the thumb close to the hand. The most usual form of full Reiki treatment in the West is based on 12 hand positions on the head and body, each of which is normally held for about five minutes, with the option of leaving the hands on longer in any position where you can feel that there is still a lot of Reiki flowing (such as feelings of heat, coldness, tingling, buzzing sensations and so on in your hands), which would indicate that the area still needs more energy. Some Reiki Masters teach a slightly different structure for the treatment, with up to six hand positions on the head and neck, and up to ten hand positions on the front of the body, including the legs and feet, and another ten on the back of the body, again including the legs and feet. This gives a total of 26 hand positions, with those on the head and body being held for about five minutes and those on the legs and feet being held for two or three minutes.

Even though I now know, and have tried out, the many different hand positions that Dr Usui apparently used, in almost every case I continue to use the 12 hand positions I was originally taught. They allow Reiki to flow into every chakra, and therefore around the whole physical and energy body, so even when I feel strongly drawn to give Reiki to some extra places, I just add them to the flow and rhythm of the traditional Western treatment. It takes just over an hour if each position is held for five minutes, allowing a few minutes for the client to turn over so that their back can be treated. If more hand positions are used, this will take longer – about an hour and a half. It is therefore very important that both you and your client should be comfortable. Holding the hands still for any length of time can be a strain if you have not got the Reiki couch, or other suitable equipment, at the right height.

It is usual to start with the client lying on their back with their arms at their sides, with the Practitioner standing or sitting behind the head for the first five hand positions. The hands are supposed to rest *gently* on the person's body, so please be careful not to exert any pressure. Most people find the gentle placing of the hands on the body very reassuring, but some people really cannot bear to be touched, or they may have religious beliefs which prohibit touch except from close family members, and you can therefore hold your hands above the body in the auric field at a height that is comfortable for you, and the Reiki will still flow into the client. This can also be useful for treating areas of the body where some form of injury means even the lightest pressure might be painful. Also, some Reiki Masters do teach people to carry out a whole treatment without touching the client – a 'hands off' approach, rather than the traditional 'hands on'. Holding your hands in the aura above the body without support can be more tiring, however, so if this is how you have been taught, please pay special attention to your stance or how you are seated to ensure your maximum comfort.

Some people, especially when they first start doing Reiki, are reluctant to place their hands on the client's body, feeling that it is in some way intrusive, so they barely allow their hands to touch the body, resulting in a hesitant, 'fluttering' feeling which most clients don't like. If the hands are placed lightly but confidently, this helps to give the client a feeling of security, and most people find it quite comforting – and as none of the hand positions is 'intimate' there is no invasion of privacy.

Be very gentle when the hands are moved from one position to another, and move one hand at a time, if possible, so that you have continuity of contact. For hand positions 6 through to 8, you will need to stand or sit at one side of the person being treated. When you have finished treating the front of the body you will need to gently rouse the client (who is usually deeply relaxed at this stage) and ask him or her to turn over on to the front. Again, make sure that they are comfortable, and help them to turn over if necessary, adjusting the pillows so that the head rests comfortably and the other pillow is placed under the ankles. Their arms don't have to be by their sides when they are lying on their front, so allow them to position them in any way they like. It is also a good idea to tell them that if they need to they can alter their position, or they can even go to the toilet part way through a treatment if they need to – occasionally Reiki has that effect! Sometimes people bravely stay in the same position despite being in considerable discomfort, because they think they are expected to, so a few words of reassurance can be helpful. Also, of course, you should let them know that if at any point they want you to stop the treatment, they only have to say so.

When the client is settled again, the treatment can continue. Hand position 9, on the shoulders, is especially good for people who hold a lot of tension in their shoulders, which is probably most of us. You then progress down one side of the body for hand positions 10 through to 12.

HAND POSITIONS FOR TREATING THE HEAD

The first few hand positions are carried out with the Practitioner either standing or sitting behind the client's head. The order of the positions on the head isn't vital – some Masters suggest starting with your hands underneath the client's head, whereas others start with the hands over the eyes, moving later to place the hands under the head. If this is what you have been taught, then rather than disturb the client, who may be very relaxed by then, the easiest way to make that transition is to gently roll the client's head to one side, supporting it with one of your hands while you slide your other hand under their head, then gently roll the client's head back and move your supporting hand so that both of your hands are fully underneath the client's head. It might sound a bit complicated, but I'm sure your Reiki Master will demonstrate this manoeuvre if this is what they want you to do! For ease and simplicity, however, I always teach students to begin with their hands under the client's head.

1 The back of the head

Very gently place both hands beneath the client's head, taking care not to pull their hair, so that your little fingers are touching each other, and your fingertips are roughly level with the base of the skull. Remain in this position for three to five minutes, and then gently and slowly slide both hands out at the same time (sideways is easiest) allowing the client's head to rest back on the pillow, and then move your hands to position 2.

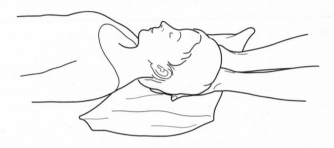

2 The eyes/brow

Place one slightly cupped hand over each eye, with the heel of each hand resting gently on the brow, but make sure that the fingertips do *not* touch the face – keep them *at least* 5cm (2in) away. After three to five minutes, move the hands one at a time to position 3.

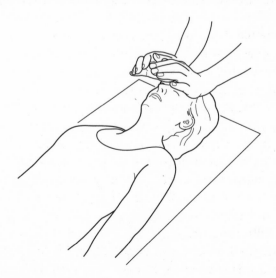

3 The ears/temples

3A *Either* place one slightly cupped hand over each ear, with the heel of each hand resting gently against the side of the head so that the fingertips are roughly level with each earlobe. Again, make sure the fingertips do not touch the face – leave them at least 5cm (2in) away. After three to five minutes, move the hands one at a time to position 4.

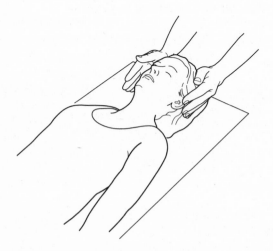

3B *Or* place one slightly cupped hand over each side of the head, with the fingers at each temple, and then move your hands one at a time to position 4.

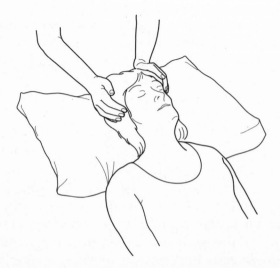

4 The neck/throat

Place one hand on each side of the neck, with palms facing the neck, and with your little fingers resting gently on the top of the client's shoulders. Your fingers should *not* touch the person's neck or throat, as this can make them feel very constricted, and even unsafe. Make sure there is *at least* 10cm (4in) between your hands and the client's neck. Remain in this position for three to five minutes, and then move the hands one at a time to position 5.

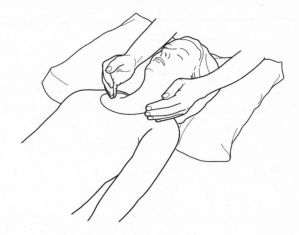

HAND POSITIONS FOR TREATING THE FRONT OF THE BODY

The first hand position, on the upper chest, can be carried out while still seated behind the client's head, or, like the following three positions, with the Practitioner standing or sitting on one side of the client (it doesn't matter which side).

5 The chest

5A *Either* from behind the client's head, place your hands in a V-shape at the top of the chest. The heel of each hand can rest gently on the person's collarbone, and the hand can be held flat on the chest this time, with fingertips pointing diagonally towards the breastbone in the centre of the chest. If you are treating a female, be aware that it is neither appropriate nor necessary to have your hands directly on the breasts, so if you have long hands or the woman has particularly high breasts, you may need to pull your hands back a little. Hold your hands in this position for three to five minutes, and then gently remove them, and move around to the side of the client.

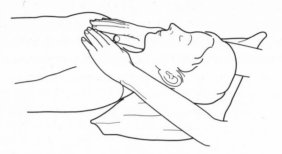

5B *Or* from beside the client, place one hand in front of the other, flat on the upper chest (avoiding contact with the throat and the breasts).

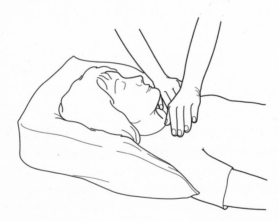

The next three positions are carried out with the Practitioner standing or sitting on one side of the client. Please ensure that you can comfortably hold each hand position for between three and five minutes, without having to stretch too much or press too hard on the client's body. Adjust your body appropriately, either by standing with your legs slightly apart with the knees soft, as in a t'ai chi or qigong stance, or by sitting on a chair. (A chair on wheels, but without arms, is excellent, because this allows for minimal disturbance as you can wheel yourself along between hand positions, rather than having to reposition the chair.) If you are treating someone on the floor, either kneel or sit cross-legged.

6 The solar plexus

Place one hand in front of the other flat on the body (resting gently, but without putting pressure on the client), with fingertips pointing away from you, on the solar plexus (below the breasts and above the waist), so that one hand is on the left side of the body and the other is on the right side. Hold this position for three to five minutes (it is OK to reposition your hands occasionally, swapping them over to different sides so that you don't get too tired) and then move them one at a time to position 7.

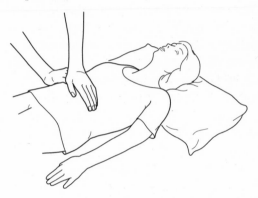

7 The waist/navel

Place one hand in front of the other flat on the body (resting gently, but without putting pressure on the client), with fingertips pointing away from you, on the waist/navel area, so that one hand is on the left side of the body and the other is on the right side. Hold this position for three to five minutes (it is OK to reposition your hands occasionally, swapping them over to different sides so that you don't get too tired), and then move them one at a time to position 8.

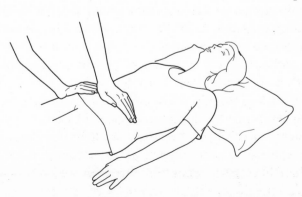

8 The pelvic area

The hand positions for treating males and females vary slightly, in order to show sensitivity with regard to the genital area.

8A For female clients, hold your hands in a V shape, with the point of the V being towards the pubic bone. This is most comfortably achieved as shown in the illustration; for example, if the client's head is on your left, then the heel of your right hand is level with her left hip bone, and the fingertips are pointing diagonally away from the pubic bone. The fingertips of your left hand are pointing diagonally towards and level with her right hip. (Any other configuration of the hands tends to be uncomfortable to hold, and to be more intrusive to the client.) Hold this position for three to five minutes and then take your hands away.

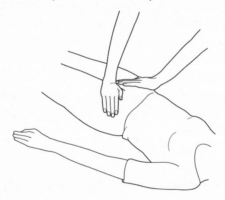

8B For male clients, to avoid contact with the male genitalia, it is usual to place one hand on each hip bone, as shown in the illustration. Again, it is more comfortable for you to have one hand with the fingertips pointing to the right, and one hand with the fingertips pointing to the left. Hold this position for three to five minutes and then take your hands away.

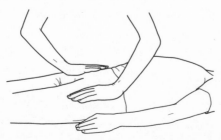

You may at this point start treating the front of the legs and feet, if needed – the hand positions for these are given on pages 144.

PREPARING TO WORK ON THE BACK

When you have completed the first eight hand positions, which cover the head and the front of the body (plus the front of the legs and feet if necessary), you will need to ask your client to turn over onto their stomach. The person will probably be very relaxed at this stage, and may even be asleep, so it is important to be kind and supportive. Very gently pat or stroke their shoulder, speak their name softly, and ask them to turn over. Assist them if they need this, and ensure that you reposition the pillow which had been under their knees – move it so that it is now under their ankles. Ensure that their head is comfortable – if you have a therapy couch with a face hole (and the towelling covered sponge ring that goes over this to make it more comfortable), the client can use this, but sometimes people don't like to feel so constricted. The head can be held on one side, or it can rest on an arm – just let the client find a position that suits them, and when they are settled again, start the treatment of the back of the body.

HAND POSITIONS FOR TREATING THE BACK OF THE BODY

You can treat the client's shoulders from behind the client's head (9A), or from the side (9B), whichever you prefer. Positions 10, 11 and 12 are all carried out with you standing or sitting beside the client's body.

9 The shoulders

9A *Either* sit or stand behind the client's head and place one hand on each shoulder so that the heel of each hand rests on the shoulder, and the fingertips are pointing down the back. Hold this position for three to five minutes, and then gently remove your hands and move around to the side of the client's body for hand position 10.

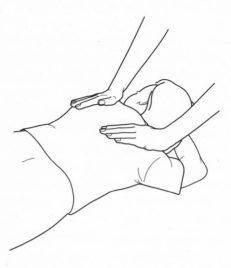

9B *Or* while sitting or standing at the side of the client, place one hand on the left shoulder and the other hand on the right shoulder. This can involve quite a stretch, so make sure you can accomplish this comfortably; otherwise revert to 9A. Hold this position for three to five minutes and then move your hands one at a time to position 10.

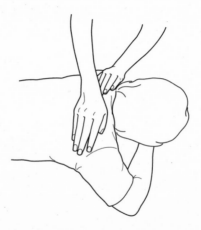

10 The back

Stand beside the person and gently, without pressure, place one hand in front of the other, with the palms flat against the back, midway between the shoulders and the waist. One hand should therefore be on each side of the body, and both sets of fingers should be pointing away from you. It is usual to leave a gap between your hands, where the spine is. Hold this position for three to five minutes, and then move your hands one at a time to position 11.

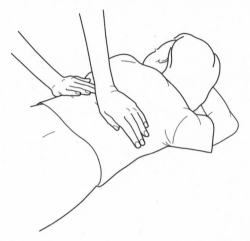

11 The waist/adrenals

Gently place one hand in front of the other as before, with the palms flat against the body and the fingers pointing away from you on the person's waist, so that each side of the body is covered, leaving a small gap between the hands by the spine. Hold this position for three to five minutes, and then move your hands one at a time to position 12.

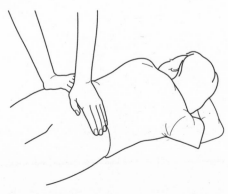

12 The buttocks

12A *Either* gently place one hand on each buttock, palms flat on the body, with each hand facing in the same direction (fingertips away from you), leaving a small gap between the hands by the spine. Hold this position for three to five minutes, and then gently and slowly move your hands away, and, unless you are going to treat the back of the legs and feet, move back to the client's head to start smoothing the client's aura (see page 147 for instructions on how to do this).

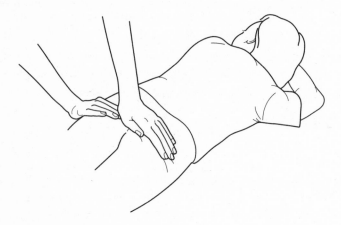

12B *Or* if you or your client prefers, you can hold your hands in the air above the coccyx so that you are not touching the client's buttocks.

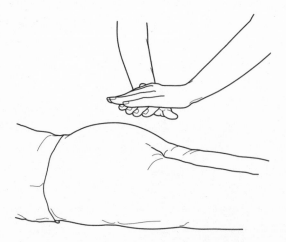

Treating Someone Lying on Their Side

If your client is unable to lie on their stomach for the last part of the treatment, for example a woman who is pregnant, then she can lie on her side instead. It is then more comfortable for you to sit at the side of the therapy couch facing her back, to carry out the rest of the treatment. If you place your chair roughly in the space between the client's waist and the middle of his or her back, you will find that you can reach all four positions on the back without having to move your chair. In each case, it is more comfortable to lay one of your arms along the couch, with the elbow of the other arm resting on the couch, so that your arms and hands are fully supported throughout. The illustrations show the client resting on her left side, but of course if she prefers she can rest on her right side and you can adjust your hand positions to suit.

9 The shoulders

Place your right forearm on the couch with your right hand on the client's left shoulder, and your left elbow on the couch with your left hand on the client's right shoulder, as in the illustration below.

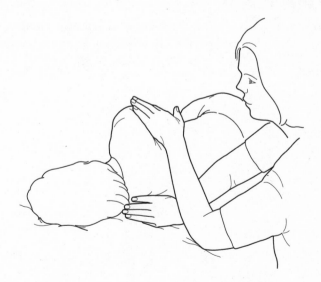

10 The back

Gently move your right hand down to the middle of the client's back, resting the side of your hand on the couch, with your left elbow resting again on the couch with your left hand on the right side of the client's back.

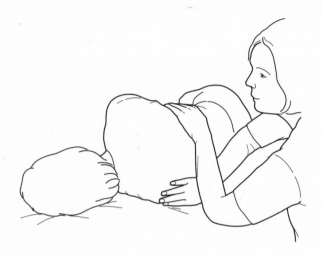

11 The waist/adrenals

Now, turn your body slightly and rest your left arm along the couch and place your left hand on the client's waist, with your right elbow on the couch and your right hand on the right side of the client's waist.

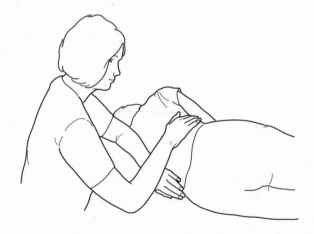

12 The buttocks

With your left forearm resting on the couch, place your left hand on one buttock, and your right elbow resting on the couch with your right hand on the other buttock.

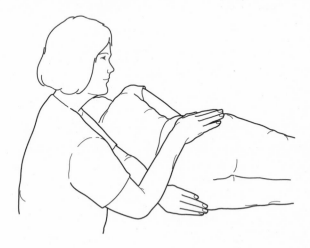

TREATING SOMEONE IN A CHAIR

Should you ever need to treat someone who cannot lie down at all, then the treatment can fairly easily be carried out with them sitting in a chair. If so, please make sure that the client's legs are uncrossed, and that both feet are on the floor (or another support), as this enables the energy to flow more effectively. You can stand or sit behind them for the head positions, and then sit or kneel at their side for the hand positions on the body. Because placing both hands across someone's body, either at the back or the front, can be quite awkward and uncomfortable for the Practitioner, it is sensible to change some hand positions slightly, and combine the back and front positions, placing one hand on each, roughly level with one another, so this would result in a treatment using nine hand positions, rather than 12.

If they are sitting on something like a dining chair, then the back-of-the-body hand positions are relatively easy. If they can only sit in an armchair or a wheelchair, however, and they are unable to lean forward a little, you can actually place your hands on the back of the chair, as Reiki will easily flow through the chair to the client.

1 The back of the head

Stand beside the client, with one hand cradling the base of their skull, and the other hand on the crown of their head.

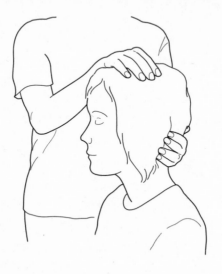

2 The eyes/brow

Move to stand behind the client with the heels of your hands resting on their upper brow, and with the rest of each hand cupped over each eye. Make sure your fingertips do not touch the person's face, as some people would find this a little claustrophobic.

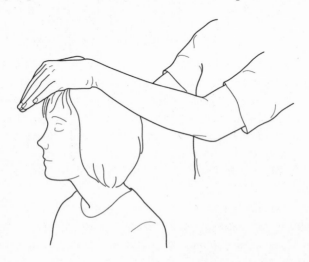

3 The ears/temples

One hand is cupped over each ear, with the fingertips pointing towards the temples.

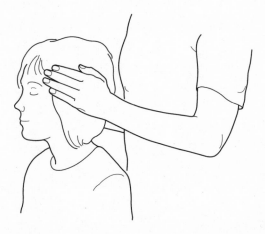

4 The neck/throat

Rest the edge of your hands on the client's shoulders, palms facing the neck about 10cm (4in) away from the neck, to prevent the client feeling threatened or as if they are about to be strangled!

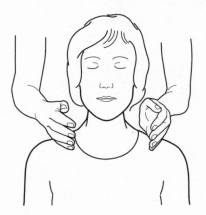

5 The shoulders

Place one hand on each shoulder, palms facing downwards.

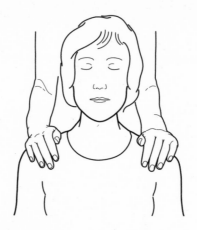

6 The chest/upper back

Move to the side of the client and, either standing or sitting, place one hand on their upper chest, ensuring that you do not touch the breasts, and one hand roughly level with it on their back.

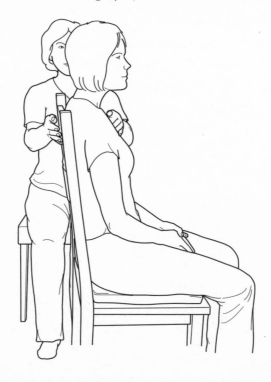

7 The solar plexus/middle back

Place one hand on their solar plexus, with the other hand roughly level with it on their back.

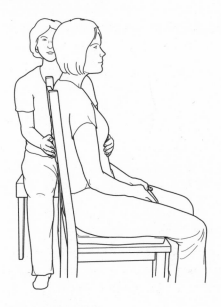

8 The waist/navel/adrenals

Place one hand on the client's waist (near the navel) at the front, with your other hand on the waist at the back.

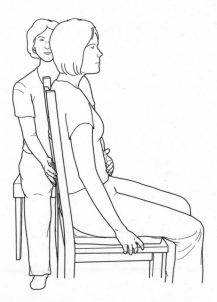

9 The pelvic area/buttocks

Hold one hand in the air with the palm focused towards the pelvic area (that is, not placed on the body, which might be intrusive), with the other hand placed at the back of (or underneath) the chair, with the palm focusing towards the buttocks.

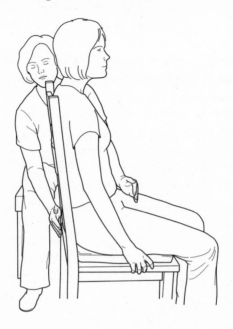

ADDITIONAL HAND POSITIONS

Because Reiki is Divinely guided, it always flows to the areas of the physical body or energy bodies that need it, and because the classic 12 (or nine seated) hand positions enable the Reiki to flow easily and effectively into all the major chakra points, other hand positions are not really essential; however, over the years many Reiki Masters have tried other hand positions, and the commonest additional positions taught are those on the legs and feet, as shown on the following pages, although these do receive Reiki when the pelvic area and buttocks are treated. If you do use any additional hand positions, such as on the legs and feet, these are usually held for only one or two minutes, but again, use your intuition, and if your hands are still experiencing a lot of sensation in a particular hand position, then continue for longer. The feet have energy zones, which correspond to all parts of the physical body, so giving Reiki to the ankles, heels, toes, and tops and soles of the feet, actually sends the healing again to every organ and system within the body.

HAND POSITIONS FOR TREATING THE LEGS AND FEET

Obviously you need to stand or sit at the client's side to carry out these hand positions, although when treating the feet (especially both soles) it may be easier to stand or sit beyond the feet, as in the composite illustrations overleaf, which show all the hand positions on the legs and feet (that is, one person in five positions, not five people!). If you decide to treat the legs and feet, you would simply continue with the first leg position – the front of the thighs – immediately following position 8 on the front of the body, the pelvic area. You would therefore only gently awaken the client after the final position on the top of the feet, asking them to turn over. Similarly, you would continue the treatment on the back, after the buttocks, by placing your hands on the backs of the thighs, progressing down the backs of the knees, calves and ankles, and ending with the soles of the feet. The hand positions are virtually the same for both, as shown in the illustrations that follow:

One hand on each thigh
One hand on each knee
One hand on each shin (or calf)
One hand on each ankle
One hand on the top of each foot (when lying on their back) or one hand on the sole of each foot (when lying on their front)

Of course, if the client has a health problem in a particular part (or parts) of the body, it makes sense to give those areas additional time, or to add a hand position if required; for example, no specific hand positions are given for the upper arms, elbows, forearms, wrists, hands or fingers, because Reiki flows down the arms particularly when using the hand positions on the chest, shoulders and middle back – but if there is a health problem there, please treat it. It is almost impossible to treat both arms at the same time when the client is lying down, so a technique I use is on page 145.

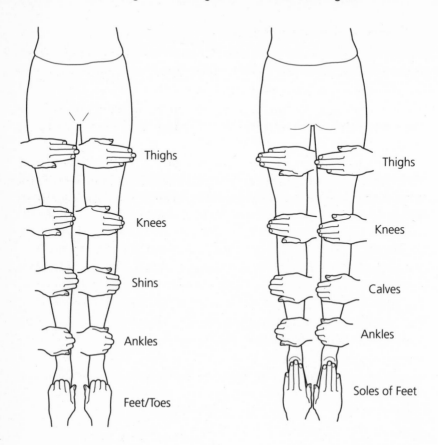

Thighs

Knees

Shins

Ankles

Feet/Toes

Thighs

Knees

Calves

Ankles

Soles of Feet

HAND POSITIONS FOR TREATING THE ARMS AND HANDS

Start with one arm, and when that is completed, move over to the other side of the body to treat the other arm. It doesn't matter which arm you start with – left or right. You can either do the arms and hands (if you have decided they need treating) immediately after hand position 5, the chest, or you can wait until you have completed the treatment on the front of the body (including the legs, if you have decided they need treating). You can then complete the front treatment by treating the arms before asking the client to turn over. Again, the illustration opposite shows a composite view of all three hand positions on each arm (that is, one person treating the client, not six people!).

Left arm, and then right arm

Place one hand on the upper arm and the other hand on the elbow. After a few minutes (not usually more than two) gently move your hands to the next hand position.

Place one hand on the forearm and the other hand on the wrist. After a few minutes gently move your hands to the next hand position.

Place one hand underneath, and one on top, of the client's hand. After a few minutes, gently remove your hands and move on to the next hand position – either the other arm or the solar plexus, or rouse the client and ask them to turn over.

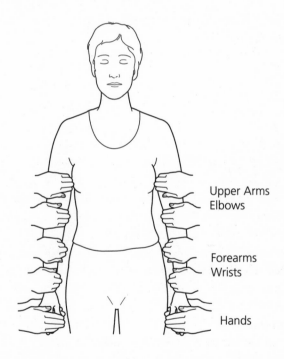

Upper Arms
Elbows

Forearms
Wrists

Hands

ADDITIONAL TREATMENT FOR THE SPINE

For people with back problems, this is especially good. It can be done when the client is lying on their stomach, or on their side, or even sitting or standing, if they are unable to lie flat. Place one hand at the base of the spine – the coccyx – and the other hand at the top of the spine, on the neck just below the base of the skull. Hold this position for several minutes, allowing the Reiki to flow up and down the spine, between your hands. This is good energetically, too, because it allows Reiki to flow up and down the central line of energy that connects the chakras, called the *Hara* line, so helping to clear blockages throughout the body and establish a better flow of *Ki*.

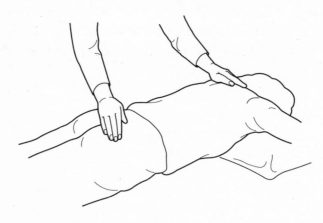

Basically, use the 12 (or nine seated) hand positions of the traditional Western full treatment as a framework, because in most cases that will be all you need; however, if you really feel it is necessary, add to them. Don't be afraid to be creative, because Reiki is a dynamic energy and a living healing system, so use it in ways that feel right to you. Both Dr Usui's and Dr Hayashi's teaching manuals showed a range of hand positions for specific illnesses, some of which used only one hand, or even just a couple of fingers, and many Reiki Masters since have also developed the idea that particular hand positions can be beneficial for certain conditions. I personally believe that as Reiki flows all around the body when a Practitioner places his or her hands on a client, then providing the Reiki continues to flow for long enough (at least an hour is preferable), every part of the physical body, as well as the mental, emotional and spiritual bodies and the whole aura, will be treated.

It is possible to give Reiki for an hour or more with the hands held in the same position – for example, with the hands on the shoulders of a person sitting in a chair – and the person will receive almost the same amount of Reiki as they would in a classic full treatment. This is neither as comfortable for the Practitioner nor as comforting for the client, but there may be occasions when it is the only alternative. But placing the hands on different parts of the body – near to each of the seven chakras – does help the Reiki to flow into the body even more effectively, and it also allows a cumulative effect.

When the Reiki begins by flowing in through the crown and brow chakras, which it does in the first three hand positions, it not only flows into the head, but also flows throughout the body, beginning the process of healing, harmonising and balancing the whole – both the physical body and the energy field. As it clears through blockages, it helps each succeeding chakra to be ready to receive even more Reiki, so maximising the flow. This means it is therefore more efficient to give a full treatment, as well as being a pleasant experience for both of you. When you try it, you will soon realise that giving a treatment feels almost as good as receiving one, because, of course, the Reiki is flowing through you as well.

Smoothing the Aura

A pleasant way to finish the whole treatment is to smooth the person's aura three times. During the treatment, the Reiki has been activating and removing negative energies from the physical body into the aura, from where they can be released, and this can have a slightly agitating effect on the aura itself if the energies are just left there. Smoothing the aura down helps the energies to settle, and can detach any negative energy which is still clinging to the inner layers of the aura. It also helps the client to begin to wake up after the deep relaxation of the treatment, which could otherwise leave them feeling a bit 'spaced out'. Always start at the head, and work down the body, as this echoes the natural flow of *Ki*, and is soothing and calming for the client. Doing it in the other direction can have the opposite effect. Start above the crown and, keeping your hands about 30cm (12in) above the body, follow the contours of the body all the way down to the feet, and then shake your hands downwards, beyond the feet, to disperse any negative energy. Repeat this whole action three times, and when you have finished, brush any remaining energy off your own hands.

AFTER THE TREATMENT

When you have smoothed down the client's aura, gently rouse them by touching their shoulder and saying their name softly. Try not to hurry the person, but if the client is still having difficulty in 'coming round', then gently massage their feet. When they are ready, help them to sit up or get off the therapy couch, and offer them a glass of water. Advise them to drink plenty of water over the next few days, to help the body flush out the toxins which may have been dislodged by the Reiki – but ask them to check with their doctor if they have any health problems that might be affected by greater water intake.

At this stage people often want to talk to you about what they experienced during a treatment, and how they feel immediately afterwards. They may also want to know what you experienced, such as where you felt any 'blocks', and whether you think you've balanced those energies. At first, you might be reluctant to offer such information, because it takes time and practice to build up your energetic sensitivity and intuition to help you understand what different sensations and energy patterns mean because, unfortunately, energetic sensations don't always mean the same thing. Each Practitioner may experience them, and interpret them, in slightly different ways, and of course there will be differences between individual clients, too.

It is important, however, to treat these issues sensibly and sensitively. You must NEVER try to diagnose any illness unless you are medically qualified, but you can have an informal chat about what areas in their body felt warm, cool, sticky, tingly, and so on – but do let them know that these sensations don't necessarily mean anything is wrong, they just reflect the different ways the energy is being used by the body. You can ask whether they have experienced any problems there, and talk in general terms about the causative issues behind illness, and the messages and lessons illness offers us, perhaps suggesting that they read some of the books recommended in the Further Reading section, to help them understand their bodies better; however, it is important to realise that *you* are not responsible for their healing, *they* are, so it isn't up to you to decide for them what is 'wrong' with them, either on a physical or an energetic level. It is also irresponsible to frighten or offend people, so please be very careful what you say and how you say it. (It can actually be very useful to take a course in counselling or NLP (neurolinguistic programming), especially if you intend to offer treatments professionally.) If you have any doubts about a person's physical (or mental) condition, especially if it doesn't seem to be responding to Reiki treatments, then of course you should recommend gently, tactfully and as reassuringly as possible that perhaps it would be best to seek medical advice 'just to be on the safe side'.

Please don't get too worried about all of this. Remember that you are not a 'healer', but simply a channel for a Divinely guided healing energy, so trust Reiki to do its work. Often days, or even weeks, after a Reiki treatment, a person can suddenly gain insight into whatever problem area they have needed help with, because the Reiki has created an energy shift that has allowed the healing to slowly permeate through the blockages until the cause reaches the person's consciousness, ready to be released.

Grounding

Some people feel energised immediately after a treatment, while others feel sleepy and incredibly peaceful. If the person seems at all 'spaced out', then make sure you 'ground' their energies before allowing them to leave. This is easily achieved by getting the client to sit with their feet flat on the floor. Take your hands and place one on each of the client's feet, and visualise the energy flowing out through the soles of the feet into the ground below – hence the term 'grounding'. It is amazing how quickly people return to feeling normal after this simple exercise. If they still seem a bit woozy, another good grounding exercise is to get them to stand up, and then march on the spot. As they lift their left knee they should touch it with their right hand, and when they lift their right knee, touch that with their left hand. This works really well to balance the two sides of the body and two hemispheres of the brain. If they also stamp their feet when placing them on the ground, this helps to throw the energy downwards. Doing this exercise for about a minute should be quite long enough – any more is a bit exhausting.

As well as helping your client after a treatment, please don't forget yourself. You will also need a glass of water, and it is sensible to carry out some self-cleansing after every treatment. I would recommend the Dry Brushing and Reiki Shower techniques in

Chapter 20. You might also like to do some Reiki on yourself, and spend a little quiet time in contemplation or meditation.

How Many Treatments?

This is rather like asking 'how long is a piece of string?' and it clearly depends upon what is being treated. For minor health problems, or to alleviate stress and encourage relaxation, one or two treatments may be enough. Major illnesses are likely to require many treatments, and afterwards it might be a good idea to have a 'top up' treatment every few months to keep the energies balanced. For very serious or chronic conditions, it is generally accepted that to give four treatments, preferably on consecutive days, is an extremely valuable way to start any treatment programme, as it begins the process of effectively breaking down the blockages in each of the four etheric bodies – physical, mental, emotional and spiritual – so that they are more prepared to receive and benefit from future Reiki treatments. If it is not possible to do the treatments on consecutive days, then at least two per week would be ideal. (After Second Degree you can combine hands-on treatments with distant treatments.)

Another recommendation for dealing with serious illness is to give a full treatment to the affected person every day for at least 21 days. This is obviously easier to achieve if it is a member of your own family or a friend who lives locally, but in other cases a combination of 'hands-on' and distant treatments (using Second Degree techniques) can be given.

Please bear in mind that in the West we are familiar with complementary health treatments lasting about an hour, so the Reiki treatment is geared to a similar time scale; however, Reiki itself is *not* geared to a specific time scale. Reiki can go on flowing – and working – for many hours, days or even weeks without stopping. We put limits on Reiki, but with Reiki there are no limits. Anything is possible. But not everything is probable. The idea of treating someone, non-stop, for 24 hours, or three days, or a week or more is not something that most of us would be willing to do, but some Reiki Masters have experimented with this using a number of Reiki Practitioners working in shifts in a 'Reiki Marathon', usually two or three at a time, with excellent results. Now, obviously a broken leg wouldn't warrant such intensive treatment, but very serious, life-threatening illnesses could.

Even with such effort, however, there is no guarantee that the person will recover, because we cannot know what is really best for someone – what their Soul/Higher Self knows is for that person's highest and greatest good. For many people, human life as we know it is all there is, and under such circumstances the client themselves, or their relatives and friends, might be desperate for their physical life to continue. Their Higher Self, however, may know that they have achieved all that they came to achieve – even if they are still relatively young – and so such intense Reiki (or indeed, any number of Reiki treatments) may have a wonderfully healing effect, allowing the person to end their days in a relatively pain-free state of tranquillity and contentment, and to make their transition peaceful. What we must continually be aware of is the rights and autonomy of every person. Each individual has the right to seek – or to turn down – the opportunity of receiving healing. What anybody else feels about the situation is irrelevant. If someone chooses to fight an illness in any way they can, that's great, and they deserve all the support they can get. But if a person feels there is no point, that they have reached the end and they want to give up, then that is also OK, and they still deserve all the support they can get. Reiki can help, either way. In all instances, you just need to follow your inner guidance and do what feels right.

WHAT IF PHYSICAL HEALING DOESN'T HAPPEN?

Reiki is not just about physical healing – it is holistic, working on many different levels, and it may be that other aspects of the person are in greater need of healing, even though we, as humans, tend to feel that physical problems should be addressed first. Another aspect I would like to mention is that not everyone wants to be healed. Of course, on a conscious level, you would expect *everybody* to choose to be healed into good health, but our motivations are often subconscious, and there may be deeper reasons why letting go of an illness, or being fully healthy, could be disadvantageous or even frightening to someone. Some people have a considerable investment in their own ill health, even if their rationale seems strange to us. Perhaps since childhood the only time they got any attention was when they were ill, or when they were sick as a child they were treated differently, or perhaps being ill means they don't have to face up to something that is going on in their lives.

Each of us is a unique individual, experiencing life in our own unique way, so it is hardly surprising that we should have complex and sometimes baffling responses to everything in our lives, including illness. Some people who try really hard to heal themselves, using all the self-help techniques available, are often puzzled and upset when their efforts are not immediately successful. Often this is because the causative levels are very deeply buried, and need to come to the surface layer by layer to be understood, so the healing has to take time. Sometimes it is because the illness itself is the lesson that has to be learned – perhaps something which affects the mobility of the person, bringing them literally to a full stop so that they are forced to look inside and pursue insight and self-awareness.

At other times it may be because they are actually trying too hard – they are so busy 'doing' things about their illness that they have forgotten how to 'be'. They may simply need to *acknowledge* the illness and its effects on them, reaching a level of acceptance of what it is like *in the present*, however painful or distressing that may be. In trying desperately to rid themselves of physical symptoms they may have actually blocked any real understanding of the lesson the illness was trying to teach them. Whatever happens, it is vital not to be critical of oneself, or to be judgemental about others, or to blame the body for not cooperating by not getting 'better'.

Confidentiality and Ethics

Needless to say, whether you are practising Reiki professionally, or simply offering some treatments to family, friends or colleagues, any person you treat should be able to rely totally on your confidentiality, as you are in a privileged position when treating them. They may regard you as a medical professional – which you are not, unless you are medically trained – and will listen carefully to anything you say. You may feel it necessary to advise someone to have further treatment(s) to maintain wellness. **Note:** As I have already said, on no account should you attempt to diagnose any illnesses. If you feel there is a serious problem, you should gently advise the person to seek medical help in addition to Reiki, but always in a way that will not alarm them. You may sometimes wish to encourage a client to examine their lifestyle and make positive, healthy modifications, but this should always be done with the utmost sensitivity, and in a positive, helpful manner, without criticism.

It is equally important not to promise a cure, or *any* particular outcome from a treatment. The amount of healing required is decided by the person's Higher Self, and the Reiki is directed by a Higher Consciousness to those areas of greatest need – so that leaves you with very little to do other than to be a channel for the energy.

Promising miracle cures is unethical, dangerous and often illegal, because you could be falsely raising hopes. Yes, miracles do sometimes happen, but no one knows when. It would be sensible to familiarise yourself with your legal responsibilities when treating people, and there is some information about this in Chapter 17. Also, if you do intend to carry out regular Reiki treatments on people, even if they are just family or friends, it can be a practical step to join an organisation like the UK Reiki Federation, as they can offer advice on professional standards, ethics and codes of practice, plus access to reasonably priced insurance. (There are similar organisations in other countries – see Resources.)

Should you offer Reiki?

Another matter to think about is whether you should offer Reiki or wait to be asked. People need to know that you do Reiki, otherwise they would not know they could ask for it, so it is fine to talk about it; however, if you always offer Reiki, rather than waiting to be asked, people could feel obliged to say 'yes', and then you would effectively be interfering in their healing.

REIKI AS FIRST AID

Giving a full treatment is clearly not the only way to give Reiki, so please don't feel constrained by the idea that you always need a therapy couch and time to do 12 hand positions. If anyone around you needs help, you have a tool available for which you only need your hands. Many minor problems or injuries can quickly be alleviated with Reiki, such as headaches, toothache, muscle strain, cramp, cuts and bruises and so on. Simply place your hands on the affected area and allow the Reiki to flow. In my experience, most such aches and pains will ease within a few minutes and will often be completely gone within a quarter of an hour. There is no specific amount of time for such events – just allow your inner guidance to let you know when the Reiki has stopped flowing. Usually this will mean that you no longer feel any sensation in your hands, but for those people who get very little sensation anyway, it may surprise you but you will still 'know' when it is right to take your hands away. Anyway, the person you are treating will probably let you know when the pain has gone.

Is it Always Appropriate to Give Someone Reiki?

There are no known contraindications with Reiki when it is used on its own; that is, when it is not used in conjunction with any other therapy. As I said in the last chapter, Reiki is very safe, and if you just use a little common sense there shouldn't be any problems; however, within the Reiki community some ideas have been circulated that perhaps need some explanation.

Some people seem to think, for example, that it isn't safe to give Reiki to anyone receiving chemotherapy or radiotherapy because Reiki is said to eliminate toxins. Actually, as Reiki always works for the greatest and highest good, in my experience it simply helps to alleviate the side effects of both types of treatment. Another similarly erroneous idea is that Reiki shouldn't be sent (that is, distant Reiki at Reiki 2) to anyone while they are under anaesthetic, in case the Reiki gets rid of the anaesthetic, but again, in my experience, it doesn't do that!

As mentioned in Chapter 6, it is sensible to wait until a broken bone has been set, or a severed finger has been reattached before giving Reiki directly to the site of the injury – it would, after all, probably be too sore! Also, if anyone is taking medication for diabetes, high or low blood pressure, or thyroid problems, they should be advised to keep a check on their condition and consult their doctor if they notice any improvement, in case the dosage needs to be adjusted. **Note:** You should *never* advise anyone to lower or stop their medication – they should always seek medical advice first.

The only other idea some Reiki people have put forward is that Reiki shouldn't be given to someone with a heart pacemaker. Of course, if you feel nervous about this, then if in doubt, don't! But as Reiki isn't an electrical force, and its action is often to bring something back into balance, there shouldn't be a problem, but if you or a client wants reassurance then they can consult their doctor. If they do this, it is best to describe Reiki as a form of spiritual healing, as some doctors won't have heard of it.

Some medical conditions, such as epilepsy, are probably best left to fully trained professional practitioners, but there is more information about various health conditions in Chapter 17.

Of course, Reiki isn't just for treating yourself or other people – there are lots of creative ways of using it with the skills you learn at Reiki First Degree, and this is what we cover in the next chapter.

Chapter 8

Being Creative with Your Reiki First Degree Skills

As well as being able to treat yourself, your family and friends, after a Reiki First Degree course there are plenty of other things you can do. In this chapter there are details of how to treat animals and plants, food and objects, how to send Reiki through the aura, and so on. In reality, it can take a lifetime to learn the full potential of Reiki, and probably even one lifetime wouldn't be enough, so the best advice I can give is: experiment and enjoy.

USING REIKI IN GROUPS

A treatment with two people

Most people consider a Reiki treatment from one person to be a lovely experience, but two Reiki people can treat one client, which obviously increases the amount of energy entering the recipient. Each Practitioner treats one side of the body, so their hand positions are complementary to each other, and both change hand positions at the same time, so there is no interruption in the flow of Reiki. The following instructions should be carried out by both Practitioners as they each progress down one side of the body. Each hand position should be held for about five minutes, so the front of the body will take 20 minutes, and the back of the body ten minutes. This means the treatment is completed in half the normal time, but because two people are channelling Reiki at the same time, the energy increases exponentially, so a half-hour treatment with two Practitioners is equivalent to more than an hour with one. As before, please ensure that your hands don't touch any intimate parts of the body, and that when treating sensitive areas such as the neck, keep your hands about 10cm (4in) away so that the person doesn't feel threatened.

Front of the body (left and right sides)

One hand over the eye and one hand over the ear.
One hand under the back of the head, and one hand by the neck.
One hand on the upper chest, and the other hand on the solar plexus.
One hand on the waist, and the other hand on the hip bone.

Back of the body (left and right sides)

One hand on the shoulder, and the other hand on the back (midway between the shoulder and waist).
One hand on the waist, and the other hand on one buttock.

THE BENEFITS OF REIKI GROUPS

Getting together with other people who do Reiki is great fun, but it also has other benefits. It can be a useful forum to discuss developments and experiences with other Practitioners, perhaps trying out new techniques or swapping tips on methods you have found useful. The more confident and experienced members can help those who are new to Reiki, or who feel shy about trying it with their family or friends without getting some more practice first, so it gives them a chance to hone their skills in a friendly and nurturing environment. The more Reiki you receive, the more you heal, and the more Reiki energy will flow through you so that you can help others to heal, so Reiki Groups – often called Reiki Share Groups – are an ideal place to 'swap' treatments with each other.

To have two, four, six or even more people treating you at once can be a delightful experience, producing an even deeper state of relaxation. (It doesn't have to be even numbers, but it is often easier that way.) Of course, the more people you have treating you, the less time it takes, as you simply share out the hand positions between you, usually with each person working on one side of the body only. If you have lots of people you can cover all of the body and the legs, feet, arms and hands as well – and of course everyone can take it in turns to receive Reiki, as well as giving it.

When treating in a large group, don't feel too constrained by the traditional hand positions. It is often more comfortable to spread out a little; for example, with the head positions it would be difficult for four people to be crowded so close together all trying to treat the head at the same time. Have one Practitioner with both their hands underneath the person's head (as in hand position 1), and then one on either side with one hand by the person's neck and the other hand by their ear. This would mean the eyes would not be treated – but with three people treating the head area there would definitely be enough Reiki to go around! Then space people out on either side, treating the body and the legs, and another at the end of the couch treating the person's feet.

If you like this idea, then why not start a Reiki Group yourself? You could contact the other people who trained at the same course as you or any other Reiki people you know. You could also find out about Reiki Share Groups arranged by local members of organisations such as the UK Reiki Federation, which usually welcome new participants.

SENDING REIKI THROUGH THE AURA

There are times when it is not possible to treat someone by laying your hands on them, but Reiki can also flow through the aura, so you don't have to be right beside the person who needs help; for example, if you are at the scene of an accident, it might be inappropriate for you to offer your help directly (unless you have first aid qualifications), but you can *intend* that Reiki should flow to the injured person(s) for their greatest and highest good. Even if they haven't asked for healing, their Higher Selves will know what is needed, and will probably draw Reiki into them to help with the shock and pain. There is no need to hold your hands out – just let the palms be open, perhaps on your lap, and simply imagine your aura expanding until it encompasses the intended recipient(s), and then mentally 'switch on' the Reiki by *intending* that it should flow for the highest and greatest good.

TREATING ANIMALS

Most types of animal respond very well to Reiki, and with many you can follow a similar format of hand positions to those on humans with good effect. Clearly, though, this depends upon the size (and temperament) of the animal. There are several methods that can be used, depending upon specific circumstances:

- Placing the hands directly on the animal

- Sending Reiki through the aura to the animal

- Placing the hands on the cage or tank in which the animal is housed

- Holding a small animal in your hands

Dealing with pets

The animals most people are keen to treat with Reiki are their pets. It seems that animals are very much more in tune with their own health and energy needs than humans, so while some will happily sit or stand for a long time to receive Reiki, and keep coming back for more, others will quickly move away. Even pets that would usually sit happily to be stroked may walk off if you try to give them Reiki, and if that happens, please let them. I have seen overenthusiastic Reiki students covered in scratches or even bite marks after determined attempts to treat their pet with Reiki when the animal clearly didn't want any!

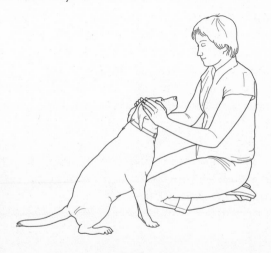

Any hand positions you choose will obviously depend upon where you can reach, and where the animal will allow you to touch, as well as where it is safe to touch. Also, remember that Reiki will flow around the whole body, even if you can only place your hands in one position. Depending upon the size, you might try one or two hand positions on the head, and two or three on either side of the body. Some animals seem to dislike Reiki being given directly onto their spine, although cats can be an exception to this. Obviously, if there is a specific injury, then that is where treatment should be concentrated, but take care not to directly touch any part which might cause the animal pain. Reiki can enter the auric field, and filter into the physical body from there, so you can hold your hands 5–7.5cm (2–3in) or more above the injury site, and the Reiki will flow in quite easily. The amount of time required for treatment will vary greatly, and will depend upon the size of the animal, as well as on the severity of any illness or injury.

Another way to help your pets, or other animals, is to Reiki their food and water to enhance its nutritional qualities and to offset the adverse effects of any chemicals or preservatives. This is simple to do. Hold the food or water bowl with one hand under it and one hand over it, and *intend* that Reiki should flow into the water. You can do this also with a box, packet or tin of food in your hands, *intending* that Reiki show flow into it – a minute is quite enough, and 30 seconds will probably do. Any homeopathic remedies or medication dispensed by a veterinary surgeon can also be given Reiki in the same way.

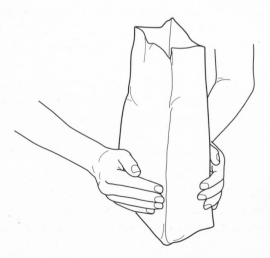

Birds, reptiles, fish, insects and small mammals

If you have a pet bird, reptile or small mammal, they may be well used to you handling them, in which case you can just hold them between your hands and let the Reiki flow. If they are likely to peck, bite or scratch you, it may be more circumspect to treat them in the cage, tank or hut where they live. Simply place your hands on or near the receptacle and *intend* that the Reiki should flow to the creature, and take your hands away when it feels appropriate to do so. Any small creatures will usually need treating for only a few minutes. Of course, if your pet needs more than one treatment, you can give it as much Reiki as you like – it is not possible to overdose on Reiki!

Farm animals and horses

With farm animals, such as cattle, sheep, pigs, goats, hens, ducks or geese, or more exotic species such as llamas and alpacas, it is often easiest to treat them through the aura from the edge of the field or beside the pen, sty or other enclosure. A horse is generally easier, as they are more used to human contact, so you could place your hands in one or two positions on the head/neck, and three or four down each side of the body; however, if treating a horse's legs do take care, as they are prone to kick, and don't stand behind a horse or approach it from behind!

Wild animals

Wild birds, or other small wild animals, are probably best placed in a cardboard box with air holes before being treated, as contact with humans can be very frightening, and the shock can even cause some to die. If you should ever need to give Reiki to an animal that might prove dangerous (for example, in a zoo), or which is too nervous to let you get near it, then it is perfectly acceptable to stand a safe distance away and send the Reiki through your own aura into the auric field of the animal.

Legal issues when treating animals

According to the Royal College of Veterinary Surgeons, in the UK the Veterinary Surgeons Act of 1966 states that anyone treating animals must be a qualified veterinary surgeon, and that no one else can diagnose problems, carry out tests for diagnostic purposes, advise or carry out medical or surgical treatment or prescribe medication.

Of course, someone treating an animal with Reiki is unlikely to be doing any of those things, and it does appear to be legal for farm workers to treat their farm animals, and for anyone else to treat their own pets, or to treat any animal in an emergency; however, if you do decide to treat any animal other than your own with Reiki it is essential that you get the owner's permission. Advise him or her to register the animal with a qualified veterinary surgeon, and take their animal to that vet for diagnosis and treatment (although the owner is of course entitled to ignore your advice, if they so wish). Regulations in other countries might be different, so I would advise you to find out what is applicable there before carrying out any work with animals.

USING REIKI WITH PLANTS AND SEEDS

Seeds and plants respond extremely well to Reiki, and I have tested this out many times. In one experiment, I kept a houseplant alive for months without water, just by giving it Reiki each day, and I have also planted seeds in identical compost and containers and given Reiki to only half the seeds. In each case those given Reiki grew much faster and more strongly than those that were not treated, and those planted in the Reiki half also had a 100 per cent germination rate.

To give Reiki to seeds, either hold the packet between your hands or plant them and hold your hands over the seed trays for a minute or two. For houseplants, hold your hands on each side of the pot for about a minute, or about 15cm (6in) away from the plant itself. If you are planting up a new garden, or moving plants to another border, any good gardener knows that plants become distressed and their growth is affected when moved, but if you Reiki them before and after uprooting them, you should find the effects of transplantation much reduced. For any of your indoor or outdoor plants, you can Reiki their water, too, by holding your hands on or over a watering can, or when holding a hosepipe, *intending* that Reiki should flow.

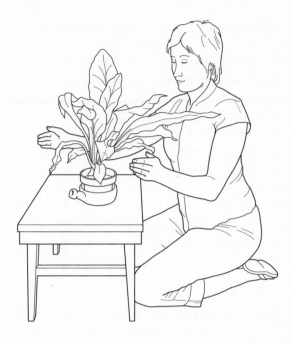

USING REIKI WITH FOOD AND DRINK

One way in which Reiki can help you to achieve a healthier life is to give Reiki to everything you eat and drink. When you give Reiki to food or drink it raises its vibration so that the energy you take in is heightened. We eat food because it is full of *Ki* – life-force energy – which we need to replenish our own reserves. Adding Reiki, therefore, not only enhances the nutritional value of the food but it can also help to balance the ill effects of any additives, preservatives and other chemicals, so bringing the food into greater harmony with your body. It is still a good idea to eat organic foods whenever possible, however, as these are grown without the use of pesticides and contain fewer harmful chemicals.

You can Reiki your food at any stage – when you put your shopping away, when you are preparing a meal, and when you are about to eat – or all three. Before you unpack your shopping bag, place your hands on either side of it for about 30 seconds, and *intend* that Reiki should flow into the contents of the bag. When preparing a meal, or making bread or cakes, and so on, assemble all your ingredients, and hold your hands near to the food for about 30 seconds

– or longer, if you wish – *intending* that Reiki should flow into it. If the food is already prepared, either at home or if you are eating in a restaurant, you don't have to hold your hands over your food overtly – you can be discreet and hold them casually by the side of your plate or around the cup or glass for 15–30 seconds, *intending* that Reiki should flow into the food and drink.

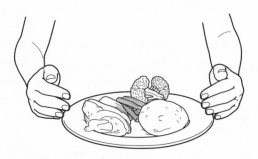

I like to use Reiki as a type of blessing, and it feels good to exchange some energy with our food, because *everything* we eat was a living thing, not just meat or fish. The vegetables, fruit, nuts and seeds we eat were also alive, and they too have given up life to provide us with energy so that we may continue to live. It is therefore in line with the Reiki principle 'Show appreciation and count your many blessings' to be grateful for what we eat. My invocation, as an example, is:

> 'Let Reiki flow into this food and drink, in grateful thanks to the earth, the plants, the creatures and the people who have helped to bring this nourishment to me. I also give Reiki to this food and drink to enhance its energetic quality and to bring it into harmony with my body, so that it helps my body to be vibrantly healthy and well.'

USING REIKI ON INANIMATE OBJECTS

So far I have only mentioned using Reiki on living things – people, animals, plants and food – but it is possible to use Reiki on virtually anything. You may think it is incredible, but Reiki can work very well on inanimate objects like cars, computers, washing machines and vacuum cleaners – but this is not really as strange as it may sound. Everything in the universe is energy, and all manufactured objects started out as natural materials. Once energy has been created, it cannot be destroyed, only transformed into some other state. Those natural materials may have changed *state* but they are still energy, so Reiki can still affect them.

My students and I have tried out this theory on many occasions, and successes include getting dishwashers, washing machines, vacuum cleaners, hairdryers, freezers, watches, clocks, cars and computers to work again after they had broken down, and even charging a mobile phone when it wasn't plugged in! Yes, it really works, although I am not suggesting that Reiki should be used in place of proper maintenance, because Reiki won't replace the oil or filters or spark plugs when they wear out, and sadly it doesn't replace gas, petrol or diesel either!

The principle is simple. Just place your hands on the machine that is not working, and *intend* that Reiki should flow into it, and keep your hands there for a while. I would suggest that you do so with good intentions, not out of anger that the machine has let you down, but from a feeling of appreciation for all the help the machine usually gives you. Your thoughts are energy, too, so on a purely functional level, resentful and angry thoughts could be counteracting the good the Reiki is doing.

USING REIKI ON PERSONAL PROBLEMS

As well as using Reiki on living things and inanimate objects, you can use it on more complex but less tangible things too, such as situations or difficulties in your personal life, or even wider issues such as world peace. Whatever type of problem you are having, from strained relationships with your partner or family, to difficulties at work or with studying, you can use Reiki to help to permeate the situation with healing. Simply write the situation down on paper – whether it needs a single sentence or several paragraphs – and then hold the paper between your hands, *intending* that Reiki should flow to the situation for the highest and greatest good. It is best to do this for at least ten minutes a day for as long as the situation exists.

Alternatively, you can visualise the situation, and imagine Reiki flowing into it for the highest and greatest good, but in both cases you need to be aware that you cannot guarantee a specific outcome with Reiki. You cannot *intend* or 'programme' Reiki to work so that it only changes the situation to the way you want it to be, because you don't necessarily know what is for your greatest good, so you have to detach yourself from specific expectations about the result. This can be challenging, because it is human nature to want a particular conclusion. But, you have to trust Reiki to bring you what you *need*, even if that is not necessarily what you *want*, because that is what your Higher Self will direct it to do.

USING REIKI ON WORLD SITUATIONS

Even in the case of sending Reiki to a world situation, such as a war or famine, we don't actually know what would be best in the long term. But you can write down or picture in your mind the major aspects of that situation, and let Reiki flow into it, *intending* that it is for the highest and greatest good. Even though we probably all believe that an end to all war and famine would be the greatest result, that may not necessarily be so; for example, perhaps a longer war might result in countries eventually collaborating or cooperating to produce a longer-lasting peace and stability, whereas a quicker solution might have broken down so that hostilities soon resumed. We simply don't know; however, it can only add to the ultimate good to send healing thoughts to such a situation, and the more of us who do so, the greater the chance of a good resolution, whatever or whenever that may be.

SENDING REIKI HEALING

Although to carry out distant healing effectively with Reiki it is more efficient to use the symbols and techniques taught at Second Degree, it is possible to send some healing at First Degree Level, although it will not be as strong. As a simile, think of distant healing at Second Degree level as being like a laser beam, where there is no diminution of strength regardless of distance, whereas at First Degree it is more like a normal torch beam which spreads out and loses light the further it goes.

Don't let this put you off having a go, though, because, as I explained in Chapter 2, we are all connected energetically. If you want to send healing and love to people, just use photographs, or write their names on a piece of paper and hold the paper or photos in your hands (or visualise them, and imagine holding their image between your hands), *intending* that Reiki should go to them for their greatest and highest good. Please remember, however, that you cannot force healing into anyone, so if the person's Higher Self knows that it would be inappropriate for some reason, then the healing will not be received, and will just dissipate.

With Reiki First Degree you have a valuable tool to use for self-healing and for helping other people, animals, objects and so on, for the rest of your life. This is a tremendous gift, and one that I hope you will enjoy. Many people find that Reiki 1 is sufficient for what they want to do, but others want to extend their healing abilities, so in Part 3 we look at what possibilities Reiki Second Degree has to offer.

Part 3

Developing Your Understanding: Reiki Second Degree

Chapter 9

Reiki Second Degree Training

Second Degree Reiki is about continued self-healing and growth, but it also broadens your knowledge and healing skills to enable you to help others to heal and grow. Reiki 2 is sometimes regarded as Practitioner Level, and I would certainly recommend it for anyone wishing to practise Reiki professionally, because it gives you a wide range of additional techniques to offer to potential clients (but see Chapter 17 for other requirements). This level is also beneficial for people who want to use Reiki more effectively on their own inner/spiritual development, so it is not simply about gaining another qualification and some additional skills in a healing technique. It is much deeper than that, because it is a significant step along your personal healing journey, and one that takes you closer to *living* Reiki – making Reiki an essential part of your daily life.

The course includes at least one further energy attunement (spiritual empowerment) which increases the amount of healing energy you can channel, and you are taught three sacred symbols and their mantras (sacred names), each of which has their own unique healing energy, together with a range of special techniques that use one or more of the symbols. These normally include a form of distant healing that enables you to 'send' a full Reiki treatment to anyone, anywhere, with the same effectiveness as if that person was with you. Other techniques might include a special type of treatment for healing deep-seated emotional or mental problems, and healing for personal or global situations.

BEFORE THE COURSE

It is equally important to choose the right Reiki Master for your Reiki Second Degree attunement, and most people attend a course with the same Master with whom they took First Degree; however, it is not essential to do so, and it should always be a decision based on what feels right to *you*, not what you feel obliged to do. As for Reiki 1, when deciding who to train with, ask questions, find out what they include in their Reiki 2 course, discover what their attitudes and beliefs are about Reiki – and about other things which might be important to you.

I would recommend that you follow the same suggestions for preparing for the course as in Chapter 5, but with the addition of making sure you give yourself a full self-treatment every day, preferably for a week or two beforehand, if it is not already a normal part of your daily routine. Also, if you can arrange it, having a day or two before the course where you can really slow down the pace of your life, maybe meditating and spending some time in nature, would be advantageous. The same applies after the course, too, if possible.

DIFFERENT APPROACHES TO TRAINING

As you would expect, it is necessary to be attuned to Reiki before attending a Second Degree course, and some Masters require you to have a gap of at least three months between First and Second Degrees, so your body has a chance to get used to the higher vibrations inaugurated by your initial attunement(s) to this healing energy. I particularly like this slow and gentle approach, and I ask my students to get plenty of practice with self-treatments (and preferably some experience with treating family and friends) before deciding whether or not they want to take a further Reiki course. There is no time limit, so it is important to take as long as you need.

There is an increasing trend, however, for Reiki Masters to forgo this requirement and allow students to take Reiki 2 very soon after Reiki 1. The course is traditionally taught over two days, but some Masters now choose to teach it in a single day, often immediately following a one-day Reiki 1 course, so that both levels are achieved in a weekend. Naturally, the approach taken by each Master depends upon how they were trained, but unfortunately some Masters who started their Reiki journey by taking both levels on two consecutive days actually believe that Reiki doesn't work effectively without using the Reiki symbols – because they never got the chance to find out for themselves.

Let me reassure you. This is *not* true. There are many hundreds of thousands of Reiki First Degree students all over the world who don't choose to go on to take a Second Degree course, because they find their First Degree skills quite enough for them. So can I emphasise – Reiki *definitely* works without the symbols, although the symbols do enhance it. Also, just because you learn the symbols at Second Degree does not mean you have to use them every time you use Reiki – you can just let Reiki flow, the same as at First Degree level.

ATTUNEMENTS AT SECOND DEGREE

Although a Second Degree Reiki course will normally include one attunement, occasionally some Masters perform two or three. Recent information from Japan makes it apparent that sometimes this level is split into several parts there, so an attunement would be given each time – see Chapter 21 on *Okuden* training. I have always found that the single Second Degree attunement is for many students an even more profound and spiritual experience than any of those received at First Degree, and many express this as if a cloud had been lifted from them, or like being reborn, so that the world looks, feels and sounds different. When observing one of my Reiki 2 classes, one of my Master students, who was very psychic, actually saw this happen during the attunement, and later described to me a misty veil being removed, leaving the students' auras lighter and clearer.

This further energy attunement also intensifies your inner healing channel, allowing far more Reiki to be channelled through – at least twice as much, and sometimes up to four times that received with First Degree – although, of course, the *quality* of the Reiki is just the same, whatever level of Reiki you have achieved. It is just the quantity that changes.

The process for a Second Degree attunement is very similar to that for First Degree, so you can expect to be asked to close your eyes throughout the procedure, and to remain silent with your hands in the prayer (*Gassho*) position. Your Reiki Master will start the attunement from behind you, then will move in front of you, and finish the process from behind you again. You will feel some gentle touching and blowing on your head and hands, and at some stage may be asked to raise your hands above your head for a few moments before they are gently placed down again. When the process is complete you should have some time to remain in a quiet, contemplative state before any further activities, and you may be given some time to yourself, for private meditation, connecting with nature, and learning the Reiki symbols.

WHAT TO EXPECT ON A SECOND DEGREE COURSE

As we have already discussed, Masters vary in the amount of time they take to teach Second Degree, and therefore there is considerable variation in what is taught; however, there are some basics that should always be included. I think my Reiki 2 courses are fairly typical of a traditional Western approach, although some Masters might put things in a slightly different order. Also, I choose to have an evening session before the course starts, which enables me to spread the course out more to give students private study time for learning the symbols, and, because I have been taught the techniques from the Japanese tradition, I include two of the most important self-cleansing methods in all my courses.

Friday

The evening session allows time for introductions, a discussion of why students have decided to take Second Degree and an outline of what the course involves. There is then a brief review of Reiki First Degree theory, including an update on the Reiki history from the Japanese tradition, which is followed by questions and answers, and a guided meditation. If there isn't a Friday evening session, these topics would probably be included on the Saturday morning.

Saturday

We begin the morning session with an opening circle, sharing Reiki around the group, followed by demonstration and practice of the Reiki Shower and *Hatsurei-ho* from the Japanese tradition (see

Chapter 20). After a short discussion of the main elements of Reiki at Second Degree – the healing practice, and personal and spiritual development – the students are introduced to the three Reiki symbols and their mantras:

1 **The Power Symbol**, sometimes called the Focus Symbol: this empowers even more Reiki to flow into whatever you are focusing on.

2 **The Harmony Symbol**, often called the Mental–Emotional Symbol: this is particularly useful for healing intellectual, psychological or emotional problems, and for creating harmony and balance.

3 **The Distant Symbol**, sometimes called the Connection Symbol: this cuts through time and space to enable you to 'send' Reiki to anyone, anywhere, at any time.

There is then a discussion of some of the ways in which the symbols and their mantras can be used for treating the self, others and animals, as well as some creative uses such as empowering goals and affirmations, healing personal and global situations and earth healing. The afternoon session begins with a reminder about what a Reiki attunement involves, and then there is a guided meditation, immediately followed by the Reiki Second Degree attunement. After this I allow my students some free time for private meditation, connecting with nature, and learning the Reiki symbols. When we meet again later, we discuss taking responsibility for our own health and well-being, and practise or discuss several different ways of using the symbols in self-treatments. We end with a short meditation and a closing circle.

Sunday

The morning begins with an opening circle and *Hatsurei-ho*, which is followed by an informal test to ensure that each student can remember the symbols accurately; this is necessary if students are to use them on each other throughout the day. There is then a discussion of the importance of energetic clearing of self and workspace in healing practice. This is followed by demonstration and practice of Second Degree techniques for treating others, including clearing and cleansing the aura, enhancing sensitivity for scanning the body for energy distortions, beaming Reiki into the aura, and carrying out a full 'mental and emotional' Reiki treatment on each other using the symbols.

In the afternoon there is demonstration and practice of distant healing techniques, including sending a distant 'mental and emotional' treatment, and how to send healing into the past and the future. Afterwards, there is a question-and-answer session, a discussion of the 21-day clearing process and the Reiki practice journals required before certification, and we end with a closing circle.

Other topics also come up in discussion at various times throughout the course, such as who and what can be treated, what to do if healing doesn't happen, what equipment is required, how many treatments are needed, confidentiality and ethics, combining Reiki with other therapies, and many of the other subjects covered in this book. Also, although I allow plenty of time to practise the techniques during the course, I think it is vital for students to put aside time over the following few months to continue their practice of both hands-on and distant treatment techniques using the symbols. I therefore do not issue a Second Degree certificate until I receive a copy of a student's practice journal, detailing their experiences when carrying out about six hands-on and six distant treatments on family or friends, plus using the symbols for healing situations.

Most traditional Reiki Masters teach a range of special techniques which use one or more of the symbols, and allow time for practising these methods, but naturally this will depend upon the length of the course. You should at least be taught the symbols, shown how to carry out some forms of distant healing, and how a hands-on treatment can be enhanced using the symbols. Other Masters also incorporate various meditations or visualisations, as well as ways of working with spirit guides and crystals, and developing your psychic abilities, although sometimes these additional techniques are taught as a separate follow-on course, together with more advanced ways of using the Reiki symbols.

DISTANT ATTUNEMENT AT REIKI SECOND DEGREE

Some Masters teach this level by offering some form of preparatory information either as a written manual including the shapes of the symbols, or as instructions on a CD or DVD, followed by a 'distant' attunement, which can be carried out in your own home at a time convenient to you. As I have previously mentioned, distant attunements do work, but the disadvantage is that you don't have the Reiki Master there with you to check that you are drawing and using the symbols correctly, nor do you have any supervised practice of carrying out hands-on or distant treatments, or an opportunity to ask questions; however, this is an option you might consider if it is difficult for you to attend a course, although if you wish to become a professional Reiki Practitioner, the National Occupational Standards for Reiki do not accept distant attunements – see Chapter 17 for more information.

AFTER THE COURSE

In the same way as after a Reiki First Degree course, you will go through another 21-day clearing process (see Chapter 4) as your vibrationary rate is heightened and you are able to tap into a higher, wider channel of Reiki. Reiki Second Degree seems to operate at an even faster vibrationary rate than Reiki First Degree, and some people experience a very profound change immediately whereas others notice slower changes over the following weeks and months. What is certain is that you will notice *some* changes. You may expect any one or more of a variety of effects, including enhanced colour consciousness, heightened sensitivity in the crown chakra area, increased intuitive capabilities, or a feeling of greater connectedness with everything around you.

In many spiritual traditions it is necessary to study and meditate for many years to reach an understanding of the meaning of your own life, yet Reiki – and especially Reiki 2 – awakens our sense of the connectedness with and Divinity in everyone and everything. It is important that you should honour this process as a valuable opportunity for spiritual growth. Be kind to yourself: commit your-self to do a self-treatment every day; drink between six and eight glasses of pure water each day, and try to spend some time in quiet contemplation or meditation. If possible, arrange to have at least one day afterwards, for gently re-entering the normal world after the powerful spiritual effects of the course.

Reiki Treatment Practice and Journal

Since one of the features of the Reiki Second Degree is that there is more to 'learn' than at First Degree, it is important to put aside some time over the following weeks and months to practise using the symbols, carrying out hands-on treatments, as well as distant treatments on people and on situations. Like anything else you learn, the more you practise, the better you get, and if you use the symbols frequently in the first few weeks and months you are unlikely ever to forget them. Even if your Reiki Master does not require it, you may therefore find it useful to keep a journal after a Reiki 2 course, detailing any of the treatments you do, and writing down any feedback you get from the friends and family on whom you practise.

As you will find in the rest of Part 3, using the Reiki symbols can dramatically expand what you can do with Reiki, both for yourself and for others. There is no limit to the power and potential of the three symbols taught at Second Degree, and it would probably take you more than one lifetime to explore all the possibilities, so there is really no need to go further with Reiki unless you are particularly drawn to teach.

Chapter 10

The Reiki Second Degree Symbols

A symbol typifies, represents or recalls something such as an idea or a quality. Symbols are in common usage, and we are probably more familiar with them than we think. For example the £ or $ signs are symbols representing money; H_2O is the chemical symbol for water; my astrological sign of Scorpio is represented by ♏, and Christianity's symbol is the familiar cross ✝.

WHAT ARE THE REIKI SYMBOLS?

There are four symbols in Usui Reiki, and each represents certain metaphysical energies. They are seen as calligraphic symbols that come from either Sanskrit, one of the world's oldest languages, or Japanese *kanji*, which is the Japanese ideographic alphabet; however, they are not flat, as if drawn in ink on a piece of paper, although that may be the way they are first shown to you on a Reiki 2 course. Their shapes are vibrational, three dimensional, having height, width and depth, and their size is unlimited – they can be as small or as large as necessary, because they are a form of spiritual energy with its own consciousness, vibrating at a very high rate. Of course, there are limits to the size the symbols can be drawn with your hand, which is how they are usually done. It is possible, however, to *imagine* any of the symbols large enough and deep enough to encompass a whole person, a whole building or even the whole planet, or small enough to fit on a postage stamp, or inside a single cell.

Reiki symbols are transcendental in nature, and they connect directly to a Higher Consciousness. Whenever a Reiki symbol is used by someone who has been attuned at Second Degree, it changes the way the Reiki energy functions. It is still Reiki, but the energy becomes empowered in different ways, depending upon which symbol (or combination of symbols) is being used. Despite their power and their spiritual nature, they are easy to use, and they work automatically, every time they are used – it is not necessary to be in an altered state, such as deep meditation. The Reiki symbols are like keys which open doors to higher levels of awareness, or like buttons; whenever you 'push' one, you automatically get a specific action. The symbols are not the power of Reiki – but they *add* power *to* Reiki, and they are an amazing and beautiful way to connect to this higher power.

Unfortunately, some people who have read about Reiki, and perhaps seen the symbols in a book or on the internet, believe that they can use Reiki, but this is *not* the case. It is the spiritual empowerment of the attunement process that activates the symbols so that they can fulfil their intended purpose. Without the attunement, the symbols do not activate Reiki. During an attunement, the energies of each symbol come down and enter the student's mind, body and spirit, so that afterwards, whenever the student uses the symbol, the same energies they were connected to during the attunement are activated and begin flowing. Therefore, even if people do get to know about the symbols, they cannot be used for healing, or any other purpose, so really it is pointless to have the symbols 'out there' where people who can neither understand them nor use them can see them. Remember, Dr Usui discovered the symbols in the sacred texts he studied, but he was not able to activate their power until after his spiritual empowerment experience on Mount Kurama. I have therefore always adhered to the traditional approach of not printing the symbols in my books, preferring to honour their 'sacredness'; however, since I wrote the first edition of *Reiki for Life* they have become so accessible, both in books and on the internet, and many of the representations are not accurate, so I have taken the decision to include them in this new edition, as I would prefer you to have the correct information.

DRAWING THE SYMBOLS

The most usual way of drawing the symbols is with the whole hand, or with the fingers – as it represents energy, it is actually drawn by the Reiki flowing from the palm chakra, but they can also be drawn with the eyes (in either an imaginary way or by moving the eyes to follow the shape of the symbol) or even with the tongue (that's a bit more difficult!), or when someone is really familiar with them each symbol can be fully visualised. Within the Reiki community there has been much debate on how necessary it is to draw the symbols correctly in order to activate them. Although it is obviously important to try to draw them accurately, rather than being slapdash and careless about it – which would not respect their spiritual nature – it is true that some slight variations were discovered between those drawn by the masters Mrs Takata taught when they first met together in 1982, although this might have been because they had to rely on memory, as she didn't allow them to take notes. They did agree to standardise the symbols' shapes, however, and it is that version that I present later in this chapter, and which I have since had confirmed by seeing the symbols in a copy of a document drawn by Dr Hayashi, who taught Mrs Takata.

The correct way for a student to draw the symbols is the way they were shown to draw them by their Reiki Master. Everyone who has received the attunement for the symbols has symbols that work, however they are drawn, because the power of the symbols does not come from drawing them perfectly, it comes from the connections made with the energies *represented* by the symbol during the initiation. Differences may exist between the symbols of each student, yet each student's symbols are correct for them, and the *essence* of the symbol remains the same. It is the *intention* to use them that activates them, and brings in the specific energies associated with them. If the Reiki symbols in this book are different from the way you draw them, this doesn't mean you need to 'correct' yours to follow the new version, unless you feel especially motivated to do so. The way your Reiki Master taught you still remains exactly right for you because, from a metaphysical perspective, 'everything is as it should be', so if you were drawn to learn from a particular Master, then that is the experience you needed at that time.

In the West we have probably become overly concerned with the symbols. From information we have received since the late 1990s from Japan, it appears that Usui began to utilise the symbols because of their specific vibrations, to try to help his students feel and detect different levels of energy that existed particularly in the human energy field. The symbols increased the students' awareness, and helped them to develop greater abilities to discern the subtle energies that would indicate physical, mental, emotional and spiritual problems or imbalances; however, the symbols were regarded as temporary tools, rather like the training wheels on a bicycle, which were no longer needed once a student had developed the necessary sensitivities, because with such increased awareness the energies represented by the symbols could be activated simply by *intending* to use them. In effect, the student would eventually 'embody' the energy of the symbol.

It is believed that Usui was motivated to teach the shapes of the symbols we use today especially for Dr Hayashi and some other naval commanders who were medically qualified and only wanted to use Reiki for physical healing. They apparently did not wish to spend the time required to 'embody' the energies by regularly chanting the *Jumon* – sacred sounds which, when practised daily, gradually allowed students to invoke the higher energies – there is more about the *Jumon* in Chapter 21.

In the 1990s, some Reiki Masters began to use various other symbols within their Reiki practice and teaching. Some of these apparently came from Tibet, and others were channelled (brought into someone's consciousness by spirit guides) for use in specific ways. Although many of these symbols can be powerful aids for healing, and form the basis for other healing systems (notably Karuna Reiki and Tera-Mai Seichem Reiki) they have very different energetic vibrations, and are not a part of the original healing system that Usui began. The Usui Reiki Ryoho used only the four symbols that were passed down through both the Western lineage of Usui, Hayashi and Takata and the Japanese lineage preserved through the Usui Reiki Ryoho Gakkai, although it is understood that the Gakkai does not now normally teach the symbols.

THE MANTRAS

A mantra is traditionally a word or sound that is repeated to aid concentration in meditation, particularly in Eastern spiritual traditions. Each of the Reiki symbols has a corresponding mantra, which some people mistakenly use as the symbol's name. The first symbol has a three-syllable mantra, but its *name* is the Power or Focus Symbol. The second symbol, the Harmony or Mental–Emotional Symbol, also has a three-syllable mantra, while the third symbol, the Distant or Connection Symbol has a five-syllable mantra, and the Master Symbol has a four-syllable mantra. Whenever a Reiki symbol is used, its sacred mantra should be repeated three times, either silently, if there are other people around, or aloud if appropriate.

Each mantra works in conjunction with its related symbol, but the mantras themselves also have power, and chanting them can bring states of energy, calm, connectedness and bliss. Originally, I chose not to print the mantras in this book because they are part of the sacred traditions of Reiki, and although they are not 'exclusive' – they are taught to every student who takes Second Degree – they are important, and should not be used lightly or without thought; however, in a similar way to the shapes of the symbols, the mantras are easily available on websites, so it feels sensible now to include them alongside the symbols in this edition.

SACREDNESS AND THE REIKI SYMBOLS

As I mentioned above, initially I refrained from including the symbols in the original edition of this book because I wanted to honour the Reiki tradition that they be kept 'secret', that is, they are only revealed to those who have taken Reiki Second Degree (or Master level in the case of the fourth symbol, explained in Chapter 18) and received the attunement which empowers them.

The 'secretness' of the Reiki symbols has probably been misunderstood in the West where the word 'secret' is seen as shameful. In contrast, in the East the words 'sacred' and 'secret' are interconnected both culturally and experientially, so it would seem unnatural to people there to openly discuss things that are part of a spiritual tradition.

During a Reiki 2 course you will be shown the Reiki symbols, usually drawn on pieces of paper which you can then copy out a number of times, to practise drawing them and to help you memorise them. Some Masters still prefer not to have them written down, and draw them in the air instead, instructing their students to copy their actions. Traditionally, the practice papers and the original copies of the symbols are taken back by the Master at the end of the course, and often these are ceremonially burned, either before the students depart, or when the Master returns home.

One of the reasons for taking back the copies at the end of a course, however, is to ensure that students are motivated to *memorise* the symbols properly, because unless they are memorised they cannot be used effectively. It may make some students feel safer to have a 'crib' sheet, but if you have to get out your copies of the symbols every time you want to use them, it will inhibit you too much. In the end, there is no substitute for learning! This is where a two-day Reiki 2 course has great advantages, because there is then plenty of time to spend practising drawing the symbols until the students feel really proficient at using them. Some Masters set a simple test on the second morning, just asking the students to take a single sheet of paper with their name on it, and draw each of the three symbols, together with their appropriate names and mantras, which they then hand to the Master for checking. If after the course you do forget how to draw any of the symbols, or are just a little unsure about whether you are doing them correctly, do get in touch with your Reiki Master – it is nothing to be ashamed of, and your Reiki Master would much rather help you to recall them correctly than have the possibility of you giving up. Alternatively, you could use the symbols and mantras from this book, if you feel comfortable doing so.

Traditionally, you are asked not to reveal the symbols (or their mantras) in any way to anyone other than people who have already done Reiki 2, although their nature and purpose can be discussed without violating this trust, and you can use their names – Power, Harmony and Distant. This means that you need to be discreet when using the symbols, preferably not allowing anyone to see you drawing them or hearing you saying their sacred mantras. The more you practise, the easier it becomes to draw the symbols subtly, and you don't need to say the mantras aloud – you can think them, instead.

Can I please remind you, however, that although the shapes of the three Reiki 2 symbols are given below, they only become active when you have received the Second Degree attunement, so there is no point in trying to use them until then!

THE FIRST SYMBOL: THE POWER (OR FOCUS) SYMBOL

This symbol comes from Sanskrit, and its shape is made up of three strokes; it is important to note that the spiral is always anti-clockwise, and that it should touch the vertical line exactly seven times, counting the place where the spiral starts as number one. It is probably the most versatile of the three given at Second Degree, and it can be used alone (it is the only Second Degree symbol that can be used by itself), or in combination with either or both of the other two symbols, usually drawn after them to bring the activating power of Reiki into their combined purposes. Its main function is to increase the power of Reiki, and to bring the energy of Reiki into the 'here and now': into the present moment. In the Japanese tradition, it is referred to as the Focus Symbol, as it focuses the Reiki on to or into whatever it is drawn over. When your body is out of balance, or you are not sufficiently 'grounded', the Power (Focus) symbol works to restore an appropriate rhythm and equilibrium, to permeate things with Reiki to clear any negative energies and bring back the natural balance and function. It therefore helps to revitalise the body, especially the first and second chakras (root and sacral) which are linked to physical and material issues. Its main functions are empowering, cleansing and protecting.

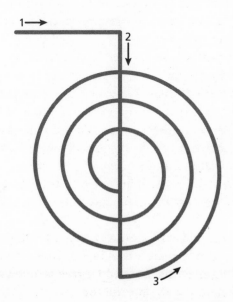

Its mantra is *Cho Ku Rei* (pronounced 'choh koo ray'), which can be roughly translated as 'the curving sword makes space by penetrating nothingness, and fills it with spirit or power'.

THE SECOND SYMBOL: THE HARMONY (MENTAL–EMOTIONAL) SYMBOL

This symbol also comes from Sanskrit, and its shape is made up of nine strokes. In the West this symbol has traditionally been called the Mental–Emotional Symbol, which is a rather long and clumsy title, so the Japanese name, the Harmony Symbol, is the one I now use, because it is so indicative of its actions. It cannot normally be used on its own, so it is usually used in combination with the Power Symbol, as it has a very gentle energy, and is quite subtle and more tenuous than the other symbols. Its main functions are to help to restore psychological and emotional balance, to raise sensitivity and receptivity, and to bring peace and harmony, and it is particularly relevant for use with the third and fourth chakras (the solar plexus and heart), as these are linked with emotional issues, and it activates the highest potential within a situation or being, bringing harmony and resolve.

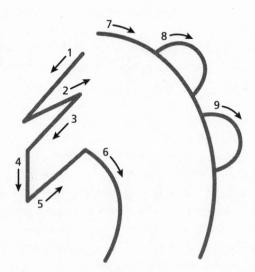

Its mantra is *Sei He Ki* (pronounced 'say heh kee') and its overall meaning is to 'make things straight', meaning to restore balance.

THE THIRD SYMBOL: THE DISTANT (CONNECTION) SYMBOL

This symbol is comprised of Japanese *kanji*, and is made up of 22 strokes. It is perhaps the most fascinating of the symbols, because it forms the bridge between worlds; for example, inner/outer, heaven/earth, transcending time and space. Its use cuts through, or goes beyond, time and space, bringing all time into the Now, and all space into the Here, so it is the key to all doors, a sort of special communicator, which connects on all levels to the Divine within. Its Japanese name is the Connection Symbol, because essentially that is what it does – it connects you to whoever or whatever you wish to send Reiki to.

To use an analogy, the Distant Symbol is an energetic equivalent of a time machine, because it enables you to connect with anything, anywhere, at any time. This amazingly powerful symbol allows you to 'send' healing to anyone (or anything) anywhere in the world, instantaneously, whether that is across the room, across town or across continents to the other side of the planet. Distance is no barrier; indeed, nothing is a barrier when using this symbol, as it enables the Reiki to connect through anything – walls, rock, lead, even through the Earth and outer space, to the intended recipient of the energy. All space is *Here*. The Reiki that is sent using the Distant Symbol loses none of its power, regardless of distance, so it is possible to 'send' a complete Reiki treatment with exactly the same effectiveness as if the person (or animal) was right beside you – because, energetically, they are.

The Distant Symbol can also be used to bridge time, connecting you with any time in the future or in the past, as well as in the present. All time is *Now*. You can therefore use it to send Reiki into the future – including a full Reiki treatment – to a point in time when you know you will need it, or to any point in the past; for example, to heal the mental, emotional or spiritual effects of a past event. Again, this symbol is not used on its own, but is always used in conjunction with the Power Symbol, and sometimes also with the Harmony Symbol. This symbol can be particularly relevant to the fifth and sixth chakras (throat and brow) as these are linked with how we connect and communicate with others.

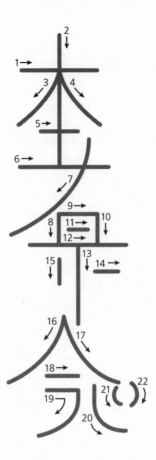

Its mantra is *Hon Sha Ze Sho Nen* (pronounced 'hon shah tzay show nen') which is variously translated as 'I unite with God', or 'The Buddha (or Christ) in me reaches out to the Buddha (or Christ) in you to promote enlightenment and peace', which in essence means that the best part of ourselves (the Higher Self) connects, through Reiki, to the best part (the Higher Self) of others.

In the next few chapters you will find out how each of the three Second Degree Reiki symbols can be used, for treating yourself, others and animals, as well as many other creative uses. I hope you will have fun with them.

Chapter 11

Hands-on Treatments Using Symbols

Reiki Second Degree equips you with increased potential for carrying out Reiki treatments, but this does not mean that your Reiki 1 skills are redundant. Using symbols when treating either yourself or other people simply adds to the standard treatment, so all the hand positions remain the same; although there is an additional hand position for carrying out a specific 'mental and emotional' treatment, and several other hand positions are suggested later in this chapter.

After Reiki 2 you may be keen to start practising as a professional Reiki Practitioner, and you will find plenty of advice on how to go about that in Chapter 17; however, this and the following three chapters will give you all the information you need to actually use the three Second Degree Reiki symbols, both for treatments and in other creative ways. Some of these techniques and ideas are common to many Reiki Masters, and others are unique, based on my many years of teaching and practising Reiki, so I hope you will find them interesting, enjoyable and useful.

TREATMENTS ON OTHERS

Preparation

Just as with Reiki 1, it is probably advisable not to do full treatments on other people until after the 21-day clearing process has been completed following your attunement. Then, before starting a treatment, it is important that you should prepare yourself and the space in which the treatment is to take place, and that you put your client at ease, so you will need to carry out all the suggestions in Chapter 7, including clearing and cleansing of the room and any equipment, self-cleansing and energetic protection for yourself, and the explanation to your client of what they are likely to experience.

There are also some additional things you can do using the Power Symbol, to cleanse the room and the therapy couch before your client arrives. With the intention that Reiki should cleanse the room of any negative energies, go to each corner of the room in turn and, facing the corner, draw a large Power Symbol, saying its sacred mantra three times while drawing an arc with your hand from the corner towards the centre of the room. When you have completed all four corners, move to the middle of the room and draw a Power Symbol above you, as if on the ceiling, and another in the direction of the floor, each time saying its sacred mantra three times.

Set up the therapy couch if you have one, and place clean pillows and a blanket ready, and then cleanse the couch (or any other suitable equipment), pillows and blanket by drawing a Power Symbol over them, silently saying its sacred mantra three times with the intention that all this equipment be cleansed of any negative energies, and filled with Reiki.

Before you start treating your client, remember to fill your aura with Reiki, *intending* that the outer edge forms a protective barrier, and the Reiki within it protects you from all negativity and harm, allowing any negative energies to be released and dispersed naturally. You can then go on to sense and scan your client's aura.

Sensing and scanning the aura

Your Second Degree attunement not only opens the chakras so that Reiki can flow even more, it also increases intuition and heightens sensitivity to subtle energies. Using the chakras in the palms of your hands, it is possible to sense where the client needs Reiki by scanning their energy field, and by scanning and healing the aura you can increase the client's ability to receive Reiki during a standard treatment. In the Japanese tradition this is called *Byosen*, and you will find details of that method in Chapter 20; however, it is possible to develop this ability quite simply.

Spend a few moments quietly tuning in to Reiki, and then sometimes it is helpful to sensitise your hands to detect the energy by rubbing them together fairly vigorously for about 10 to 15 seconds – with the intention of sensitising them, not just to make them warm! You can further enhance your ability to scan intuitively by drawing a Power Symbol over each hand, and a Harmony Symbol in front of your third eye chakra, but this is optional.

Then silently ask Reiki to show you the places that need healing, and with your left (or non-dominant) hand between 15–30cm (6–12in) above the body, start at the head and very slowly move your hand down the body, keeping your hand the same distance away.

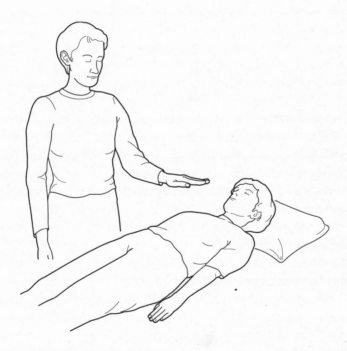

Closing your eyes can help you to heighten the awareness in your palm so that you can recognise different types of sensation. Also, it may take quite a lot of practice before you can easily identify what feelings indicate a healthy energy field, because this varies so much from person to person, but gradually you will find that you will intuitively 'know' what each type of sensation means. There is likely to be a 'background' sensation common to most of a client's body, such as an overall warmth or very slight tingle, and often the location of a chakra is indicated by what feels like a cool breeze on your palm. Distortions or irregularities in the energy field mean you have detected a place that needs Reiki, and you may feel these as a coldness, warmth, heat, tingling, pressure, slight 'stickiness', or little electric shocks, pulsations or a pulling on your hand. Your hand may also simply be guided to the right spot, and you will often 'know' where the distortion is before your hand gets there. You might also find that you develop the ability to 'see' or sense the energy field, and even the inside of the client's body – rather like X-ray vision – identifying areas that need special attention. These sensations and impressions may be so slight at first that you may think it is your imagination. Trust your experience. As you practise, your ability to scan the aura and sense imbalances will improve.

When you find an area of distortion or imbalance, either make a mental note of where it is and move further down the body to continue scanning, or deal with it directly by moving your hand up and down in that spot until you find the height where you feel the most distortion. Using both hands, palms facing downwards, channel Reiki into the aura for a minute or two, so that Reiki can heal both that part of the aura and the areas of the physical body connected to it. Continue to channel Reiki at this spot until you feel the flow of Reiki subsiding, and then go back to scanning by moving your hand slowly down the body, stopping as before when you detect an area of imbalance, until you have scanned and healed the whole energy field.

As you work within your client's energy field, you may intuitively become aware of the cause of the distortion and any personal problems connected to it. You may also gain insight into how the problems were created and what the client can do to facilitate healing. This development may initially alarm you, if you are not used to receiving such intuitive information; however, it actually shows that you are reaching another stage in your spiritual development and growth with Reiki, so it is a good sign. Share this information with the client only if you feel guided to do so, and then only with loving kindness and great sensitivity, and without judgement. Always treat the client and the process with great respect, and remember that unless you are a medical doctor (some Reiki Practitioners and Masters are) it is not permissible for you to diagnose any conditions.

A SPECIAL MENTAL–EMOTIONAL HEALING TREATMENT

Few Reiki Masters teach this very powerful treatment technique from the Western tradition that uses all three symbols, but I learned it from my Reiki Master, a member of The Reiki Alliance, when I did Reiki 2 in 1992. It can be carried out immediately before a standard hands-on treatment using the 12 hand positions. If you use this method, you can then reduce the timings of the standard hand positions afterwards to about three minutes (as opposed to the normal five minutes), which should still result in a treatment lasting approximately one hour. This procedure effectively floods the whole body and aura with waves of Reiki, and connects it to the Source, allowing pure love and deep healing to flow down directly into the person in a profound way.

Because this is such a spiritually intensive treatment, it is especially important to prepare yourself fully first – for example, with the *Kenyoku-ho* technique and a Reiki Shower (see both in Chapter 20). Another very important aspect of this treatment is that it is absolutely crucial to concentrate fully on the client for the duration of the 'mental–emotional' part of the treatment, which lasts for between five and ten minutes. Using the symbols in this way effectively 'opens up' the client's crown, heart and solar plexus chakras, in order to facilitate really deep healing. This means, however, that they are particularly susceptible to receiving your thoughts on a subconscious level, so it is imperative that you think positively, rather than negatively, and that you don't let your mind wander off to think about your own concerns, problems or irritations. The visualisation technique, which is described on page 196, actually helps you to concentrate on the treatment, so it will not be as hard as it sounds. If any negative thoughts do drift into your mind, just let them go (you might like to see them drifting away inside pink bubbles). If your mind wanders off a little, just bring it back, and consciously project some positive thoughts to the client, such as 'I am healthy, fit and well' or 'I am calm, relaxed, and all is well in my world', and then allow your concentration to return fully to your client.

Additional hand position for the mental–emotional treatment

This method also utilises a new hand position, which is held for the whole of the 'mental and emotional' part of the treatment. Your non-dominant hand (usually your left hand) should be placed beneath the client's head (assuming the client is lying down) so that the palm of your hand cradles the base of the skull comfortably. Your dominant hand will then be free to draw out the three symbols (instructions below) in the air in front of the crown of your client's head, and will then be placed directly on the crown, as shown in the illustrations below. It is more comfortable to be seated slightly to one side of the client's head, so that your arms and hands can be reasonably relaxed and well supported – if you sit in an uncomfortable position, it will slow the flow of Reiki because you will tense your muscles, which also tends to constrict the energy channels.

1   Before starting the treatment, ensure that both you and the client are comfortable, and then ask the client to relax and close his or her eyes.

2   Sit quietly with your hands one on top of the other on your heart chakra. Reiki yourself for a few moments, breathing deeply and evenly to centre yourself. Then draw the Power Symbol in front of you from the top of your head down to spiral over your solar plexus so as to clear, protect and empower you, silently saying the Power Symbol's sacred mantra three times. (Remember that the Reiki symbols are sacred, so it is better if you ensure that no one else can see the symbols being drawn or hear their mantras.)

3   Draw the Power Symbol on each of your palms, silently saying its sacred mantra to yourself three times, and then scan the client (see above), noting any particular areas that may require additional attention.

4   When you are ready to begin the treatment, sit down next to the client and gently slide your non-dominant hand underneath their head – it is OK to ask them to lift their head slightly to facilitate this, as the treatment hasn't yet started, so they will

not be disturbed by this action. Ensure that this hand position is comfortable for both you and the client.

5 With your dominant hand (usually the right) begin by drawing the Distant Symbol in the air beside the client's crown chakra, 5–10cm (2–4in) away from their head (see below). Silently say its sacred mantra three times, and then say the client's name three times. This establishes the link between you, Reiki and the client.

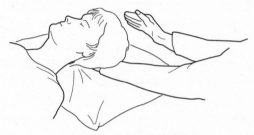

Preparing to draw the symbols

6 Then draw the Harmony Symbol beside the client's crown chakra, silently saying its sacred mantra three times and the client's name three times. This opens up the client's energy field and subconscious mind to receive all the benefits of the healing.

7 Draw the Power Symbol beside the client's crown chakra, silently saying its sacred mantra three times to bring the Reiki energy in. Imagine each symbol going through the crown, brow and throat chakras and into the heart, and think, believe and *intend* that this Reiki energy is channelled with love and light for the highest and greatest good.

8 Finally, place your right or dominant hand onto the client's head over their crown chakra.

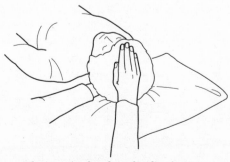

Placing your hand on the client's crown

9 **The visualisation sequence** Now, with your inner eye, visualise Reiki as soft white light flowing out of the palm of your
dominant hand until it is filling the client's head, and then see
or sense it swirling slowly down through the whole of the body
– into the neck and shoulders, down each arm, into the chest,
waist and abdomen, into the hips and legs, right down to the
toes. When you can visualise the client's body completely filled
with soft white light, then, leaving the white light filling the
whole body, slowly turn your attention back to the client's head.

10 Now imagine that Reiki, as a rainbow of coloured light, is
flowing out of the palm of your hand until it fills your client's
head, and slowly take this rainbow of coloured light through
their whole body right down to their fingers and toes. Leaving
the rainbow light filling the whole body, allow your visioning
to come back once more to their head. (You may 'see' all seven
colours, or just a few – accept whatever comes as being exactly
right for your client at this time.)

11 Now visualise Reiki as brilliant, sparkling white light flowing
out of your palm, becoming brighter and brighter, and imagine
this brilliant white light once more flowing through the whole
of your client's head and body, until every part is completely
filled with brilliant, sparkling white light.

12 As soon as the client's body is filled with this brilliant white light,
imagine that light spreading out of the client's body to fill the
whole of their aura. Imagine it flowing into the first layer and,
when that is full, see or sense it spilling over into the second
layer, and then on into the third layer, and then the fourth
layer and the fifth layer. Sense it spilling over into the sixth
layer and then on into the seventh layer, so that the whole of
the client's aura is filled with shimmering, sparkling white light.

13 Next, imagine that brilliant white light expanding still further,
until it flows out beyond your client's aura, swirling upwards
and outwards until it fills the whole room with Reiki as sparkling white light.

14 Now visualise a strand of that Reiki, as brilliant white light,
coming up out of the client's solar plexus chakra or heart
chakra (or both), and in your imagination, take that strand of

brilliant white light, still connected to your client's body, and let it lengthen until it goes through the ceiling, and then stretches up above the building, right up into the sky, and then higher and higher, through the clouds and up into the atmosphere, until it reaches the very edge of the Earth's atmosphere.

15 Now, pause for a moment, and let that strand of Reiki white light gradually expand outwards, see it growing and spreading out across and around the whole world, sense it meeting up with other strands of Reiki light until the whole world is covered in a fine mesh of Reiki, holding the Earth in a web of healing.

16 Then take your attention back to that narrow beam of Reiki light, and let it flow up beyond the Earth's atmosphere, further and further through space, past the planets of our solar system, between the stars, heading towards the centre of the Universe, towards the Light, the Source, the All That Is. Feel it connect with the ultimate Source of love and light and healing, and sense some of that love and light and healing flowing back down that strand of Reiki light. This ultimate love and healing may appear as golden light, or as any other colour, or it may seem like a liquid or a mist – again, accept what comes as being right for your client – but gradually it flows down the strand of Reiki light, back through space, back through the Earth's atmosphere, back down through the sky, through the roof and the ceiling and into the client's body. Visualise that love, light and deep healing flooding throughout the client's body, until every part is completely filled with this beautiful, peaceful, loving and deeply healing energy.

17 When you intuitively sense that this process is complete, slowly take your attention back up to the connection of the strand of Reiki light with the Source and, with a sense of gratitude and respect, gently detach the strand and begin to bring that narrow beam of Reiki back down through space, back between the stars, back through the solar system, down towards the beautiful blue planet Earth, through the Earth's atmosphere, through the ceiling, until it is once more inside the client.

18 Now seal in this special healing by imagining a Power Symbol being drawn over the solar plexus chakra and/or the heart

chakra, saying its sacred mantra silently three times, and *intending* that this unconditional love and deep healing be sealed into the client's body.

19 Finally, take your hand away from the client's head and draw the Power Symbol once more in the air beside the client's crown chakra, and silently say its sacred mantra three times, with the *intention* of closing the client's chakras and ending this part of the treatment. Closing this part of the treatment properly is very important. It seals in the Reiki and closes the crown chakra, protecting the client's aura, which allows you to relax a little and return to a more normal level of concentration. You might like to end with a little blessing of your own, such as, 'I seal this treatment with love and light, and wish you joy, insight and healing through Reiki.'

20 You can now begin a standard Reiki 'hands-on' treatment. Since one hand is already underneath the client's head, very gently slide the other hand underneath the client's head until both hands are next to each other. (You may have to move your body to facilitate this, as it will now be more comfortable if you are directly behind the client's head.) Try to do this without disturbing your client, who will probably be deeply relaxed by this stage.

21 Proceed with the rest of the hand positions – 2, 3, 4, and so on – in the normal way, but you can reduce the time for each hand position to about two and a half or three minutes. (If you choose to include any additional hand positions, such as on the arms or legs, between 30 seconds and one minute each will be enough after a mental–emotional treatment.) You may find it useful to draw with your hand or visualise the Power Symbol, then say the mantra three times over any areas that need special attention (such as those which you identified during the scanning process). Most of the time you should do all 12 hand positions, but as the mental–emotional treatment is so powerful, you may sometimes sense that the client does not need to turn over for the four hand positions on the back – use your intuition to decide on this – so you can spend longer on other positions.

22 End the full treatment by sealing the client's whole energy field by drawing a large Power Symbol and saying the mantra three times over the whole body, *intending* to seal in the Reiki healing.

23 Then remove your hands from the recipient and place them at mid-chest height in the *Gassho* (prayer) position and mentally give thanks for the Reiki, bowing slightly as a mark of respect.

24 Finally, gently smooth the client's aura down three times, starting at the head and ending at the feet. To help to 'ground' your client, it can be useful to end by gently massaging the soles of their feet – but with a reasonably firm pressure, so that you don't tickle them!

Allow the client to 'come round' slowly, and give them some time to discuss their feelings or reactions to the treatment, or to ask questions. Always make sure that they are given a glass of water, and encourage them to drink about 2 litres (3½ pints) of water a day for the next three days, to help to flush any toxins out of the system which have been loosened by the Reiki. If the person seems at all 'spaced out', then make sure you ground them before allowing them to leave. Ask them to stand, or sit with their feet on the floor, and place one of your hands on each of their feet and visualise the energy being drawn down into the earth – 15–30 seconds should be enough. If they are still not grounded, get them to stamp their feet on the floor, or to perform a cross-over balancing action, marching on the spot, so that when they lift their left knee, they touch it with their right hand, and the right knee with their left hand, for about a minute.

After the client has gone, sit quietly for a short while doing Reiki on yourself. I recommend that you carry out the *Kenyoku-ho* again, and/or the Reiki Shower, to cleanse and clear yourself of any unwanted energies that may have attached themselves to your energy field. Visualise or draw the Power Symbol on the walls and in the centre of the room to clear and protect the room, and clear the therapy couch with a Power Symbol, too. You may also find it is a good time to carry out some Reiki projects, such as distant healing, immediately after completing such a treatment, as your Reiki energies will be flowing especially well.

QUICK TREATMENTS

Sometimes it is not possible to do a full treatment, so over the years I have discovered a number of ways in which you can perform a quick chakra balancing treatment or energy boost (the Reiki Sandwich technique), which can be helpful.

Chakra clearing and balancing

This can be done with the client either lying down or sitting upright in a chair. By working directly above or next to the chakras, in the aura, the Reiki is able to clear the chakra of blockages and to balance the energies. Ask the client to close their eyes, and then quietly centre yourself by breathing deeply and evenly for a few moments, and *intend* that the Reiki should flow for the highest and greatest good.

1   When you feel ready, prepare yourself for the treatment by standing a little away from the client, then draw a Power Symbol over each of your palms and a large Power Symbol down the front of your body, saying its sacred mantra three times each time you do so. This empowers your whole energy field with Reiki, so that when you approach the client again, both of you will be encompassed in a field of Reiki.

2   Starting at their head, draw a Power Symbol with your right (or dominant) hand in the air about 15–30cm (6–12in) above their crown chakra, silently say the mantra to yourself three times and hold your hand there for approximately one minute.

3   Then move your hand to hold it above the brow (third eye) chakra (or in front, if they are seated), again about 15–30cm (6–12in) away from the head. Draw the Power Symbol in the air above (or in front of) their brow chakra, silently say the mantra three times and hold your hand there for about one minute.

4   Repeat these actions in exactly the same way for each of the remaining chakras – throat, heart, solar plexus, sacral and root – holding your hand still in the air above (or in front of) each chakra for about one minute.

5   When you have finished, take your hand a little further away from their body, draw a large Power Symbol in the air over (or

in front of) the whole of their body and silently say the mantra three times *intending* that this seal in the Reiki.

6   Then move away from the recipient and place your hands at mid-chest height in the *Gassho* (prayer) position and mentally give thanks for the Reiki, bowing slightly as a mark of respect.

7   Finally, either click your fingers, or clap your hands, or shake your hands vigorously, to end the connection.

8   Remember to cleanse yourself afterwards with Dry Brushing (*Kenyoku-ho*) or the Reiki Shower.

Quick chakra and aura balancing

If you don't have time to carry out the technique above, a quick alternative is to draw the Power Symbol on each of your hands, and then stand behind the person (who can be sitting or standing) and draw a very large Harmony Symbol (saying its mantra silently to yourself three times) in the air starting behind their head and ending roughly level with their coccyx, and follow this by drawing a very large Power Symbol (mantra silently three times), starting above their crown and then continuing the rest of the symbol down their spine, finishing roughly level with their coccyx, *intending* that this harmonises and balances the person's chakras and aura. Then stand back, and clap your hands a couple of times to break the connection, and follow this by cleansing yourself with a Reiki Shower.

The Reiki Sandwich

If you don't have time to do a full Reiki treatment on someone, you might find the following technique useful. It provides a quick, energy-lifting vibrational shift in the auric field. You don't have to place your hands directly on the individual, but they can remain in the aura, just beyond the body itself, so that the client is 'sandwiched' between your hands. One or two minutes in each position is usually enough, because holding out your hands can be quite tiring. Prepare yourself for doing this quick treatment in the usual way (see above).

1   Ask the client to either stand with their feet apart (level with the hips) or to sit up straight on a chair with their feet flat on the floor, and their eyes closed.

2 Draw a Power Symbol on each of your palms, saying its sacred mantra silently to yourself three times, and then draw a large Power Symbol in front of their body and then another at the back of their body, each time saying its sacred mantra silently three times.

3 Stand so that the client is sideways in front of you.

4 Place your hands, palms facing each other, roughly 20cm (8in) apart, just above the crown chakra. Hold this and each following position for about one minute (or more, if you feel this is necessary and you and the client are still reasonably comfortable).

5 Palms still facing each other, move your hands down to the third eye chakra, one hand 15–20cm (6–8in) from the front of their head, and the other the same distance away from the back of their head, both palms facing towards the client.

6 After a minute, move your hands down to the throat chakra, one facing the front of the throat and one facing the back of the neck, the same distance away as before.

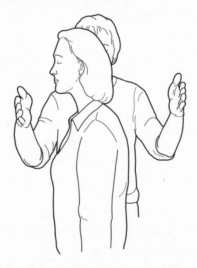

7 Next move your hands down to the heart chakra, one hand facing the centre of the chest, and the other hand at the same height facing the middle of the back, the same distance away as before.

8 Repeat with the solar plexus chakra, above the waist.

9 Repeat with the sacral chakra, just below the navel.

10 Repeat with the root chakra, at the base of the spine.

11 Next, turn your palms to face downwards, and keeping them about the same distance away from the body as before, push your hands downwards until they almost touch the floor, letting the energy flow down towards the feet, to ground it. (If you cannot bend easily, then just let your palms face downwards for a few seconds, and *intend* that the energy flows down towards the feet.)

12 Then turn your palms to face upwards, and move your hands a bit further away from the body, say 25–30cm (10–12in), and slowly lift the energy as you move your hands up the whole body to the crown.

13 When your hands are above the crown chakra, briefly bring them together until your fingertips touch, and then pull them apart again, letting the palms face downwards. With your hands at least 30cm (12in) away from the body, sweep the aura quite quickly downwards as your hands move down from crown to feet.

14 Then move away from the recipient and place your hands at mid-chest height in the *Gassho* (prayer) position and mentally give thanks for the Reiki, bowing slightly as a mark of respect.

15 Finally, snap your fingers or clap your hands, or shake them vigorously to break the energy connection. (You can also cleanse yourself energetically with the Dry Brushing or Reiki Shower techniques afterwards.)

TREATMENTS ON YOURSELF

At Second Degree level, self-healing is still one of the most important aspects of Reiki, not only as a part of the spiritual discipline of Reiki (see Chapter 16) but also because it is an act of self-love to give yourself a Reiki treatment every day, and a simple and sensible way to help your body to maintain good health. If you wish, you can draw the Power Symbol on each hand before you start self-scanning (described below) or a self-treatment, or simply visualise it in front of you before commencing. Alternatively, you can draw the symbol, or imagine it, over each area that you are treating. Each time you use the Power Symbol, say its sacred mantra three times silently to yourself.

Self-scanning

The scanning process described earlier in this chapter (see pages 190–2) can also be done on yourself, and it is an excellent way to get to know yourself and your energy body. If you do get any intuitive ideas, please accept whatever is shown to you without judging or blaming yourself – you have simply reached the right time to increase your self-awareness in this way, and you are being shown deeper levels of yourself that need healing. Allow the Reiki to flow into that area of your body, and your energy field, and ask Reiki also to flow into your consciousness to help you to let go of this problem area, both consciously and subconsciously. Following this procedure regularly helps your personal and spiritual awareness and growth, and increases your sensitivity so that you become even more skilled at identifying blockages in any other people you treat.

Standard self-treatment enhanced with symbols

A self-treatment can be made even more effective by using the Power Symbol. Before you start, empower your whole energy field by drawing a Power Symbol on each palm, and a large Power Symbol in front of your whole body, silently saying its mantra three times each time you use it. Then before placing your hands in each of the 12 hand positions, either visualise a Power Symbol in the air above that position or draw a Power Symbol directly on the body in the area that is being treated, each time silently saying its mantra three times.

Using a mental–emotional treatment for self-healing

You can considerably enhance the effectiveness of your Reiki self-treatment by carrying out a 'mental–emotional' treatment, which is exactly the same as that detailed previously for using with other people. This does require considerable concentration for about five minutes or so, but you can then shorten the length of time you spend on the other hand positions, if you wish.

1 Start by sitting or lying quietly with your hands on your heart chakra, doing Reiki on yourself for a few moments. Then draw the Power Symbol from the top of your head down to your solar plexus so as to clear, protect and empower you, silently saying its sacred mantra three times. (Remember at all times that the Reiki symbols are sacred, so it is best if no one else can see the symbols being drawn or hear their mantras. It is possible to draw them very small with practice.)

2 Next, draw the Power Symbol on each of your palms, say the mantra three times and then place one hand under the back of your head so that it covers the occipital bone at the base of your skull.

3 With the other hand draw all three symbols in the air over your crown chakra, starting with the Distant Symbol, saying its sacred mantra three times, and then say your own name three times.

4 Then draw the Harmony Symbol, say the mantra three times and your name three times.

5 Finally, draw the Power Symbol, say the mantra three times, and imagine each symbol going through the crown, brow and throat chakras and into the heart, and think, believe and *intend* that this Reiki energy is channelled with love and light for the highest and greatest good.

6 When you have finished this, place the hand that you have used to draw the symbols onto your crown chakra, and begin the visualisation sequence, with soft white light filling your head and body.

7 Continue with the whole of the visualisation sequence (steps 9 through to 17) as in the full mental–emotional treatment on pages 196–7.

8 When you have completed the visualisation, seal in this special healing by drawing a Power Symbol over your solar plexus chakra and/or the heart chakra, say the mantra three times, *intending* that this unconditional love and deep healing be sealed into your body.

9 Finally, draw the Power Symbol once more over your crown chakra, say the mantra three times, with the intention of closing your chakras and ending this part of the treatment. Closing this part of the treatment properly is as important for you in a self-treatment, as it is when using the mental–emotional treatment with a client. It seals in the Reiki and closes the crown chakra, which means you can then reduce your level of concentration. You can, of course, end with a statement of gratitude to Reiki for its many blessings and healing.

10 You can now continue your self-treatment in the normal way, placing your hands in each of the 12 hand positions, but you can reduce the time for each position if you wish.

Although you have the 'mental–emotional' visualisation sequence written in full earlier in this chapter on pages 194–9, you might find it helpful to listen to it on a CD, either when self-treating, or when treating a client. There is no reason why a client cannot listen to it, as it can be a lovely experience for them too, as it takes them on a beautiful inner journey, which may lead to important insights. You can either record your own version, or buy my CD (which includes other useful visualisations too) from my website (see Resources).

The Reiki symbols are powerful and versatile, and as you have seen from this chapter, they further empower and enhance the effectiveness of any hands-on treatments, so people who have received a Reiki treatment from you before you took Second Degree may notice a difference afterwards. They may remark on an increase in sensations, or a deeper feeling of peacefulness, and you will probably gradually notice differences too, especially in your ability to 'tune in' to the areas that need the most Reiki and in your capacity to interpret any sensations you feel. In the next chapter we take a look at distant healing, where you can send one of the above treatments to anyone anywhere in the world, and it will be as effective as if you were placing your hands directly on them.

Chapter 12

Distant Healing Techniques

The techniques taught at Second Degree level enable you to send very powerful healing to anyone, anywhere, at any time, including in the past and the future. Using the Distant (Connection) Symbol allows you to connect to the person (or animal) to whom you wish to send healing, forming a 'bridge' which cuts through time and space, and along which the Reiki can flow. When you further empower the Reiki by using the Power (Focus) symbol, this means that it is not only possible to send general healing, that is, simply allowing Reiki to flow to a person, animal or situation, but also to use these techniques to carry out a complete Reiki treatment on a specific person (or animal) at a distance. This will have the same effectiveness as if they were with you, receiving a hands-on treatment. This ability to 'send' powerful and effective healing into the past or into the future can even be 'programmed' (rather like a video or digital TV recorder) to be delivered at a particular time.

There are a few points which need to be made clear before we discuss any of the specific techniques for distant healing. I use the term 'send' when referring to the Reiki flowing from you to the recipient; however, apart from the initial connection, which is carried out by the Distant Symbol, it is the recipient who has to 'pull' the Reiki once the connection has been made, although no conscious effort is required, as this is decided by the recipient's Higher Self. As I pointed out earlier, you cannot force healing into anyone, and that includes anyone who is far away. The person or animal who is receiving the Reiki has to want it, at least on a subconscious level, otherwise the Reiki will simply come back to you.

The Ethics of Distant Healing

First, a reminder that distant healing is something that can be sent by someone with any level of Reiki, as described on page 166, and one of the really good things about Reiki for most of us is that we have something we can use to help other people, so of course we will want to 'send' healing and love to people we know are ill or in distress. Sending distant *treatments*, however, is only possible after Second Degree with the use of the Reiki Distant Symbol, and is much more powerful and effective; however, there are ethical considerations for both distant healing and distant treatments, because ideally they should only be sent with the permission of the recipient.

One point to consider is that when sending healing or treatments our motives and intentions may be good, but there is also something of a controlling element in these motivations – we want someone to 'get better' or 'be happy'. That might be *our* perception of what is for their highest and greatest good, but as I have pointed out before, we may *think* we know what that is but most of the time we probably don't.

If a person comes to you for a full hands-on Reiki treatment or asks you to put your hands on their head for some Reiki to help get rid of a headache, for example, then they obviously know what they are doing. By asking for the Reiki they are taking some responsibility for their own healing. It is equally important that the person who is to receive a distant treatment actually knows about it – other than in exceptional circumstances, such as someone in a coma. Otherwise, by sending Reiki to that person you are intruding on their personal space without permission.

Imagine if someone suddenly grabbed you by the shoulders, thrust you on a therapy couch and began giving you Reiki, without so much as a by-your-leave! You would regard that as an unwanted interference, and an infringement of your right to choose. Well, the same is true for distant healing. You have no right to 'send' a Reiki treatment to anyone, even if your motives are good and you just want to help. It has to be their choice.

Sometimes, a well-meaning relative or friend of a sick person will ask you to send that person a distant Reiki treatment – but be wary. Make sure they have asked that person's permission, first – unless, of course, that person is unconscious or too young or too ill to be able to make such a choice. Under those circumstances it is acceptable to attempt sending a Reiki treatment – and if the Reiki flows then their Higher Self has given permission, but if it comes back you will know that it was not appropriate at that particular time.

When I say the Reiki 'comes back' that might sound strange – and indeed, it can feel a bit strange. What I mean is that you make a connection with the person by using the Distant Symbol, and when you start 'sending' the Reiki – or a more accurate description would be *intending* to allow it to flow – it reaches its destination instantaneously. This is because the Distant Symbol brings all time and space into the here and now, so it is just as if you have placed your hands on the person and the Reiki has 'switched on' and started to flow into them. If the recipient is unwilling to receive the Reiki, however, it has nowhere to go, so it comes straight back across the bridge formed by the Distant Symbol and 'hits' you – fairly gently, but quite definitely – in the heart chakra, solar plexus or third eye (brow chakra).

If this happens then please close down the connection between you and the intended recipient and redirect the Reiki – you can say or think that the Reiki can flow into the planet, for instance, to heal the Earth, or you can allow it to flow into your own body to heal you. To close down the connection, you can just draw the Power Symbol again, saying its sacred mantra three times, the person's name three times and the location once, *intending* to end the connection between you and the person concerned. Alternatively, you can visualise the Distant Symbol as a long bridge between you and the person, and visualise a Power Symbol flowing lightly across that bridge to close the connection, then gently and respectfully disconnect the end of the bridge from that person and draw it back towards you. Wherever it enters you, draw a Power Symbol over that chakra, and *intend* that the process be over.

DISTANT REIKI FOR GENERAL HEALING

It is fairly easy to use the symbols to send healing and love to people – remembering the ethics above.

1   Write the person's name on a piece of paper and hold the paper in your hands.

2   Draw the Distant Symbol in the air over the paper, saying its sacred mantra three times, the name of the person three times and then the name of their location once (the town, area or even country will be sufficient if you don't know exactly where they are – on an energetic level, your *intention* to connect with a specific person is enough).

3   Then draw the Power Symbol, say its mantra three times and *intend* that Reiki should go to the person for the highest possible good – about five minutes is usually long enough. You can also use a photograph of the person, holding it in your hands in the same way, or you can even imagine the person lying between a huge pair of hands receiving Reiki to the whole of their body or simply visualise them bathed in light.

4   To finish, clap your hands, or shake them vigorously to end the connection.

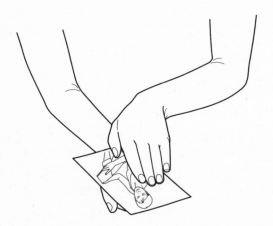

Sending distant healing to several people simultaneously

You may sometimes wish to send distance healing on a regular basis to people – perhaps several at a time – such as friends or relatives who are ill or who are having difficulties with their studies, jobs or relationships. Again, remember that it is best to have their permission.

1   Write all their names on a piece of paper with the towns, districts, counties or countries where they are situated, and hold this paper in your hands.

2   Draw the Distant Symbol in the air above the paper, say its sacred mantra three times and then say each person's name three times with their location once.

3   Then draw the Power Symbol, say its mantra three times, say that Reiki is sent with love and light to these people for their highest and greatest good, and then hold the list between your hands for between five and 15 minutes. Use your intuition – you will know when the Reiki has stopped flowing.

4   When you finish, draw the Power Symbol again and say its mantra three times with the *intention* of ending the healing.

5   To conclude, clap your hands, or shake them vigorously to end the connection.

Note: When sending distant healing to a number of people at the same time, it is not usually advisable to use the Harmony (Mental–Emotional) Symbol. This can potentially have the effect of opening up someone's energy field, so it would be better to use it only when you are concentrating specifically on one person at a time. If you need to use this symbol, then you need to do a full distant treatment on that person individually.

DOING A DISTANT FULL REIKI TREATMENT

Using this technique enables you to send a full Reiki treatment with exactly the same effect as if you were carrying out a hands-on treatment on that person or animal. It is very simple to do, and takes much less time than a hands-on treatment, but it does require a considerable amount of concentration, so before starting you need to be somewhere quiet where you will not be disturbed for 20 minutes or so.

Because this treatment works in the same way as if the person was with you, it is particularly important that you should have their permission before sending the treatment, and ideally you should arrange a convenient time when that person can be sitting comfortably or lying down somewhere quiet where they will not be disturbed for at least three quarters of an hour. (This amount of time is to allow them some relaxation after the treatment.) After all, if you were going to give someone a 'hands-on' treatment you would need to suggest a suitable appointment time, so the same should apply to a distant treatment.

Although Reiki always works for the highest and greatest good, it is probably sensible to avoid sending a full treatment when you don't know what the person is doing, as Reiki often makes people feel very relaxed or even a bit drowsy. If they were driving or operating machinery, for example, this could potentially make it more difficult for them, so in situations where you are not sure what they are doing you can 'programme' the treatment for when they are asleep at night – more details later in this chapter.

As Reiki is always Divinely guided, however, it will 'know' when it is safe for someone to receive it; I know of several instances similar to the following: a distant treatment was sent at an agreed time, but the person who was due to receive it had to deal with an emergency and was up a ladder fixing a roof. Obviously, at that point, receiving Reiki might have been inappropriate, so the Reiki 'waited' until the person had finished and was putting the ladder back in his garage, at which point he actually felt the Reiki 'descend' so was able to quickly go into his house and sit in a comfy chair to receive it properly.

Using a 'correspondence'

You can also use a 'correspondence' – something you use to represent the person and on which you can place your hands during the treatment 'as if' they were on the person. This could be your own knee and thigh or a pillow, or even a teddy bear or some other cuddly toy. This works because everything is energy, and therefore everything is connected, so when you use an object to represent (correspond to) something else, your intention transmutes the energy esoterically, so that for a period of time the correspondence 'is' the body of someone else. (Yes, I know it sounds a bit weird, but it does work!)

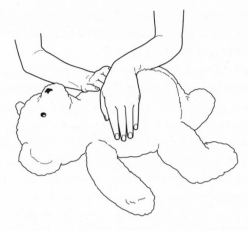

You don't have to use an object as a correspondence. Photographs and names written on pieces of paper also act as correspondences, as do images that you visualise. When visualising a person you can imagine them to be life-size or the same size as a pillow or teddy bear, or really small so that they would fit onto your hand. You could then use visualisation to imagine your hands in different positions on the body – or you could visualise the person held between huge hands, so that all parts of their body would be receiving Reiki at the same time.

One word of caution: when using the Distant Symbol, you create a really powerful connection, and when they are receiving a distant treatment many people who are energetically quite sensitive actually feel as though the Practitioner's hands are on their body, and they can feel when the hands move to be placed elsewhere. Although this is excellent, it does mean that you must be as careful when doing a distant treatment as when doing a hands-on treatment, so make sure all your hand movements are gentle.

The main caution in this case, however, is about imagining the person turning over (or physically turning over whatever you are using as a correspondence) to have their back treated. Please do this *very slowly and gently* as the energetically sensitive person can become very disturbed by this, and can sometimes feel the need to actually turn over, so you must give them time to do this. I know of people who have fallen off a sofa or out of bed in the middle of receiving a distant treatment when the Practitioner 'flipped' them too quickly onto their stomachs – even though they were many miles apart at the time!

DISTANT TREATMENT METHODS

1 A standard distant treatment

1   Prepare yourself for doing the treatment. You should sit some-where comfortable and quiet, where you will not be disturbed – switch the telephone off, ask the family to leave you alone for half an hour, and so on. You might choose to light some incense or burn some aromatherapy oil and have some gentle music on in the background. Spend a few minutes meditating – doing the *Hatsurei-ho* (see Chapter 21) is a good way to prepare yourself, as it will also cleanse your energy field.

2   Picture the person to whom you wish to send the Distant Reiki treatment. You can use a photograph or write their name and address on a piece of paper, or you can just visualise them. You can also use a 'correspondence' as explained above – a pillow is especially good, because it is long enough to fit your hands on. Just imagine that whatever you are using as a correspondence is the person, so spend a few moments deciding which part rep-resents their head, which represents their body, and legs, and so on.

3   Draw the Distant Symbol over the photo, paper or body of the correspondence, say its mantra three times, the name of the person three times and their location once (either their whole address or just the town, area or country they are in, if you don't know exactly where they are). Just imagine the Distant Symbol going out like a huge bridge between you and the person to whom you are sending a distant treatment.

4   Then draw the Power Symbol over the photo, paper or body of the correspondence, say its mantra three times, the name of the person once and their location once. Imagine a large Power Symbol over the body of the person, and then let it descend so that the person is completely encompassed by the symbol, so that its healing energy can flow throughout the person during the treatment.

5   Then say that this Reiki is sent with love and light, for the highest and greatest good. You may also mention any spe-cific parts of the body, or illnesses or situations that you know

need special attention, and ask that they receive healing if this is possible at this time, but it will be the person's Higher Self who decides how to use the energy, so try not to have specific expectations, that is, it is important to take your ego out of the healing process.

6   You can then carry out a standard treatment by placing your hands as if they were in each of the 12 standard hand positions, either actually on the correspondence or in the air above a photo, etc. Start with hand position 1 under whatever represents their head, and hold that, and then each following hand position for two or three minutes for those on the head and body and for between half a minute and one minute on any other hand positions you choose to do, such as the arms, hands, legs and feet.

7   When you have finished, close the whole treatment by smoothing down the person's aura with your hands (in the air or over the pillow, etc.) and then draw a Power Symbol over the whole of their body (starting at the head) again saying its sacred mantra three times, with the *intention* of closing the person's chakras and ending the treatment.

8   I like to end with my hands in the prayer position (*Gassho*), to show respect and mentally thank the Reiki, and then clap my hands together firmly (usually three times) to break the energy connection. Afterwards I spend a few minutes in quiet contemplation, and then carry out some self-cleansing – either the Reiki Shower or Dry Brushing or the whole of *Hatsurei-ho*.

2 A mental–emotional distant treatment

This is an even more powerful way of doing a distant treatment, as it works deeply on the psychological or emotional causative levels, helping blockages to rise to the surface to be healed and released, so this is the method I usually use. The visualisation helps to keep your mind really focused on the person receiving the treatment, which is essential, as their chakras are opened by the Harmony Symbol in order that they can receive the maximum amount of Reiki. Just like the hands-on treatment of the same name (see previous chapter) it is important to project only positive thoughts during the sending of this treatment.

1   Carry out the same preparations as in steps 1 and 2 of the standard distant treatment on page 214.

2   When you are ready, place your non-dominant hand underneath the photo, paper or correspondence (whichever part you have decided represents the head), and draw the Distant Symbol in the air above the photo, paper or correspondence, say its sacred mantra three times followed by the name of the person three times and their location once, and direct its energy to whatever represents the crown of the recipient.

3   Draw the Harmony Symbol, say the mantra three times, name of the person three times and direct its energy to the crown of the person.

4   Draw the Power Symbol, say the mantra three times, directing its energy to the crown of the person, and *intend* and say that this powerful Reiki healing is sent with love and light, for the highest and greatest good of [name of person].

5   Carry out a full mental–emotional treatment on the person, using the visualisation in steps 9–17 on pages 196–7 in Chapter 11 (see also my website in Resources for a CD of this visualisation), remembering to maintain your full attention on the person. When this has been completed, draw a Power Symbol and say the mantra three times over whatever represents the person's crown chakra, *intending* that the mental and emotional part of the treatment has ended. Remember, it is really important to end this part of the treatment properly. You can then relax your concentration for the next part of the treatment.

6   Next, carry out a shortened standard distant treatment, as in step 6 of the previous treatment, reducing the timing of the hand positions on the head and body to one or two minutes each. (The shortened standard treatment can even be omitted, if necessary, although it is clearly better to include it whenever possible.)

7   Finally, smooth the aura, close the treatment with the Power Symbol, and carry out your own cleansing, as in steps 7 and 8 of the previous treatment.

PROGRAMMING THE TREATMENT FOR A FUTURE TIME

If you are unable to agree a particular time, or if you have another commitment at the time, which is suitable to a potential recipient, then it is possible to 'programme' the treatment to go to them either at a specific time arranged between you or while they are asleep, rather like setting a video, DVD or digital recorder to record a TV programme at a particular time. To do this, follow the instructions for carrying out a standard distant treatment until you have completed number 5, and then say 'This Reiki is to be received by [name of person] at [date and time agreed/when they are asleep tonight/ when it will be most beneficial].' You can also pre-programme a mental–emotional distant treatment in exactly the same way.

Programming for repeat-healing treatments

If there is a requirement to send a person lots of treatments – say, for example, someone needs 21 consecutive treatments to help with some chronic or life-threatening condition – it will take you about 15 to 20 minutes a day to carry these out. However, there may be times when you have a few daily treatments to do on other people, or perhaps you have some serious commitments and are unsure of being available to carry out the distant treatments at the right time. It is possible to 'programme' a treatment to be received regularly at the same time each day, without you having to sit there doing it every time – again, rather like programming a video/DVD/digital recorder to record the same TV programme daily at the same time. Remember that the Distant Symbol cuts through time and space, so this is no problem.

Carry out either the standard distant treatment or the mental–emotional distant treatment in exactly the same way as the above sections, but when you reach step 5, add the following instruction 'This Reiki is to be received by [name of person] at [time agreed]/ [or] when they are asleep [today or tonight] and for the following six days [or nights].' Then, after one week, you can either get back to doing the distant treatment on a daily basis or if the same conditions exist for you, you can reprogramme the treatment for another seven days.

If someone is very ill, or perhaps is unconscious or experiencing some other dangerous health crisis, a useful tip is to programme a treatment to go to them every hour or every two hours. For this you would carry out either of the above distant treatment instructions up to step 5, and then say 'Let a full Reiki treatment flow to [name of person] every hour [or every two hours] for the next 48 hours.' Again, after the two days you can review the situation, and see whether you need to reprogramme it in the same way or reduce the number of treatments and so on.

Before programming a number of distant treatments to go to someone, it is important to first find out how they reacted to a single distant treatment. Occasionally, a person can experience some pain or discomfort while receiving either a hands-on or a distant treatment, and while usually this discomfort doesn't last very long, it would be disconcerting, and perhaps even a bit frightening, if the person knew they would perhaps have to go through that every day if their distant treatments were programmed for a week!

SENDING DISTANT TREATMENTS TO SEVERAL PEOPLE SIMULTANEOUSLY

Wherever possible it is obviously best to put aside the time needed for an individual distant treatment, but where time is short, or if you have a number of close friends or relatives who need regular distant treatments, this can involve a considerable time commitment on your part, as each treatment (particularly the mental–emotional treatment) can take 20 minutes or more. It is therefore possible to send a full distant Reiki treatment to a number of people at the same time, provided you have their permission to do so and have agreed a suitable time when they can receive it. It is *not* appropriate to send the mental–emotional treatment to several people at the same time, though, as this really does require all your attention to be on one individual.

1   I would suggest you limit this to a maximum of three people. You can use a single correspondence, such as a pillow, on which to place your hands, and then have photographs of each person nearby or their names and addresses on pieces of paper. (You

can visualise them, but it is difficult to keep all their images in your mind.)

2 Draw the Distant Symbol over one photograph (or name) saying its mantra three times, the name of that person three times and their location once, and then over the same photo (or name) draw the Power Symbol and say the mantra three times.

3 Repeat this process with each of the other photos or names, and then place your hands over the correspondence you are going to use.

4 Draw the Distant Symbol again, say (aloud) that 'this pillow [or whatever else you are using] represents each of the following people [say each name and location three times, e.g. Joe Bloggs in London], so that a complete Reiki treatment now flows to all of the people I have named, for their highest and greatest good.'

5 Then draw the Power Symbol over the correspondence, say the mantra three times and commence the treatment by placing your hands in position 1 for a couple of minutes, then moving them gently to position 2, and so on.

6 Finish the treatment by smoothing the aura three times (from head to feet).

7 Draw the Power Symbol again over the pillow and once over each photo or name, say the mantra three times for each and *intend* that the distant treatment be over.

8 To conclude, clap your hands three times or shake them vigorously, to end the connection, and then mentally thank the Reiki, and finish by carrying out some self-cleansing.

Please note that I am *not* suggesting the use of the Harmony Symbol in this multiple-treatment, but as your *intention* is for each person to receive a full Reiki treatment for their highest and greatest good, they will all receive whatever Reiki they need individually. As I said earlier, if you feel the person would benefit greatly from a mental–emotional treatment, then you need to do a separate treatment on that person.

In this chapter, we have been concentrating on distant healing for people, but there are also some other ways of using distant healing techniques, such as for personal problems and world situations, and other creative ideas too, and these are given in the next two chapters.

Chapter 13

The Reiki Symbols as Part of Daily Life

There are so many things you can do to enhance your life when using the Reiki symbols in addition to treating yourself and other people. The symbols are so versatile that the list is almost endless, but I have written down some of the most useful ideas in this and the next chapter. There are techniques for using the symbols around the home and at work; using them for clearing, cleansing and creating sacred space; using them for healing bad habits and other situations, and more. I hope you have fun trying them out.

USING SYMBOLS WHEN TREATING ANIMALS, BIRDS, REPTILES, FISH OR INSECTS

With the Second Degree symbols, you will find it even easier to treat animals, birds, reptiles and fish. You can use the Distant Symbol to connect to any type of creature anywhere and at any time, and the Power Symbol to bring the Reiki powerfully to it; you can do this from any distance away.

Another way to help animals is to draw the Power Symbol over their food and water (saying the mantra three times) to enhance its nutritional qualities and to offset any adverse effects of any chemicals or preservatives. Any homeopathic remedies or medication dispensed by a veterinary surgeon can be treated in the same way.

USING THE SYMBOLS WITH PLANTS AND SEEDS

When you walk past any of your houseplants, occasionally draw the Power Symbol over them, saying its mantra three times and *intending* that the Reiki flow for the plants' highest good. The same applies to plants in your garden, yard or patio, to the crops in your allotment or fields and to seeds or cuttings. You can also treat plants using the Distant Symbol before the Power Symbol – if you are away on holiday, for instance.

USING THE SYMBOLS WITH INANIMATE OBJECTS

Using symbols, especially the Power Symbol, enhances any Reiki you might give to machinery or equipment that is not working. Either draw the Power Symbol in front of or over the machine, or draw the Power Symbol over each of your palms before placing your hands on the machine. For an object far away, simply connect with it using the Distant Symbol, saying its mantra three times and the name of the object three times and its location once. Then use the Power Symbol, say the mantra three times and *intend* that Reiki should flow into the object for the highest possible good.

USING THE SYMBOLS WITH FOOD AND DRINK

The Power Symbol and its mantra can be used over all food and drink: the food on your plate and all your ingredients when you are cooking, too.

USING THE SYMBOLS ON PERSONAL PROBLEMS AND SITUATIONS

Whatever kind of problems you are having, from strained relationships with your partner or family to difficulties at work or with studying, you can use Reiki to help to permeate the situation with healing. Here is one method, and you will find other ideas later in this chapter.

1   First, write down the details of any problem area you are working on and hold the paper between your hands. Examples could be 'Allow Reiki to flow into the situation of my relationships, for the highest and greatest good' or 'Let Reiki flow into the situation of my money issues, for my highest and greatest good.'

2   Then draw the Distant Symbol over the paper, silently saying its mantra three times, and *intending* that the Reiki connect with the situation.

3   Next, draw the Harmony Symbol over the paper, say the mantra three times, asking that Reiki flow to harmonise and heal the situation in whatever way is for your highest and greatest good.

4   Then draw the Power Symbol over the paper and say the mantra three times, *intending* that Reiki flow into this situation for the highest and greatest good.

5   Maintain this position for five to ten minutes, and when you have finished, thank Reiki for its help, draw another Power Symbol, say the mantra three times over the paper, *intending* that the healing is sealed in, and the treatment is over.

6   Do this each day, and continue to work on this situation until some resolution to the situation appears.

EMPOWERING GOALS WITH REIKI SYMBOLS

You can use a similar method for working on your goals and dreams with Reiki.

1   Write down *all* the aspects of what you are seeking, so if you want a cottage in the country, put down how many bedrooms and bathrooms you want, what kind of kitchen, whether you want central heating or open fires, a small garden or acres of farmland, and so on.

2   Then draw the Distant Symbol over the paper and say the mantra three times to connect with your goal.

3   Now draw the Harmony Symbol and say the mantra three times to help your goal to be harmonious and in balance with your life.

4   Finally, draw the Power Symbol to bring the Reiki in. Say the mantra three times, and then hold this piece of paper in your hands and *intend* that Reiki should flow into that goal for the highest and greatest good.

5   Give it Reiki for at least ten minutes a day until you achieve what you want.

Beware: be sure you *really* want it before you ask for it, because if your goal is in harmony with your highest good, you will achieve it; however, your highest good can sometimes be served by going through negative experiences, as well as positive ones, so sometimes the outcome might not be as rosy as you expected. For example, lots of people dream of winning millions of pounds or dollars, but when they do they find it a dreadful responsibility, causing friction in the family and huge changes in their lifestyle that do not make them happy after all, perhaps because their friends don't want to be around them so much, because they feel uncomfortable about not being able to keep up with their spending power. But those are valid life lessons too. See what I mean?

It is also necessary to think of whether what you are asking for is ethical. For example, if you have a specific house in mind but it is not actually for sale and there are people already living there, there are any number of reasons – pleasant and unpleasant – why the current owners might have to put it on the market. It is therefore much better to describe the type of home and location you are seeking, rather than a specific property. Another ethical question is about relationships. You may have a specific person in mind with whom you would like to develop a close, intimate relationship, but even if that person is free and single, it is *not* appropriate to work with Reiki in this way. It would be an infringement of that person's rights, and would be interfering with his or her emotional choices.

Empowering affirmations with Reiki symbols

If you are working with affirmations – positive statements which can help to reprogramme your thinking – then these can be made even more effective by writing them down, drawing the Reiki symbols over them, holding the paper in your hands, and then saying them over and over to yourself while giving them Reiki. (You can use all three symbols for this, together with their mantras, in the usual order: Distant, Harmony and Power.)

This can be a really powerful method for change, so make sure that your affirmations are always really positive, with an intention for your highest and greatest good and are fully in the present. So, for example, use 'I have a wonderful, loving relationship with a man/woman who loves me' even if this is not the case right now, rather than 'I will have . . .' or 'I would like . . .', and 'My body is healthy and full of vitality' rather than 'I am not ill any more'. This is important, because what we think, say and feel *now*, at this moment in time, is what is creating our future. In that context, our minds and bodies see no difference between 'real' or 'imagined' reality, so, for example, some research in Japan reported in the *Kyushi Journal of Medical Science*, 1962, found that blindfolded children who were told that poison ivy was being brushed against their arms produced swelling, redness and itching on their skin, even when the plant used was perfectly harmless. Their beliefs produced what they expected would happen. When we use affirmations we are affirming what we want to be true, and feeling and acting upon it as if it were true, and this creates the right positive climate to manifest and make it real for ourselves.

Try the power of words for yourself. To demonstrate it more dramatically, you can start with a negative statement, so stand up straight and say aloud, 'I feel sad' at least ten times, and you will find that your shoulders will start to droop, and your voice will become quieter and sadder. But then immediately afterwards use a positive affirmation by saying, 'I am happy' between 10 and 20 times, and your body begins to straighten up again, your voice lifts, and eventually it is hard to suppress a smile!

Because Reiki will always work for your highest and greatest good, it will help you to achieve your ideal, but it may first produce results that force you to face up to the blocks that are currently preventing you from having what you want. For instance, if you are desperate to form a loving relationship, this might be because you don't feel you are a whole person without a partner. This could indicate that you need to work on your self-esteem and ability to love yourself, so it is likely that these issues would arise first. So you get what you need, rather than what you want – but at least you will be a step closer.

Using symbols to heal unwanted habits or addictions

The Harmony Symbol can be used to help you to change or eliminate habits or addictions which are no longer useful to you, such as smoking cigarettes, drinking alcohol, taking non-prescription drugs or even overeating. It is important, however, that you should actually *want* to give up the habit that you are working on, because you recognise the benefits to you and acknowledge those benefits as being more advantageous than whatever it is that the habit gives you. Reiki can be of considerable assistance, but it cannot force you to do something you don't want to do, or something you are only doing to please someone else.

The Harmony Symbol works on the psychological and emotional causes underlying things, and each of the aforementioned habits has its root in at least one, and probably both, of these potential causative issues. Using the Harmony Symbol will help to bring those causative issues to the surface – such as rejection, fear, anxiety, self-loathing, the need for affection, and so on – so that they can be examined and healed. Such self-realisations can, of course, be very uncomfortable, so if you don't really want to tackle the problem, you will simply push it back under the surface and nothing will be achieved. But if you really do want to work on the problem, then Reiki can help you to change to better, healthier habits as well as helping you to heal and let go of whatever issues have been underlying your habit. It can also allow you to let go of the problem enough to feel a sense of gratitude for the lessons it has taught you, because every experience has value in the insights it offers and its contribution to who you are right now.

1   Write your name on a piece of paper, together with a suitably positive statement such as, 'I am now choosing a healthier lifestyle, so I choose to heal and let go of my need to smoke/drink alcohol/overeat/take drugs.'

2   Then, in the air above the paper, draw a Harmony Symbol, silently saying its mantra three times and repeating aloud three times the statement you have written.

3   Next, draw a Power Symbol and say its mantra three times.

4   Hold the paper between your hands, treating it with Reiki for 15 to 20 minutes a day. Continue to do this until you feel that you have really let go of this unwanted habit.

CLEANSING AND CREATING SACRED SPACE

Any space can become contaminated with negative energy, or negative energy can simply collect and stagnate in corners. The more you become involved in your spiritual path, the more important it is not to be surrounded by negativity, so use Reiki everywhere, all the time, to create positive space around you.

1   The simplest and easiest way of clearing negative energy from your surroundings is to place Power Symbols all around you – in all the corners and sides of any room, plus the ceiling and floor.

2   Draw the Power Symbol (as large as possible, if no one is watching, otherwise draw it discreetly) and say its mantra to yourself three times in each place.

3   *Intend* that the Reiki should clear and cleanse the room and seal it in light, making it a sacred space.

This is good not only for any room in your home but also in your workplace, in hotel bedrooms, hospital wards or anywhere else you are staying.

You can cleanse just about anything with Reiki, using the Power Symbol and *intending* that the Reiki cleanse whatever you are directing it at. You can try it on your bed, your clothes or your car – in fact anything in your life that might attract or hold negative energy.

Cleansing yourself

You can also use the Power Symbol to cleanse yourself if you have been somewhere that you feel was energetically rather negative, such as after visiting people in hospital or after attending a funeral.

1   Draw a Power Symbol (discreetly) in the air above your crown chakra, saying its mantra to yourself three times, and *intending* that the Reiki cleanse your whole energy field.

2   Then, imagine the Power Symbol growing and extending until it fills your aura. Visualise it moving downwards towards the ground, taking with it any negative energy until the negativity flows into the Earth with the Reiki, which will heal it and transmute it so that it is useful energy for the planet.

USING THE SYMBOLS FOR PROTECTION

The Power Symbol can be used for protection, and because Reiki works on all levels, the protection it provides is also on all levels and includes protection from physical harm, verbal and emotional confrontations and psychic attack. It can be used to protect your car, your home, your children or anything else you value, and you can use it to protect you and your family when you are travelling, too.

There are a variety of ways of using Reiki for protection, and I have given some of the most popular ones below. Please be inventive – you may think of other ways.

Self-protection

(This is best repeated on a daily basis, and again in any situations that call for it.)

Either draw a large Power Symbol in front of you and step into it, silently saying its sacred mantra three times, imagining it encompassing you and *intending* that it forms a protective barrier around you.

Or draw (or visualise) a Power Symbol in front of you, and on each side of you, and imagine drawing one behind you, saying its mantra three times, and *intending* that it forms a protective shield around you. You can also add a Power Symbol over your head and beneath your feet, if you like.

Your car, home or other objects you care about

(This is best repeated on a weekly basis.)

1   *Either* physically draw, *or* imagine drawing, a large Power Symbol over the object, saying its mantra three times.

2   Then imagine the Power Symbol expanding until it covers the object above, below and on all sides.

3   *Intend* that the Power Symbol protects that object for as long as is necessary.

4   If you are away from the object, then use the Distant Symbol to connect with it first.

When travelling

1   If you know your destination, discreetly draw a Distant Symbol, saying its mantra to yourself three times, and imagine it forming a bridge of light connecting you with your destination.

2   Then, imagine a large Power Symbol over your car or the bus, train, ship or plane you are travelling in, say its mantra three times and imagine the Power Symbol spreading until it covers your means of transport above, below and on all sides.

3   *Intend* that the Power Symbol protects all the occupants of that means of transport for the duration of the journey.

4   You can then imagine a Power Symbol travelling ahead, clearing the way for you along the bridge of light formed by the Distant Symbol.

For children

There may be occasions when your children are not with you and you sense that they may need protection. You can connect with them using the Distant Symbol, and then imagine a large Power Symbol encompassing them, *intending* that it protect them for their highest and greatest good.

Please be sensitive to the fact that this is actually a controlling and potentially intrusive thing to do – you are deciding what is best for them, because you love them and want them to be safe. This is natural enough, but their highest good may not be best served by being so protected – children need challenges to help their personal and social development. If they are old enough to understand, I think it is always best to ask their permission first. Then, if they want Reiki protection, they are choosing it rather than having it thrust upon them.

USING THE SYMBOLS FOR MOTIVATION, MEMORY AND SELF-GROWTH

The symbols can be used to enhance various aspects of mental performance, such as the following:

For self-motivation

Draw a Power Symbol over your forehead, saying its mantra three times, *intending* to increase your motivation in general or for specific tasks.

To help your memory

Either draw a Power Symbol over the top of your head *or* the Harmony and Power Symbols on your crown and brow chakras, saying their mantras three times, and *intending* that Reiki should help you to remember whatever it is you need to remember.

To help you learn things (such as for exams or interviews)

Use the Harmony and Power Symbols on your crown and third eye chakras, and also draw them over the passages, chapters or information you need to learn, silently saying their mantras three times and *intending* that Reiki helps you to learn.

For self-growth and increased understanding

Draw the Harmony Symbol followed by the Power Symbol on both palms, and then hold your head with both hands either on your brow and the back of your head, or on both sides. Imagine the symbols entering your head, and as you silently say the symbols' sacred mantras *intend* that the Reiki helps you with your self-growth and understanding.

For achieving goals, dreams and ambitions

Draw the Harmony Symbol on both hands followed by the Power Symbol, and then hold your head with one hand on your forehead and the other hand on the back of your head, saying the sacred mantra three times and *intending* that Reiki helps you to achieve your goals, dreams and ambitions.

USING THE SYMBOLS WITH EMOTIONAL AND RELATIONSHIP ISSUES

The Harmony Symbol, when used together with the Distant and Power Symbols, is the most useful for helping you to improve all kinds of relationships, from family to friendships and business contacts. Of course, you cannot determine the outcome because the Reiki will still be acting for your highest and greatest good. But, generally, you will find that there is some improvement as the people involved will be aware, on an energetic level (and through their Soul/Higher Self), that you are trying to create greater harmony for the good of you all. Do remember, however, the ethical principles discussed on page 208, and always ensure that you state and *intend* that the Reiki flows for the greatest and highest good of all concerned.

For relationships of all kinds

(This can be repeated as often as necessary – even on a daily basis, until the relationship shows signs of developing greater harmony.)

1   It is helpful to imagine the pairings or groups of people (such as you and your partner; or you and your work colleagues, and so on) all together.

2   Draw the Distant Symbol to connect to the group.

3   Then the Harmony Symbol to bring peace and harmony.

4   And then the Power Symbol to bring healing energy to the situation, saying each of their mantras three times and a description of the group once (for example my wife and I; or Bill, Wendy, Jean and myself at work, and so on).

5   Then, imagine the Harmony Symbol as if it is hovering above the group, and watch it gently descend until it encompasses the whole group.

6   *Intend* that it bring its peaceful, harmonious energies to the group for the greatest and highest good.

7   Hold this image for about five minutes – you can turn it into a visualisation if you want, seeing the people involved getting on better and perhaps ending with a hug.

8   Then draw the Power Symbol, say its mantra three times and *intend* that the healing is complete.

9   Finally, clap your hands or shake them vigorously to break the connection.

For meetings of all kinds

1   Do the same as above, but perhaps imagine the appropriate group of people sitting around a table.

2   If you don't know all their names, or don't know what they look like, it doesn't matter, just specify 'all the people at my interview' or 'all the people at the Council meeting' etc.

3   As you are using the Distant Symbol you can also specify the time of the meeting or interview.

4   When you hold the image of the group you can perhaps 'see' the meeting ending with everyone smiling and shaking hands.

For emotional issues of all kinds

This can be repeated as often as necessary.

1   To deal with nervousness, fear, depression, anger, sadness, restlessness, impatience, stress or tiredness, draw or imagine a large Harmony Symbol over your crown chakra. Then visualise the symbol expanding until it encompasses the whole of you.

2   Say its mantra three times and ask and *intend* that it brings its gentle, healing, peaceful and restorative energy to fill your physical and energy bodies, to bring greater harmony and balance to your life.

3   Then use the Power Symbol to bring the energy in to support the Harmony Symbol.

4   Let yourself stay in a meditative state and imagine being surrounded and encompassed by Reiki for at least five minutes, but preferably for about 15 minutes, or until you feel much calmer and more content.

5   Then draw a Power Symbol to seal in the peaceful energies, saying its mantra three times.

6   Finally, clap your hands or shake them vigorously to break the energy connections.

For letting go of blocked feelings or unhealthy attachments

1   In a similar way to the method above, draw (or imagine drawing) a large Harmony Symbol over your crown chakra.

2   Then imagine the symbol expanding until it encompasses the whole of you.

3   Say its mantra three times, and ask and *intend* that it brings its gentle, healing, peaceful and restorative energy to fill your physical and energy bodies, to bring greater harmony and balance to your life.

4   Then use the Power Symbol, saying its mantra three times, and ask and *intend* that it works with the Harmony Symbol to unblock and release any deeply held feelings (such as resentment or hatred) or that it unblock and release any unhealthy attachments (such as to a former husband or wife, boyfriend or girlfriend).

5   It is helpful if you can visualise something like a small cloud of grey energy, representing all your old emotions related to this situation, actually being detached and floating up through your energy field to be released – imagine it going 'pop' as it moves outside your aura – to be healed by Reiki.

6   When you feel calmer and more content, draw a Power Symbol to seal out the old, useless emotions, saying its mantra three times.

7   Finally, clap your hands or shake them vigorously to break the energy connections.

SENDING REIKI INTO THE PAST

You can send Reiki into the past, to allow it to heal past events or hurts. It will not necessarily physically alter what has happened

– although it can have an impact energetically – but it can allow healing and forgiveness to permeate that time, which will gently alter the way you feel about it.

For example, if you had a difficult or traumatic experience in the past and you know the approximate date, you can use the Distant Symbol to send Reiki back to that time to heal the problem or trauma. It often helps if you have a photograph of yourself close to the time of the event in question, but if you don't know the date or don't have a photo, it will still work by simply naming the problem and asking that Reiki go to the cause to heal it.

1   Write down the situation and roughly the timing (e.g. a broken relationship when you were 20 years old) and draw or imagine the Distant Healing Symbol over the paper (and photograph of you at that age, if you have one). Silently say its sacred mantra three times, sensing it connecting the you of today with the you of that time.

2   Then draw or imagine the Harmony Symbol over the paper/ photo, say the mantra three times, sensing its healing flowing to the hurt and upset and to the root cause and the lessons you were meant to learn from the event.

3   Then draw or imagine the Power Symbol over the paper/ photo, say the mantra three times, sensing a strong flow of Reiki moving into that time, for the highest and greatest good.

4   Allow the Reiki to flow for 15 to 20 minutes, or longer if it feels appropriate. Then draw the Power Symbol over the paper/ photo, say the mantra three times, *intending* that the healing be sealed in.

5   Finally clap your hands to break the connection, and let go of that event in your thoughts.

If, in the days following this activity, you get a sense that the healing is not complete – perhaps you have dreamed about the event, or it unexpectedly enters your thoughts quite a few times – then repeat the above instructions, sending Reiki again to the same situation. You can do this as many times as you feel is needed, but once is often enough. Sometimes, however, it is the way you have worded the situation that is preventing the healing from being completed;

for example, perhaps you are trying to send the Reiki to the other person involved, which ethically is not the correct way to do this.

You can only have responsibility for your own self-healing, but by healing your own reactions and thoughts about a particular time or event, that healing automatically flows outwards rather like the ripples made by a pebble thrown into a pond. It gradually permeates through the energetic signature of the whole situation, including allowing any other people involved to receive whatever healing their Higher Selves deem is necessary. So, healing your own part in the event can have some extraordinary effects; I have known cases where family members, who have not spoken to each other for years because of a family feud, have suddenly got in touch again when students of mine sent Reiki to the original situation. Healing their *own* feelings about it helped others to recognise this on a subconscious, energetic level, so that they too could heal their own part in it.

SENDING REIKI INTO THE FUTURE

It is just as simple to send Reiki into the future. If you know you will be involved in an important event, situation or activity in the future with which you feel you need Reiki's help, such as a job interview, a visit to the dentist or a potentially difficult business meeting, then again write down the event or situation and the approximate date and time. Proceed in the same way as above, sensing the Reiki flowing into the future to wait for you there.

It is also possible to 'bank' Reiki so that you can draw on it as and when you need it, by imagining some sort of container – it could be a box, a jug or a fun container like a big piggy bank.

1   Draw the Distant Symbol to connect to the container, saying its sacred mantra three times.

2   Then draw the Power Symbol, saying its mantra three times.

3   Visualise the container filling up with Reiki, for the highest and greatest good.

When it is used in this way, the Reiki energy stores up like a battery. When the time comes, its healing energy descends to surround you and help you. People have used this technique to help them with all sorts of events, including driving tests, trips to meet their potential mother-in-law, hospital appointments – basically anything that might be difficult or frightening, or that would make them feel nervous, as well as happier events like weddings, parties, the first day in a new job, and so on. Just try it out for yourself.

EMPOWERING EVERYTHING IN YOUR LIFE

There is really no limit to the ways in which you can use the Reiki symbols to enhance and empower your life. The simplest and easiest thing to do is to use the Power Symbol regularly over just about everything, with the intention of filling it with Reiki so that not only will it function even more effectively but it will also emanate Reiki, so that as you walk around your home or other spaces you regularly use, you are always soaking up Reiki. The following is a sample list, but you can probably think of even more. Just be creative, and enjoy it:

Bath water/shower head
Light bulbs/heaters/central heating boiler
Television/DVD/Blu-ray/digital recorder/gaming consoles
Oven/hob/microwave
Toiletries/cosmetics
MP3 player/iPod/CD/cassette player/radio
Washing machine/drier
PC/laptop/electronic notebook/printer/scanner/e-book reader/
    satnav
Dishwasher/vacuum cleaner
Clothes/shoes/handbags
Telephone/mobile phone/pager/iPhone
Camera/camcorder
Kettle/coffee-maker
Jewellery/clocks/watches
Car/caravan/motor bike/bicycle
Food processor/juicer
Bed/bedding/pillows
Chairs/sofa/dining table
. . . and anything else!

Now you have lots of practical ways of using the symbols to enhance your life, and I hope you will find them really helpful. Now, however, it is time to be a little more adventurous, so the next chapter has some very creative ways of using your Second Degree skills to have fun with Reiki. Enjoy!

Chapter 14

Creative Uses for Your Second Degree Skills

Now is the time to start having fun with Reiki! The symbols are so versatile that the only limits will be how much imagination you can bring to using Reiki.

ENHANCING INTUITION AND PSYCHIC ABILITY

Everyone has some form of psychic ability that they can choose to develop or block. Being attuned to Reiki can often unblock this ability or allow you to develop it further than you would otherwise have done. This isn't anything to be nervous about because, as always, Reiki works only for the highest and greatest good, so if it is the right time in your spiritual journey for you to develop your intuitive skills, you will be able to do so.

There are three types of psychic ability:

1 **Clairsentience**, meaning 'clear sensing', such as to feel or sense subtle energies or spirit.

2 **Clairaudience**, meaning 'clear hearing', such as in mediumship or channelling.

3 **Clairvoyance**, meaning 'clear sight', such as being able to see into the future and the past, and being able to see subtle energies like auras.

Clairsentience

Many people who practise Reiki find their ability to sense subtle energies greatly improves as their experience with Reiki increases. They can detect different layers of people's auras and sense imbalances, and they can also check whether those imbalances have dispersed after giving Reiki. Also, they become more aware of any 'atmosphere' in a room or between people. Some people build up their skills so that they can sense the presence of spiritual beings, including spirit guides and angels, even to the extent of being able to feel their touch.

Clairaudience

Other people find that they become mediums – hearing messages from discarnate beings (that is, people who are no longer living on the physical plane) – or they develop the ability to 'hear' guidance from their spirit guides (discarnate beings in a higher dimension who wish to share their wisdom to help us). They may also be able to 'channel' information from highly evolved teachers from spiritual realms (sometimes called ascended masters). Some actually hear real voices that seem to come from outside their head, but most just find that the words appear inside their head, like thoughts – and yet not quite like thoughts. I know that may be confusing, but it is quite difficult to describe. One way to tell the difference is that when a question is being asked – even if you are doing the asking yourself – the answer from spiritual guidance appears in your head before you have even finished formulating the question.

Clairvoyance

Quite often, people develop the ability to 'see' other realities, such as being able to see inside someone's body to tell what is wrong with them physically. The first time this happens can be a big shock: I remember my first occasion, which was seeing someone's cardiovascular system in full moving colour, with three blockages clearly apparent – and wow, was I surprised! However, it did mean I could position my hands directly over the blockages, and that I could check afterwards to see if the blockages had gone – which they had. Other clairvoyant abilities include seeing colours or blockages in auras and chakras; 'seeing' the energy representations of a person's life within their aura, such as what their home looks like, or being able to describe their family members; and being able to see visions of things that have happened in the past or which might happen in the future. (Please note that I said 'might' happen in the future. Your future is not fixed, as it is being created by your own thoughts, words and actions. So if you change your mind, you will change your future too.) Some people also develop the ability to see angels and spirit guides.

How to Develop Your Psychic Abilities

If you wish to develop your psychic awareness and intuitive skills further, then work with the Reiki symbols on your third eye (brow chakra), the seat of your intuition, inspiration and insight.

1   Draw both the Power Symbol and the Harmony Symbol onto each hand.

2   Hold one hand on your forehead, and the other hand behind your head at approximately the same level.

3   Alternatively, draw both symbols actually on your forehead, or in your aura, about 5cm (2in) away from your third eye chakra.

4   *Intend* that Reiki should flow into your third eye to awaken and enhance your intuitive ability safely and easily, for your highest and greatest good.

5   Then hold your hands on your head for a few minutes, allowing the Reiki to flow.

Don't do this too often or for too long, as you may get headaches. If you don't feel comfortable doing this, then write on a piece of paper, 'I wish to develop my psychic awareness safely and easily for my highest and greatest good.' Hold the paper between your hands and place the symbols over it or put it in the centre of a crystal grid (see pages 245–8).

PSYCHIC PROTECTION

It is very important to protect yourself psychically as you become more sensitive and intuitive, because, as the vibrational frequencies of your energy body are raised, they become more attractive to some of the lower energies. This can make you more vulnerable than usual to psychic drains (people who drain your energy, whether they know they are doing this or not) and psychic attack (harmful thoughts from other people, again, whether they know they are doing this or not). Here are some suggestions for self-protection, and it is a good idea to carry out at least one of them at the beginning and end of every day. As you will see, the techniques get progressively more protective, so the first and second methods can certainly be used on a daily basis, but fortunately you're unlikely to need the level of protection in the third or fourth methods very often, so save those for whenever you really feel you need them!

1   Draw a large Power Symbol in front of you and step into it, saying its mantra three times. Imagine being wrapped inside the Power Symbol so that it is in front, behind and each side of you, and *intend* that the Reiki protect you from any negativity or harm.

2   Imagine yourself in a bubble of white or golden light that is filled with Reiki; *intend* that the edges of the bubble are permeable only by love, light, Reiki and positive energies.

3   Imagine yourself inside a bubble of Reiki light, and imagine that the bubble is closely surrounded by a fine mesh made of gold which is only permeable by love, light, Reiki and positive energies.

4   If you ever feel really threatened, then do all of the above. Outside your bubble of light filled with Reiki and covered with gold mesh, imagine a ring of fire, and outside that imagine a shiny eggshell made of mirror or shiny silver, with the mirrored side facing outwards. This effectively forms an energetic boundary around you, so that any negativity or psychic attack sent your way will only rebound back to the sender, because it is reflected by the mirror or silver.

USING SYMBOLS FOR EARTH HEALING OR FOR WORLD SITUATIONS AND DISASTERS

The Earth really needs as much healing as we can give her, and with Reiki you have a wonderful tool to use both for planetary healing and for sending healing to world situations or to help in crises or disasters. There are many methods for Earth healing, some of which were mentioned in Chapter 8, but here are some other suggestions, which can all be enhanced by using the Reiki Second Degree symbols.

1   Go to a place of power, such as an ancient stone circle, and *either* visualise a huge Power Symbol over the top of the circle, *or* sit in the middle of the circle, or place your hands on one of the stones, and allow Reiki to flow into the stone and then around the circle and into the Earth itself.

2   Another good thing to do at a stone circle or ancient cairn is to 'walk' the shape of the Power Symbol into the earth – although of course you really need to be alone to do this, as the symbol's shape is meant to be kept sacred.

3   Sit or stand either outdoors or indoors and draw or imagine a large Power Symbol over the floor or earth. Then, with your palms facing downwards, allow Reiki to flow into the Earth, *intending* that it flows for the Earth's greatest and highest good.

4   Imagine that you are holding a small version of the world between your hands, and send it Reiki. (Use the Distant Symbol to connect you to the Earth, and then the Power Symbol to activate greater healing.)

5   Hold something in your hands to represent the Earth, such as a globe, or even a stone, and draw the Power Symbol over it, filling it with Reiki, and *intending* that the Reiki should fill the planet.

6   To send Reiki to global situations, such as famines, ecological disasters or war zones, write down the situation and hold the piece of paper in your hands. Draw the Distant Symbol, then the Harmony Symbol and then the Power Symbol, saying each

of their sacred mantras three times and *intending* that Reiki should go to that situation for the highest possible good. In this way the Reiki is not being constrained to go to only one aspect of the situation, such as the people affected by the famine, but to the whole, so that it can also permeate the aid agencies, the governments, any warring factions and so on.

It really is gratifying to feel that you can do *something* to help, because so often we are too far removed from such situations to either fully understand them or to offer practical assistance; however, by sending Reiki we cannot predetermine the outcome, but must trust Reiki to work with the Higher Consciousness to heal, harmonise and balance the situation for the highest and greatest good.

USING REIKI WITH CRYSTALS

Crystals and gems have been regarded in many cultures as having magical powers and have been used throughout history for their healing qualities and beauty. Each crystal has different energy balancing and vibrational qualities. These can interact with the human energy body to promote healing, which is enhanced even more by filling them with Reiki. Using Reiki with crystals is not a part of traditional Reiki, but many Masters and Practitioners find crystals a useful and attractive addition to their healing work.

Most of the popular crystals are forms of quartz, and their unique crystalline structure seems to be ideally suited to holding healing energy. There are many different types and shapes of crystal, and most can be used as a vibrational tool to dislodge negative vibrations, the most commonly used for this purpose being clear quartz, rose quartz and amethyst. When choosing your crystals, hold the intent or purpose of 'healing' in your mind as you select them.

Clear quartz

This is the most versatile and most easily programmable crystal. It receives, activates, contains, amplifies and transmits energy, balancing the chakras and dispelling negativity from your own energy field and in the environment. When used as a tool for therapy it is an excellent channeller of healing energy. It is also known to promote clear-sightedness and inspire communication with your Higher Self, and it works well with any area of the body.

Rose quartz

This is known as the 'love stone', because its energies promote forgiveness and compassion by helping you to let go of stored anger, resentment, guilt, fear and jealousy. It eases emotional and sexual imbalances and enhances awareness of your true self, helping you to learn to love yourself. It works particularly well with the spleen, kidneys, heart, circulatory system and reproductive system.

Amethyst

This is known as 'the elevator' because it is a powerful aid to spiritual enhancement, cutting through illusion and inspiring healing, Divine love, inspiration and intuition. It also strengthens the endocrinal and immune systems and has a good effect on right-brain activity (the creative and intuitive side), the pineal and pituitary glands, and is believed to be an exceptional blood cleanser and energiser.

Some crystals can be found in their original rough state, while others have been shaped or polished. For healing, I don't think it matters what shape you use, but I do find crystal pyramids, crystal balls and crystal wands particularly useful, as they seem to concentrate healing energy more effectively.

Cleansing crystals

When you first bring the crystals home, it is important to cleanse them thoroughly. This is because they absorb energy easily, and you don't know what kinds of energy they have been absorbing before you bought them. Cleansing rids them of any negative energetic vibrations. There are various methods, such as holding the crystal in clean running water (not salt water) and letting them dry naturally afterwards by leaving them in bright sunlight or moonlight so that they absorb a full charge of masculine (Sun) and feminine (Moon) energies. I use this method, but I also use Reiki. Simply hold the crystal in your hands and/or draw the Power Symbol over it, say the mantra three times and *intend* that Reiki should cleanse the crystal. If you have a crystal with a number of facets, while holding it in one hand you can draw the Power Symbol over each facet with your other hand, and as you say its mantra three times, 'pull' any negative energy downwards, away from the crystal, and throw the negative energy towards the floor.

Empowering and programming

To empower and programme your crystals once they have been thoroughly cleansed, pick up each crystal individually and draw all three Reiki symbols over them, saying their sacred mantras and *intending* that the crystals be filled with an unlimited supply of Reiki. This will then be held within the crystal and released when required to be used for healing. You can carry the crystal around with you to aid your own healing or you can give it to someone else who needs healing energy. I don't use crystals during a Reiki treatment, but some people like to place charged crystals (that is, filled with Reiki) near to a client, or even on the client's chakras, during a treatment. If this is something you would like to try, I would recommend you attend a course on crystal healing to find out more about them, and of course it would be important to ascertain if the client was happy with using them, and you should remove the crystals before smoothing the aura down.

You can also write down any problem you are experiencing on a piece of paper and place it under a programmed crystal, *intending* that the Reiki flows constantly into the problem to promote healing for the highest and greatest good. Cleanse the crystal and reprogramme it once a week to maintain the strength of the energy.

CREATING A CRYSTAL GRID

Placing charged crystals in a grid formation magnifies their power in a similar way to many people treating one person with Reiki: the energy increases exponentially. There are a number of ways in which you can create crystal grids, but all have a central crystal and a number of crystals surrounding it. Clear quartz crystals normally have one end where the facets end in a point, so these are the ones I usually use. Placing the points facing towards the centre concentrates the energy in the centre of the grid, whereas placing the points facing outwards allows the energy to dissipate over a wide area. Sometimes it is possible to obtain crystals with points at both ends so they would transmit energy in both directions.

Crystal grids, therefore, create a powerful space for healing, and they can be any size you want, but the most useful size is up to a diameter of 30cm (12in) for indoor use. You can create a small crystal grid almost anywhere, but it is best to keep it out of sight or out of reach of other people once it has been set up, because its energy will dissipate if it is disturbed. The crystals can be placed on a cloth, a board or a tray if you want them to be portable, or on a high window ledge or shelf, if they can stay in the same place for a long time. To permeate or protect a sizeable area with Reiki, you can create a large grid by placing crystals in the corners of a room, or in each corner of your home, or buried in the ground at each corner of your garden, for instance; however, just because the grid is large it doesn't mean that the crystals have to be large as well. For most purposes, crystals about 5–10cm (2–4in) in length are fine.

Before setting up the grid I would always cleanse the area first, physically and energetically, and it is important to do this regularly. To allow the grid to become dusty would be disrespectful of the healing properties of both the crystals and the Reiki.

Once a crystal grid has been set up, it can be left where it is for a long time, providing you remember to clean and cleanse the area and the crystals regularly and to re-empower the grid with Reiki when you put the crystals back in place. The American Reiki Master, William Lee Rand, has placed 12-point crystal grids fixed on copper plates at the North and South Poles, designated for earth healing and world peace. They will presumably stay there for as long as the copper and crystals continue to exist. Even though they may now be under many feet of snow or ice, they can still be regularly recharged with Reiki using the Distant Symbol to connect with each of them.

The main way to use a crystal grid is to place under the central crystal something that represents what you want the healing to go to, such as a photograph or a piece of paper with a name on it, or details of a situation or problem that needs healing. It will then receive continuous Reiki – although you will need to 'top up' the Reiki regularly and will also need to gently cleanse all the crystals regularly. You can therefore use the grids to empower affirmations; to send distant healing to an individual or to a list of people; to send healing to a single situation or multiple situations; to send Reiki to a future or past event.

The four-point crystal grid

This simple grid is especially good for Earth healing, as the four crystals can represent north, south, east and west, and the central crystal can represent the whole Earth – a crystal sphere would be particularly appropriate here. The grid can also be used for other healing purposes: placed around your home or your therapy room to create a healing environment, or as a small grid to use for distant healing of people, places or situations.

Cleanse and empower each crystal as above, placing a crystal in the centre (any shape will do, but apart from a sphere a pyramid is particularly good as its base has four sides) and place the other four crystals with their pointed end facing the centre. Then draw the Power Symbol over the grid, making sure you encompass the whole grid, say its mantra three times and *intend* to empower this grid with unlimited Reiki energy (you can add the other two symbols as well, if you wish). *Intend* that whatever is represented by what is placed in the centre should receive healing (that is, a photograph or a piece of paper with a name on it is obviously a representation of the person, rather than the actual person).

The eight-point crystal grid

This grid can be any size you choose and is also very good for earth healing or for world situations, as it has a crystal in each of the eight directions (that is, including south-east, south-west, north-east and north-west), but it can be used for more general healing too. Cleanse all your crystals and then place a crystal in the centre and eight evenly spaced crystals around it with points facing inwards towards the central crystal. *Intend* to create a healing crystal grid, and empower the grid first with the Distant Symbol to enable the grid to connect even more effectively with whatever is placed within it; then the Harmony Symbol, to generate deep healing and harmony; then the Power Symbol to bring in the Reiki, saying their sacred mantras three times each. Top up the grid with the Power Symbol every day if possible, and cleanse all the crystals thoroughly at least once every three weeks. (The grid can then be set up again.)

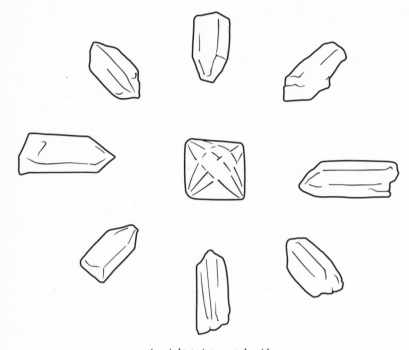

An eight-point crystal grid

The 12-point crystal grid

This is especially good for distant healing where you want the healing to continue to go to someone (or several people) for a number of days or even weeks. Place a crystal in the centre and then 12 equally spaced crystals in a circle around it, like the numbers on a clock face. Empower the grid with the three Reiki symbols, as in the eight-point grid above. But, when placing a photograph or name of a person in the grid, as you draw the Distant Symbol, say its mantra three times, then the name of the person three times, their location once and the number of days or nights the healing is to flow. Then draw the Power Symbol over it, saying its mantra three times. Always remember to add 'for the greatest and highest good' for all distant healing.

As you can see, there is a lot of scope for using your Second Degree skills in all sorts of creative ways. In Part 4 we look at the need for energetic cleansing and the importance of spiritual development, as well as how to become a professional Practitioner, or a Reiki Master.

Part 4

Your Continuing Steps Along the Reiki Path

Chapter 15

Energy Cleansing for Yourself and Your Environment

As you progress on your spiritual path with Reiki you can become increasingly sensitive to other people's energies, and one of the possible consequences of this is that you can 'pick up' energy – particularly negative energy – from other people and from your surroundings. Of course, you can protect yourself from this, as I have discussed in Chapter 13, but it is almost impossible to energetically protect the whole of your aura, as it can be quite large, and I'm sure you don't want to be a kind of psychic blotting paper, walking around absorbing everybody else's rubbish! It is therefore *vital* to cleanse yourself (your whole energy body as well as your physical body) every day, and often several times a day, depending upon what you are doing.

My initial impression when I was trained was that the Reiki channel created by an attunement could not become blocked, but after many years of experience I have revised my opinion on this. I now realise that unless people work on themselves by using a regular energy-cleansing routine and carrying out a self-treatment each day, plus working on their spiritual awareness and development, the Reiki channel does seem to get smaller, which affects the amount of flow. Energy meridians are, in this way, not dissimilar to a water pipe, which can become clogged by a build-up of residues on the inside, slowing down the flow. If the residues continue to accumulate and nothing is done to clean the pipe out, it could eventually become completely blocked.

I am convinced that this is one of the main reasons why, in Japan, students are encouraged to follow a daily spiritual practice and receive regular *Reiju* empowerments (see Part 5 on the Japanese tradition), not only to increase the amount of Reiki they can channel, but also to help to keep their energy channels free flowing. Reiki itself will cut through negative energy and other blockages, but it needs as clear a channel as possible to work effectively, and most of us have plenty of negative 'stuff' stored in our bodies. Some of this could possibly adhere to the Reiki channel as it is loosened and brought to the surface to be eliminated over the weeks, months and years of using Reiki. Negativity in the form of thoughts and emotions is pretty stubborn stuff!

Eventually, our energy channels can become really clean and free flowing, but how long this takes will depend upon how much 'baggage' we have been collecting during our lifetime(s); however, the process is ongoing and continuous. Having Reiki does not shield us forever from susceptibility to collecting negative thoughts and emotions. Our initial attunement starts the purification process, but afterwards we really need to continue with self-treatments, a sensible energy cleansing routine and spiritual practice, and, if possible, regular *Reiju* empowerments.

One of the main aspects which has been missing in the Reiki traditions in the West has been self-cleansing, and of course it is clear to us now that Dr Usui would have been well aware of the need for energetic cleansing because of his knowledge of martial arts, with the consequent emphasis on keeping the *Ki* healthy and free-flowing. With hindsight it is probably not surprising that he included in his healing system a number of techniques which are similar to those from the chi kung (*ki-kou*) traditions for energy raising and balancing.

TECHNIQUES FOR SELF-CLEANSING FROM THE JAPANESE TRADITION

In this chapter we cover self-cleansing techniques more commonly used in the Western Reiki traditions, but in Part 5 you will find several techniques for self-cleansing from the Japanese tradition, particularly *Hatsurei-ho* (pages 354–5), and a part of the *Hatsurei-ho*, called *Kenyoku-ho* but also known as Dry Brushing (pages 355–6), which can be used on its own as a way of brushing off negative energies. Another technique called the Reiki Shower (pages 333–6) floods your energy field with Reiki to cleanse and revitalise it. Essentially, any of these methods can be used as and when they are needed. If you are treating clients, however, I would suggest you carry out a full *Hatsurei-ho* before the first client and after the last client, and do the Dry Brushing technique or the Reiki Shower technique between each one, so please do read through Chapters 20 and 21 to discover more about these methods.

None of these techniques requires you to use the Reiki symbols, so anyone with any level of Reiki can use them; however, if you have Second Degree you can draw a Power Symbol over each hand before you start, *intending* that Reiki should flow to clear and cleanse your energy body, which can enhance the process.

WESTERN REIKI TECHNIQUES FOR SELF-CLEANSING

There are various techniques for self-cleansing which come from a variety of sources, mostly within the West, that you might like to try.

Cold showers

To cleanse your physical and energy bodies fully I recommend a cold shower. Yes, I know it might be an unpleasant thought, but it really works! **Note:** If you have any health condition that might make you particularly susceptible to shock from the cold water please ask your doctor before adding this technique to your cleansing routine.

In many Eastern cultures, cold water is believed to have a particularly vibrant cleansing energy, so when it flows through your energy field and over your physical body the 'shock' of it shakes loose the negative or 'sticky' energy that is trapped in and around your body. Although a warm or hot shower or bath is good for cleaning your physical body, and can also be very relaxing, it has the effect of expanding your aura. This can potentially make the negative, sticky energy enter further into your energy body so that it becomes harder to remove. This therefore means that it is important to *start* your shower with cold water rather than ending with it, which some people like to do to close the pores in the skin, although you can do *both* if you wish.

The important thing is to let the cold water flow over all your chakras, so that they are cleansed. You do not necessarily have to stand right under the showerhead with the cold water flowing over all of you at once, unless you want to, and you can wear a shower cap unless you want to wash your hair. Your crown chakra will still be cleansed by the water flowing over the cap. Also, it is only necessary to be under the cold water for about 10 to 15 seconds in total.

The parts that need the water to flow over them are all your major chakras at the front from the crown down to the root chakra and the same down the back, plus the minor chakras and major points on your meridian system, including your shoulders, elbows, wrists, hands, hips, knees, ankles and feet. You might find it easier to hold the showerhead in your hand and direct the water quickly, always in a downward flow – I usually start with my feet, just to get used to the temperature, then each arm (and under each arm) and down each side of the body. Then I let the water flow from the crown of my head down the centre of my back, and then from the crown down the front of my face, throat and body, finishing with both legs and feet again. As soon as this is accomplished, you can turn the water up to the nice, warm temperature you usually shower with, and I guarantee you will feel wonderfully clean, invigorated and refreshed.

If you don't have a shower in your home, you can buy shower attachments which will fit onto most bath taps, or you can use a jug: just fill the washbasin with cold water, stand in the bath, and pour the water over your chakras. Afterwards, you can fill the washbasin with comfortably hot water, to warm yourself up, although a vigorous towelling or wrapping yourself in a towelling robe will do the job too.

I recommend at least two cold showers a day – one in the morning, to wash off any negative energy you have picked up during the night (there are theories that at least a part of our spirit rises out of our body during our sleep, but even if this does not happen, any negative thoughts or dreams can 'pollute' our energy field). Then another one before bed, to wash off the negative 'stuff' we pick up during an average day – including the energetic residue of any arguments or disagreements, negative comments and thoughts from people we have met, even the misery and violence we have seen on a TV news programme. If you work in any of the caring professions or as a therapist, counsellor, or other profession where you are dealing with negative people, I would really recommend a cold shower as soon as you get in from work, otherwise the negative energy you have been absorbing all day from your clients will slowly seep into that nice, comfy chair into which you flop as soon as you get home. Much better to wash it all off, put on nice clean clothes and feel refreshed and ready to enjoy your evening.

If after reading this you suddenly think of all the negative energy that you must have brought into your home over the years – don't panic! There are suggested techniques to help you cleanse your environment in a later section.

Using Reiki with your normal cleansing routine

In addition to the above cold showers, I am sure you will continue with your usual cleansing routine – nice, relaxing hot baths and exhilarating hot showers are one of life's great pleasures, I think; however, to energetically cleanse yourself as well, you can draw the Power Symbol over the showerhead, or hold it in your hand and *intend* that Reiki flows into it, if you don't have Second Degree, so that as the water flows through it picks up Reiki to cleanse and heal you as you shower. You can also draw the Power Symbol over your bath water, before you step in (or when you are sitting in it, if you forget) or place your hands in the water and let the Reiki flow for about 10 seconds, if you don't have Second Degree, so that you are bathing in cleansing, healing water. Add a few drops of lavender oil, light some candles and you have the perfect remedial, relaxing retreat. (Remember, you should never leave a burning candle unattended.)

USING VISUALISATION FOR CLEANSING

Another way of energetic cleansing is to use your thought energy in a visualisation – when you consciously and deliberately imagine something. It isn't as effective as a cold shower (sorry, there's no getting away from that!) but it will help when a real shower isn't available, and it is also a gentle and relaxing thing to do. Here's one for you to try. You may find it useful to record this visualisation on a CD or tape, speaking slowly and rhythmically, in as relaxing a way as possible, or there are visualisation CDs I have recorded available from my website, www.reiki-quest.co.uk.

1 First, make yourself comfortable, either sitting or lying down, somewhere you can remain undisturbed for at least 20 minutes. Spend a few minutes tensing and then relaxing each group of muscles in turn, from your toes right up to your facial muscles. When you are fully relaxed, you are ready to go on to the next stage.

2 Close your eyes and concentrate on your breathing. Let your breathing become slower and deeper, and begin to count your in-breaths: 1 and 2 and 3 – let your breath come in as deeply as possible; 4 and 5 and 6 – make sure you are expelling every bit of air on each outbreath; 7 and 8 and 9 – your breathing is really deep and slow now; and 10 . . . let your breath out with an audible sigh, but continue breathing in this slow, deep way.

3 Now, I want you to imagine that you are standing on a path at the edge of a beautiful wood, and I want you to connect with all of your senses to bring this scene to life. You can feel the warmth of the sun on your skin, and feel a gentle breeze ruffling your hair. You can hear the leaves on nearby trees rustling in the breeze, and the songs of birds, too. Looking around you, you can see a beautiful blue sky, and the green of the grass, and the bright colours of flowers and butterflies. You can smell the sweet grass, and the breeze smells of pine and other woodland fragrances from the trees ahead. You can even imagine putting out your hand to touch a nearby leaf, or the bark of a tree.

4 Now begin to walk along the path into the wood, where the sun is streaming down through the trees, and as you walk, you hear the sound of running water, and the path seems to be leading you closer and closer to the sound.

5 Suddenly you come out of the trees into a sunlit glade, and at the far side of the glade is a beautiful waterfall, where the water runs into a deep blue pool that is surrounded by colourful flowers and long grasses. You walk towards the waterfall, and you feel the need to wash yourself clean in its sparkling water.

6 Quickly, you remove your clothing and step into the cool, sparkling water, letting it wash over your head and face and neck,

over your shoulders and arms and hands, over the front and back of your body and legs, feeling it cleanse you and refresh you.

7   When you feel really clean, you notice that the ribbons of water in the waterfall turn into ribbons of rainbow colour, and your body is washed with red, orange and yellow light, and then with green and blue and indigo and violet light. And, as the rainbow colours fade away, you walk out of the waterfall, and take a dip in the beautiful blue pool.

8   The water of the pool feels warm and relaxing, and it makes you feel playful, so you splash around for a few moments, enjoying the feel of the warm softness of the water.

9   Then, as you climb out of the pool, you find a pile of lovely fresh, clean clothes waiting for you, which you put on, and then you turn towards the waterfall and the pool again, and you acknowledge with thanks that you have been cleansed and purified, and with a little bow of gratitude, you turn and walk back along the path, towards the entrance to the wood where you first started.

10 When you reach the edge of the wood, you spend a few moments just experiencing again the warmth of the sun, the scent of pine and fresh grass, and the sight of the blue sky, enjoying it for a few moments longer.

11 Then the images begin to fade, and slowly your awareness begins to return, and you can sense again the chair or bed beneath you, and any sounds in the room. As your awareness fully returns, you can open your eyes, and you will be back in the room where you first began this visualisation, feeling peaceful, cleansed and refreshed.

TECHNIQUES FOR CLEANSING YOUR ENVIRONMENT

Where do you need to cleanse?

Because you can potentially pick up negative energies anywhere, then the answer should probably be 'everywhere', but obviously that isn't practical! Basically, you need to regularly clean and cleanse all the areas in which you spend any substantial amount of time, and for most people that means their home and their workplace, or at least their immediate surroundings at their place of work.

At home, the areas you need to concentrate on are the corners of each room, where negative or stagnant energy can collect, and places where you sit often, and especially where you sleep, so your bed and favourite chair are important. In the rest of this section I give a number of ideas on how to cleanse your environment, and you can try out any or all of them, and find which you prefer.

You can also minimise the amount of negative energy that is brought into your home, and one of the easiest ways is to remove your shoes (and ask guests to remove theirs) and leave them by the front (or back) door. This isn't just an attempt to avoid dust or dirt soiling your carpets (although that is an added benefit!), but negative energy tends to be dense and 'heavy', so it is generally thickest at ground level. This means that in areas where there are lots of people, especially paved areas such as city streets, shopping centres, supermarkets and so on, which have the greatest potential for being negative because of the numbers of people who use them, there is a layer of 'sticky' negative energy lying around at ground level. Therefore, when you walk in such areas, you are virtually wading through a 'soup' of negative energy that could attach itself to your shoes, so if you take them off by the door, you are limiting the effect of such negativity in your home.

One helpful way of getting rid of some of that negativity is to walk on a patch of natural earth – an area of grass would be ideal – *intending* that any negativity leaks back into the earth where it can be transformed and used, before you actually go back into your home. You can also stamp your feet vigorously a few times on a patch of grass, and this will help to shake loose much of the negative energy. It is also a particularly good idea not to have outdoor shoes in your bedroom, as you can be more susceptible to negative energies when you are asleep. Even better, would be to take off your shoes when you get home, and walk barefoot or in slippers straight to your bathroom and have a cold shower, thereby getting rid of all the rest of the negativity you've picked up during the day!

Using Reiki for clearing, cleansing and creating sacred space

You can use Reiki to clear, harmonise and protect any spaces you occupy, and the most effective way is to place Power symbols in each corner of each room, and on the floor and ceiling, and also on any furniture where you spend lots of time, such as your bed or favourite chair or sofa, your office desk and computer, or any other place you work, such as your taxi if you're a taxi driver. That could be pretty useful, as I would guess you might get quite a few negative passengers each day! Draw the Power Symbol, say its mantra to yourself three times, and imagine and *intend* that the whole area be filled with Reiki. If you don't have Second Degree, you can still use Reiki for cleansing. Just sit quietly, and visualise and *intend* that Reiki flows from your palms to clear and cleanse the area of any negative energy and fill the whole room with healing energy and light, perhaps imagining the light of Reiki flowing like a soft mist until it fills the whole space. You can then visualise the Reiki spreading like a white light until your whole home or office or workplace is filled with it. Over a period of weeks you will gradually sense a lighter and more peaceful feel as the Reiki peels away layer upon layer of negativity that has just been lying around for ages.

Don't limit your space clearing only to your home or workplace, though. Use Reiki to cleanse anywhere you spend time, such as your car, a hotel bedroom or anywhere else you are staying, from the spare bedroom in a friend's house to a caravan or holiday cottage, or even your cabin on a cruise liner!

Using sounds and scents for cleansing

Certain sound vibrations can have a cleansing effect, and a good way to use sound to cleanse rooms is to make 'noise' in the corners, to break up stagnant energy. This can be as simple as clapping your hands together firmly a few times, or you can bang on a drum, or use a Tibetan bell or singing bowl, for example. Your own voice can also be used, and 'toning' an 'om' is a good way to do this, but even shouting or singing loudly can work too – just have the *intention* that what you are doing is cleansing the area.

Scents are also vibrational, and you can use aromatherapy oils or incense sticks to help with cleansing. I find that a few drops each of lemon oil and lavender oil in water in an oil burner is the best for cleansing spaces, and the smell is both pleasant and refreshing. One or two lit incense sticks, wafted into the corners of the room, is another nice way of cleansing a space, and if you have Second Degree you can combine the lit incense sticks with drawing out the shape of the Power Symbol, *intending* that Reiki lightens and clears an area of all negative energies, which is an excellent cleansing technique.

The ceremonial use of smudge

Another way of using a combination of scent and smoke for cleansing is to use a smudge stick or smudge mix. 'Smudge' is the name given to a combination of herbs that the Native Americans use for cleansing physically and spiritually. The herbs most commonly used are sage (usually *Salvia apiana*, white sage), cedar (Western red cedar, *Thuja plicata*, or California incense cedar, *Calocedrus decurrens*) and sweetgrass (*Hierochloe odorata*). The sage is used to banish negative energies, cleanse and purify; the cedar is used to balance male–female energies, and sweetgrass is said to bring sweetness, beauty and forgiveness into one's life and surroundings. Occasionally, other herbs are included in the mix, such as lavender, to bring spiritual blessings, but it is best to avoid mixes that include juniper, as that can have contraindications for pregnant women.

The dried herbs can either be in a wand, where long strands of the herbs are tied into a bundle, or are available as a dried mix of seeds, leaves and small pieces. Sweetgrass is usually braided into a long plait, tied at each end. The ceremonial use of smudge involves setting light to the herbs so that they smoulder and produce a cleansing smoke, which is then wafted around the area which needs cleansing, or around and through a person's auric field. The wands are the easiest to deal with, as they catch light fairly quickly and smoulder for several minutes, which is usually enough time to waft the smoke into each corner and along each wall of a room.

To smudge someone, get them to stand with their arms held out at the sides, level with their shoulders, and take a smouldering smudge wand and, making sure you keep it 5–10cm (2–4in) away from their body to avoid burning them (or their clothes!), pass it over the top of the head and shoulders two or three times. Then pass the smudge wand along the top and underneath each arm, and then gracefully zigzag the smoke down the front of the face, body and legs, and then again at the back of the head, down the back of the body and legs, finally asking the person to lift one foot at a time, as you waft the smudge smoke under the sole of each foot. You may need to relight the smudge stick several times to keep it smoking.

To smudge yourself, the traditional way is to waft the smoke towards you using a large feather – preferably one that you have found specifically for that purpose. Hold the smouldering herb wand in one hand, and the feather in the other, and 'brush' the smoke towards you with the feather, from the top of your head down to your feet, and then waft the smoke over your shoulders so that it flows down your back. You can also do this under each arm, again making sure that you hold the smudge stick far enough away from your body so that it doesn't burn you or your clothes. I find this a very relaxing thing to do, and the smell is lovely, too! Many people can really notice the difference in their energy field after smudging – it feels light and clear, and this often has an energising effect, so it's good to do this in the morning, or whenever you're facing a difficult task, for instance. But, for safety, do remember when you've finished smudging to put out the smudge – putting it into a metal container like a saucepan with a lid is the easiest and safest way, as when it is starved of oxygen it will go out quite quickly.

The self-cleansing and environmental clearing techniques in this chapter are excellent ways of keeping your energy body clear so that Reiki can flow through you more effectively, and ideally you can integrate them into your daily Reiki practice. In the next chapter we look at how important the spiritual aspects of Reiki are for your development.

Chapter 16

The Importance of Spiritual Development

As we know, the roots of Reiki as it is practised today began in Japan and came from a Buddhist tradition, and there will be more information about this in Part 5. Therefore, with its lineage based in the Mystery Schools of the East, Reiki is also a spiritual discipline – a tool to encourage personal and spiritual awareness and growth, and to develop a more spiritual and meaningful way of life. But, unlike most other spiritual disciplines it doesn't take years of study and dedication before you are granted access to it. Anyone can take Reiki, at least at First Degree or *Shoden* level, regardless of their age, gender, nationality, spiritual background or beliefs, because Reiki is not a religion and, despite its Buddhist origins, it can fit into anyone's spiritual practices.

The attunement to Reiki starts a process that continues throughout life: a process of slowly raising awareness of our life purpose, of what we are here to achieve and how we can achieve it. This is working on a very subtle level, and many people who don't use Reiki regularly on themselves are unaware of it. But Reiki works as a catalyst for change, bringing to the surface those aspects of life that are blocking our spiritual progress. Sometimes this can seem a challenging process, but it is always beneficial, as Reiki is Divinely guided and always works for our highest and greatest good. By this I mean that Reiki helps to bring forward in our lives what we *need*, but of course that is not necessarily always what we *want*. We still have a choice, however, because Reiki respects our right to free will.

The more you use Reiki and the more you progress by taking further training and experiencing more attunements, the more the Reiki is able to clear your energy channels and the easier it becomes for Reiki to raise your energetic vibrations to the next appropriate level. This effectively raises your consciousness, so that your connection with your Soul/Higher Self becomes closer and therefore its guidance becomes more easily accessible to you. You may feel guided to meditate more, to explore aspects of spirituality that had not previously interested you. You may feel the need to let go of restrictions in your life that are stifling your personal and spiritual development. This might mean a real urge to change your job, see less of certain friends, take more time for yourself despite family commitments or even end a relationship that has become unhealthy or oppressive.

In addition to using Reiki, in this chapter we examine various other ways in which you can work on your personal growth and spiritual development, including meditation, visualisation, and working with spirit guides and angels, but first we take a look at the tenets which Dr Usui believed would help his students to progress spiritually – the Reiki Principles.

THE REIKI PRINCIPLES

Dr Usui identified a need to help his students with their personal and spiritual development, so he adopted a set of Reiki Principles, sometimes called the Reiki Ideals or the Reiki Precepts. You will find further information about their Japanese origins in Chapter 20. There are several versions of the Reiki Principles commonly used in the West, but the most familiar are these two:

From The Reiki Alliance and some independent Reiki Masters:

> *Just for today do not anger*
> *Just for today do not worry*
> *Honour your parents, teachers and elders*
> *Earn your living honestly*
> *Give thanks to every living thing.*

From The Radiance Technique (set up by Dr Barbara Weber Ray):

Just for today I will let go of anger
Just for today I will let go of worry
Today I will count my many blessings
Today I will do my work honestly
Today I will be kind to every living creature.

The Western versions are obviously all based on what Mrs Takata taught, but recently discovered forms in Japan, when translated, are also very similar. The following is a quote from a translation of part of Dr Usui's memorial:

> *When it comes to teaching, first let the student understand well the Meiji Emperor's admonitory, then in the morning and in the evening let them chant and have in mind the five admonitions which are:*
>
> > *Do not get angry today*
> > *Do not be grievous*
> > *Express your thanks*
> > *Be diligent in your business*
> > *Be kind to others.*

You can see that there is some disparity – for example 'honour your parents, teachers and elders' does not appear to be in the Japanese version, so it may have been something which Mrs Takata instituted, but because it is so familiar to many Reiki people I have included it in the following section.

LIVING WITH THE REIKI PRINCIPLES TODAY

Although Usui asked his students to live by these Principles more than 90 years ago, they are as relevant to Reiki students – and others – today. Working more closely with the Reiki Principles is a valuable part of the spiritual discipline of Reiki, absorbing them into your everyday life so that they become an ordinary aspect of living. Using meditation and the Reiki symbols will help you to develop an even deeper understanding of their meanings.

Just for today – living in the present

One of the most important aspects of the above principles is the phrase 'Just for today'; living in the moment and being aware of what is going on around you, forces you to live in the present, in the Now, which is the only time over which you have any control. Living in the present gives opportunities for appreciation and wonderment, for truly experiencing whatever you are doing at any given moment. It is a Buddhist precept – being mindful. In other words, having your mind right here, right now, not allowing your thoughts to wander into memories of time gone by or imaginings of time to come.

Just for today, do not anger

Anger is such a destructive emotion, and often we use it against those people we care about the most, so it hurts us as much as it hurts them. Anger is often generated when someone or something fails to meet our expectations – or even more importantly when we don't come up to our own expectations. But anger rarely achieves anything other than to make you and others feel bad. Anger is actually a conscious choice, a habitual response you have developed, so you have probably been reacting in a similar way to similar circumstances for years, but you can break that cycle and choose a different response instead. Then you can choose not to be angry – just for today. Use Reiki and meditation to help you to develop forgiveness and understanding of yourself and others.

Just for today, do not worry

Worry is linked with our fear of the future and the unknown, and is our usual response to a 'what if' scenario – to something that might occur, but which nine times out of ten does not. Worrying is another habit we get into, yet no matter how much of it you do, the worrying itself will never achieve anything or change anything. Whatever problem or situation you are worried about – even issues such as serious health problems – if there is some action you can take to improve matters, then take it, but if there is nothing you can do about it, then there is really no other option than to 'let go and let flow'. Doing Reiki on yourself can help you to achieve a less anxious and more positive frame of mind.

Although we continue to struggle and strive to control a situation, we are just creating an energy cycle which makes things worse – *'what you resist, persists'* – whereas when we let go and stop worrying about the situation, something good often comes along to sort it out. That 'good' may be a person, some useful advice, a new form of treatment or just the amount of money you need. It is amazing how often just the right thing turns up. So you can choose not to worry – just for today. Use Reiki and meditation to help you discover and calm your fears, and to develop hope and trust.

Be kind to others – honour your parents, teachers and elders

This doesn't just mean honouring and being kind to older people! It really means that we should honour, respect and be kind to *everyone*, because they all play a part in our lives – partners, friends, neighbours, colleagues, children, shop assistants, bus drivers – in fact, every person we meet under any circumstances. All the people with whom you interact throughout your life are your teachers, whether you love them or loathe them, and every interaction is a potential learning experience, because from a soul perspective all experiences, pleasant or unpleasant, contribute to the soul's growth and development.

And of course, there is a saying 'what goes around, comes around', so as you honour, respect and are kind to other people, they will do the same for you, too. Therefore, it is important to honour and respect everyone you meet and value *yourself* for the important difference *you* make to the Universe too. Use Reiki and meditation to connect with the people who have been important in your life so far, to help to heal any past hurts or misunderstandings and to permeate all your future communications. All people, animals, birds, insects and plants – and even the planet itself – have a vital role to play and should therefore be valued, respected and treated with kindness. So, just for today, honour and be kind to every living creature – including yourself.

Be grateful/show appreciation/count your blessings

We need to value and appreciate many things in our lives and to be grateful for our many blessings; however, sometimes we need to recognise those blessings first, because if life is a struggle and if we are going through a 'bad patch', this colours our view of life until we assume that everything in life is bad. Even when we are happy and healthy we are often not aware of it and take it very much for granted. Yet most of us are living very good lives, even if they aren't perfect.

Take time out of every day just to stand and stare at the beauty of a flower or the happiness of a child at play. Develop an awareness of life and what it means to live it. Of course there will be ups and downs, happiness and sadness, but every experience is valuable because it helps to make you who you are. So, just for today give thanks for your many blessings. The world is a wonderful place in which to live a physical life, so use Reiki and meditation to help you to develop an 'attitude of gratitude' to discover and trust in the abundance of the Universe and to develop your own belief in your deservingness of love, beauty, peace and anything else you need or desire.

Earn your living honestly/devote yourself to your work

Earning a living in this sense means all types of work, from paid employment or voluntary work to everyday tasks, like housework and cooking a meal for ourselves or our families. We often confuse what we *do* with who we *are*, taking our sense of identity from the kind of job we have – or do not have. What we need to remember is that we are human *beings*, not human *doings*! We are *all* valuable and special; every life, every person has a role to play in the whole and we all impact on each other in many different ways, so it is important to respect any work that we have chosen for ourselves and honour ourselves by doing our best to create a feeling of satisfaction in it.

All work is valuable to the extent that we choose to value it, so take satisfaction from even the simplest tasks, and do everything to the best of your ability. Also, Dr Usui's intention with Reiki was that it should be a tool for spiritual growth, so this Principle is about working towards personal growth and spiritual development each day with Reiki, and perhaps also with meditation, energy cleansing, reading self-help books, and so on. Remember that *you* are your life's work!

There is an old Zen Buddhist saying:

> *Before enlightenment, chop wood, carry water;*
> *After enlightenment, chop wood, carry water.*

No matter how spiritual your life may become, you will still need to work in some manner to feed yourself, clothe yourself, keep yourself warm and live comfortably. Doing your work honestly also means being honest with yourself, as well as with others – it means accepting yourself for who you are. So, just for today, do your work honestly. Use Reiki and meditation to discover your life's purpose, so that you can *live* what you *love*.

As Reiki begins to fill your life, you will start to feel more and more connected to 'All That Is'. As your consciousness is raised, you become more aware that every living thing is a part of you, and that you are a part of it and that everything is a part of the Divine, God, the Source, or whatever you choose to call it. The realisation will come that there is no place for prejudice, judgementalism, cruelty or indifference in a world where we are all connected, all a part of the whole, all One. (You will find more about the Reiki Principles and how to live with them in today's busy world in my book *Living the Reiki Way*.)

WHAT IS MEDITATION?

Incorporating meditation into your daily routine can be a simple and effective way of enhancing your personal growth and spiritual development. Meditation is an altered state of consciousness that results in a deeply relaxed state of being that can be used to either increase or decrease your awareness of the world around you; however, people sometimes worry about whether they can meditate, because they have heard that you need to empty your mind, and maybe also that it has to be done with your legs crossed in the lotus position. Neither supposition is true! Firstly, it isn't really possible to completely empty your mind – we all have about 60,000 thoughts crossing our mind each day – but it *is* possible to quieten your mind by using one of the methods below.

Secondly, the lotus position isn't a requirement, although if you can do it, that's fine, but it is best to meditate with your back straight and your shoulders relaxed, so sitting upright in a comfortable chair, or on the floor, if you prefer, is ideal.

In all forms of meditation there is some sort of focus that aims at first simply to reduce and eventually to eliminate the chatter of daily life and the stresses of the environment in which we live, providing a haven within which we are free to connect with our inner being. It helps us to overcome the problems and illusions we create for ourselves and which we allow others to create for us, and it also helps us to overcome those habits that we have formed which hold us back. Meditation allows us to go beyond the everyday into who we really are. The art of focusing and awareness of being in the moment changes brain activity, which leads to an opening up of ourselves to the joy of the Universe. There are many methods of meditation, including:

- Chanting or singing using repeated simple phrases or mantras – such as chanting the Reiki symbols' mantras.

- Meditation on symbols (such as a cross), icons (such as a picture of Jesus or the Buddha) or mandalas (beautiful circular designs) – or, of course, the Reiki symbols.

- Meditation on the four elements – earth, air, fire and water (this occurs in both Eastern and Western spiritual traditions).

- Meditation with sound, such as Tibetan gongs or the sounds of nature.

- Guided meditation, usually called visualisation, which takes you on an inner journey into your deeper self.

All methods of meditation are equally valid, so you might wish to try out a few in your search for the one that fits you the best, or you may find that a combination of forms of meditation is the way for you to develop. You can start by finding somewhere quiet and comfortable where you will not be disturbed so that you can sit or lie still for a while. It is best to have your spine straight, as this aligns the chakras and enables your *Ki* to flow properly, and you might like to have one or two candles lit and burn some incense or relaxing essential oils. (Remember, you should never leave a burning candle or incense unattended.)

When you are ready, just centre yourself by beginning to breathe deeply and evenly, and allow your whole body to relax. Sometimes this is best achieved by tensing your muscles first and then letting them go, starting with your feet and legs, then the trunk of your body, your shoulders and arms, and finally your neck, face and head. Allow yourself to fall into a slow, regular pattern of breathing (in through your nose, and out through your mouth) and then begin to count each in-breath 1, 2, 3 and so on up to 9. After the ninth breath return to 1, 2, 3 and up to 9 again, continuing like this for about five minutes. When you are more used to meditating, you can continue for much longer, but five minutes, twice a day, is a good way to start. Once you have established a habit of meditation, you can try other methods, until you find one or two that you like. If you look in your local newspapers or on the internet, there are often groups advertising meditation classes or there are plenty of books and CDs available on the subject, so if it is not something you are familiar with, do give it a try.

Here is a beautiful meditation for you to try, which was given to me by my friend and fellow Reiki Master, Helen Galpin. It engenders a wonderful feeling of peace, and spreads a loving and forgiving energy to the people and the world around you, so it is ideal as a spiritual practice every day.

Blessing meditation

1   Sit in a quiet place, close your eyes and focus on your breath, and imagine that you are breathing in a wonderful golden light, and that this light is cleansing and healing as it moves through your body.

2   When you are ready, move your hands into *Gassho* (prayer position), and say the following aloud, quietly. Begin with your own name, and then say:

> *'I bless you*
> *I honour you*
> *I love you*
> *I bless you.'*

3   Now, slowly go through all the people you are closely connected with. Start with all the members of your family, one by one, and then your friends and work colleagues, and anyone else who pops into your mind. For each person, speak the words, and feel the words:

> *'I bless you*
> *I honour you*
> *I love you*
> *I bless you.'*

4   When you are ready, lower your hands so that they are open in front of your heart, with your palms facing upwards.

5   Say out loud all the places on Earth that you feel might need healing, such as areas where there are wars, or where there have been natural disasters, and then say:

> *'I bless you*
> *I honour you*
> *I love you*
> *I bless you.*
> *I hold this love, peace, healing and light in*
> *my hands for you, and I share it with you.'*

Feel the words as you speak them, and sit for a while feeling and sharing the healing and love.

6   Next, imagine the Earth in your hands, our wonderful blue planet, and say out loud:

> *'I bless you*
> *I honour you*
> *I love you*
> *I bless you.*
> *I hold this love, peace, healing and light in*
> *my hands for you, and I share it with you.'*

7   When you are ready, place your hands on your lap and sit for a while in the wonderful healing energy you have created.

8   Finish by placing your hands in *Gassho*, and give thanks.

WHAT IS VISUALISATION?

In visualisations you either consciously and deliberately imagine something, like the visualisation used in the Mental–Emotional Treatment in Chapter 11, or you allow your Soul/Spirit/Higher Self to influence your mind and present you with new ideas and new concepts, or a different way of looking at things. Often we will encounter a long-forgotten object, or smell something that reminds us of a special time, or hear someone say a particular word which jogs us out of our limited realities and allows our mind to go somewhere else – a state we might describe as 'daydreaming', which is another 'altered state of consciousness'. Visualisation is a more structured, supportive and effective vehicle for doing this, and it is easier to do than you might think.

When you begin visualisations you may have an expectation that you should 'see' things very vividly, but few people do. As an exercise, close your eyes and try to remember what your bedroom looks like. Can you 'see' how the furniture is arranged? Do you 'know' what colour the curtains are? That's visualising! At first you might see only part of an image or see it for only a few moments and find that the 'seeing' is more a 'knowing' what is there or imagining what is there, or it may be a feeling or even appear in words. All of these 'sensings' are valid parts of visualisation. With practice, the more often you take yourself on visual journeys the more the focus of what you 'see' will become clearer, more defined and more definite.

There are many CDs available of visualisations or guided meditations, and my particular favourites are those by Gill Edwards detailed in Further Reading, and I have also produced a number of CDs of meditations and visualisations that are particularly relevant to Reiki practice – see my website www.reiki-quest.co.uk for details. Of course, you can make up your own CDs or tapes, or just let your mind lead you where it wants you to go. Choose a beautiful place to imagine to start with, such as a sunlit glade in a forest or a sandy bay with the sound of gentle waves in the background, and then just 'go with the flow' and enjoy it.

Working with guides and angels in visualisations

Some people feel called to work with angels and spirit guides (or aspects of their Soul/Spirit/Higher Self which they choose to call guides and angels) when they do Reiki, either actually when they are using the healing energy or when they are meditating, perhaps even sensing their presence around them as a form of energy. If you wish to call upon angelic beings or guides during healing, then include them in your initial intent and invocation when you start to use the Reiki, asking your angel or guide to help you with the healing work you are about to do, and please remember to thank them afterwards. You can also connect with a spirit guide or angel in a visualisation, and there are many ways of doing this. You can ask and *intend* at the beginning of a visualisation to meet a guide or guardian angel, and then imagine yourself meeting them in a forest glade, or on top of a spiritual mountain, for example.

If you have Second Degree, you can enhance that connection by using the Reiki symbols. There follows a very powerful connection meditation I have devised, which I hope you will enjoy trying out. (This is also available on one of my CDs.)

A visualisation to meet an angel or guide

1 Make sure you are sitting or lying comfortably where you will not be disturbed for at least 20 minutes, and then allow your body to relax, centring yourself by breathing deeply and evenly for a few minutes.

2 Then protect yourself for your visual journey to the spiritual realms by imagining a Power Symbol in front of you and another Power Symbol behind you and on each side.

3 Draw or imagine a Distant Symbol, silently saying its mantra three times, and sending it like a bridge or rainbow up to the spiritual realms.

4 Then imagine yourself walking over that bridge, and draw or imagine a Harmony Symbol flowing across in front of you, silently saying its mantra three times to harmonise your energies with the higher vibrations of the spiritual dimension.

5 Now see or sense your guide or angel coming to meet you. You might see them as beings or as beautiful light, or just sense their loving presence.

6 Let your guide or angel lead you to a place where you can communicate with them, and ask your guide or angel to provide you with helpful insights on any problems, difficulties or questions you have at this time. Give yourself plenty of time to experience this.

7 After the communication has finished, your guide or angel will lead you back to the start of your Distant Symbol bridge and may give you a sign or a gift to take back with you to the physical realms.

8 When you are about to leave, thank your guide or angel for their loving help and inspiration, and turn, taking any gift or

sign with you, and walk back along the Distant Symbol bridge to the place where you are sitting or lying.

9 In your imagination, withdraw the Distant Symbol bridge or rainbow, and then go over in your mind what you saw or experienced, including examining and trying to interpret the significance of the sign or gift you were given.

10 Spend some time just doing Reiki on yourself, and meditate on the insights or inspiration you have received.

REINCARNATION, KARMA AND HEALING PAST LIVES

Our Soul/Spirit/Higher Self is that part of us which is directly connected to God/Goddess/All That Is. The soul is spiritual energy, and just as everything else in the Universe is energy, once that energy has been created it can only be transformed, not destroyed. Therefore the soul energy, which is the core of our being, is eternal, and it grows and develops through its experiences during each incarnation. When the physical matter, which has been its body during a single life, wears out and expires, the soul moves on, eventually reincarnating into another body with which to experience physical life.

This is where the expression 'past lives' comes from. Each of us alive on the planet today has probably had hundreds, if not thousands, of physical lives as humans, and we may have had some lives as other species too, such as animals or birds, and so on. Some people believe these can occur between episodes of human life, whereas others believe they were at a time before our individual soul energy started to live human lives.

There is also a belief in the East that during every incarnation each soul gathers Karma, meaning that the sum of a person's actions in previous states of existence decide his or her fate in future existences. Each good thought or action is said to build up a bank of positive Karma, and each bad thought or deed builds up a debt of negative Karma, which then has to be worked out or repaid during many subsequent lives until that soul achieves Enlightenment.

In-between lives, or when the soul has evolved sufficiently so that it no longer needs to experience physical life, it can still have a connection to the physical by acting as a spirit guide. This is a soul energy existing in another dimension, often referred to as the etheric or spiritual realms, whose remit is to help humanity with guidance, inspiration, healing and so on, which is channelled through a human; however, some people believe that such spiritual guidance comes from aspects of our own infinite Soul/Higher Self which are always connected to the God-consciousness/All That Is, so that the collected wisdom of the whole Universe is always available to us, if we choose to seek it.

PAST-LIFE HEALING TECHNIQUES

If you believe in reincarnation and past lives, you might like to try these two past-life healing techniques. Method A can be used after First Degree, but Method B requires the use of the symbols.

Method A

Write on a piece of paper that you wish to heal any negative Karma you may have collected in past lives. Hold this paper between your hands for about ten minutes, and *intend* that Reiki should flow into those past lives for the highest and greatest good. You can repeat this exercise any number of times, until you intuitively feel that the healing has been successfully carried out.

Method B

This technique is one I have developed which can produce some very powerful healing and is probably best done during meditation. (Please remember to say each symbol's mantra to yourself three times each time you use it.)

1 Make sure you are sitting or lying comfortably where you will not be disturbed for at least 20 minutes, and then allow your body to relax, centring yourself by breathing deeply and evenly for a few minutes.

2 Start by asking your spirit guides and angels to help to heal any past life (or lives) that may be producing Karma for you in this life. Those angels or spirit guides who will help you with this task may appear to you in your imagination or you may simply sense their presence.

3 Then protect yourself by imagining a Power Symbol in front of you and imagine another Power Symbol behind you and on each side.

4 Now visualise connecting to that life on a bridge made by the Distant Symbol, and send the Harmony Symbol and the Power Symbol ahead of you as you imagine yourself walking over the bridge.

5 Visualise yourself standing on the threshold of that life and, knowing that you are protected by your guides, angels and Reiki, ask to be shown in a form that is easy for you to understand any insights which might be helpful to you now in your present life. Give yourself some time to 'see' those aspects of a past life (or lives) that are affecting you now.

6 Then *intend* that Reiki produce deep healing in that life (or lives), healing any Karmic wounds in yourself and in any people whom you affected in that life, for the highest and greatest good.

7 Then, thanking your guides and angels for their help, turn and walk back across the Distant Symbol bridge and step off, turning back to face the bridge.

8 Send a Power Symbol across the bridge to seal in the healing, and then imagine the Distant Symbol drawing back and getting smaller or fading until it disappears, so that it no longer connects you with that life.

9 Next, draw a Power Symbol again in front of you to cleanse and clear the energies.

10 Finally, put one hand up in the air and bring it down forcefully in front of your body, like a Karate chop, to finally sever any further links with that life's Karma. Heal the cut with another Power Symbol, love and light.

11 Give yourself some Reiki for about ten minutes, and don't worry if you feel very emotional, as this is quite normal. Allow those feelings to wash over you and then let them go, releasing the emotions with gratitude for the lessons they have helped you to learn.

LIFE-LONG HEALING

You can therefore incorporate Reiki into all aspects of your life, using Reiki for your physical, mental, emotional and spiritual well-being. Reiki can lead you towards a deeper, more meaningful and fulfilling life. Reiki is an energy, a tool for healing, a vehicle for learning and a catalyst for change. It contains unlimited love, joy, peace, compassion, wisdom, abundance and even more. Reiki is the Divine love and light that powers the whole Universe; it is a gift of incredible power and sometimes daunting complexity, but Reiki is available to everyone when they are ready to take that next, exciting step on their spiritual journey.

For some people, that next step is to become a professional Reiki Practitioner, and that is what we deal with in the next chapter.

Chapter 17

Becoming a Practitioner

Becoming a Reiki Practitioner can be a rewarding and interesting step to take, but if you are considering it, you need to know the latest requirements for professional practice in the UK, and in other countries if you practise elsewhere. In Britain there are now National Occupational Standards (NOS) for Reiki Practitioners who are offering Reiki treatments to the public. (It is not necessary to comply with these requirements if you only use Reiki to treat yourself, family and friends.) The NOS give guidance on the minimum levels of knowledge and understanding required, and they are appropriate for all styles and types of Reiki. There is also a Core Curriculum, which covers what should be included in a Reiki Practitioner's training before they can be accepted for inclusion in the National Register of Reiki Practitioners (currently held by the GRCCT – General Regulatory Council for Complementary Therapies). I cover all of this in depth in my book *The Reiki Manual*, but I will try to summarise the essentials in this chapter.

THE CORE CURRICULUM

Most Reiki Masters cover the basics of what you need to know about how to treat other people in their Reiki 1 and Reiki 2 courses, but few, if any, will offer the full range of what is required by the Core Curriculum, so you will probably have to 'add on' other training to cover the rest. The main recommendations from the Reiki Council are:

- Potential professional Reiki Practitioners (which can be at either Reiki 1 or Reiki 2) should carry out 75 full treatments (in person), which should be properly recorded on each client's treatment record card, and five of these need to be supervised by someone occupationally competent in Reiki; for example, an experienced and qualified Reiki Practitioner.

- The training period for potential registrants from beginning to completion of the required elements should be a minimum of nine months.

- The training should include at least 45 hours' in-person (that is, face-to-face contact) learning.

- The total training hours should be a minimum of 140. This should be made up of in-person training and distance learning (using manuals, DVDs, emails, telephone conversations, and so on) as follows:

	In-person	Distance	Total
Reiki – theory and practice	15	35	50
Practitioner skills	20	40	60
Practice management	10	20	30
Total	**45**	**95**	**140**

It will also be necessary to complete a minimum of 12 hours' CPD (continuing professional development) each year after registration, at least six hours of which should be Reiki specific (see pages 296–7).

In terms of fulfilling the requirements, a normal two-day Reiki 1 course probably takes about 14 hours, and will cover in that time probably much of the Reiki theory and practice you need, plus some practitioner skills, and a Reiki 2 course of a similar length will cover more Reiki theory and practitioner skills, and possibly some information about practice management. You can see that you would still be short of the necessary hours of in-person training, and would not at that stage have covered any of the distance learning – and if your Reiki 1 and 2 courses had been only one day each, you would need quite a lot of additional training hours to comply. It should also be noted that distant attunements would not be considered sufficient – you do need to attend at least one course where the Reiki Master is present; however, other 'in-person' training could be less formal, such as attending 'Reiki Share' evenings, where a Reiki Master gives some instruction.

This might look really daunting, but it doesn't have to be, as some Reiki Masters will offer 'top up' courses and pre- or post-course distance learning materials, and organisations such as the UK Reiki Federation also put on additional workshops, plus your local college might have suitable courses that you could join for topics such as first aid, anatomy and physiology, health and safety, or how to run a business.

THE NATIONAL OCCUPATIONAL STANDARDS

These were developed through a process of discussion and consultation between the RRWG (now the Reiki Council) and Skills for Health, the UK's health sector Skills Council. They outline the minimum knowledge and understanding you need in order to fulfil your obligations as a professional Reiki Practitioner. They currently cover three main areas of practice, two of which are common to all complementary therapies:

1 **CNH1** Explore and establish the client's needs for complementary and natural healthcare.
2 **CNH2** Develop and agree plans for complementary and natural healthcare with clients.
3 **CNH12** Provide Reiki to clients.

The relevant knowledge, training and experience you need can be roughly divided into the following topic areas:

Knowledge of Reiki: What style of Reiki you practise, including its history and your lineage, what 'healing' is, how to carry out self-treatments and treatments on others, and how to provide Reiki to clients, including preparation, initial discussions, after-treatment advice, and when it would be inappropriate to give Reiki.

Anatomy and physiology: Basic knowledge of the skeletal structure, the functions and locations of major organs, common illnesses, and the ability to identify 'red flag' symptoms and notifiable diseases.

Communicating with clients: Basic understanding of verbal, non-verbal and written communication, such as discussing a client's needs, questioning and listening skills, interpreting body language, plus writing information in client records.

Practice management: Providing suitable premises and equipment, being aware of health-and-safety needs, appropriate pricing, marketing and publicity, making appointments and keeping records, and looking after yourself.

Professional standards, ethics and codes of practice: Dealing with all clients ethically, respectfully and professionally, understanding the need for integrity and confidentiality, and creating good therapist–client relationships.

Legal requirements: Complying with all relevant laws, including discrimination (age, religion and beliefs, disability, gender, race, sexual orientation), working with minors or vulnerable adults, not diagnosing or offering medical advice, health, safety and security legislation, data protection legislation, financial and other record keeping requirements, insurance requirements, advertising and marketing restrictions, complaints procedures and restrictions on treating animals.

GETTING STARTED AS A PRACTITIONER

Hopefully, you haven't been put off by all of the above requirements! In essence they are just intended to make sure that all Reiki Practitioners are properly trained so that they are able to give clients a really good experience. Another benefit is that this helps to make the practice of Reiki more professional and therefore better respected by the general public and by other health professionals.

Initially, it is probably best to begin in a small way, integrating your practice into your life slowly, perhaps by doing treatments one or two evenings a week. That way you can start building up a regular client base and find out if you really enjoy it. First, though, it is sensible to get plenty of practice and experience with family and friends because any potential clients will expect you to know what you are doing, and if you feel unsure so will they. Another

reason is because the more you practise the better able you will
be to understand and detect subtle energies and to give each individual client what they need. Although it is possible to become a
Reiki Practitioner after Reiki 1, there are obvious advantages in
waiting until you have acquired the additional skills taught at Reiki
2; I would then recommend at least six months of regular treatments on family and friends before setting up in business to take
clients on a professional basis. A target to aim for in the six months
would be to have carried out as many of the requisite 75 treatments
as you can, making sure you keep proper written records of each,
and these should be spread among as wide a variety of people as
possible. Ten or 20 treatments on one person doesn't actually give
you much varied experience. Also, ask your friends and family to
give you some honest feedback, because this information will be
really valuable to ensure you treat clients well right from the start.

What is important, however, is that you develop – and stick to –
your own high standards of behaviour and professional practice,
ensuring that you do everything you can to treat people politely,
sensitively and with great care and attention. You should also
ensure that each client has as comfortable and comforting an experience as possible, so you will need to pay attention to the environment you are providing as well as to the way in which you talk to
the client before and after the treatment, and the way you carry out
the treatment itself.

Where to set up your practice

To start your practice in a small way it is sensible to use your own
home, but it is much better if you have a room you can set aside for
the purpose, so that it can always be kept clean and tidy. Of course,
you can set up a treatment couch in your living room, but it tends
not to give you such a professional feel, and if you share your living
space with other people this could be tricky; however, you will need
to check the legal position regarding working from home or the
change of use of one of the rooms. Also, your household insurance
may have to change or there may be clauses in your mortgage or
rental agreements that have to be complied with.

An alternative is to take your therapy couch to clients' homes and
treat them there. This does have the advantage that the client will
probably feel comfortable within their own environment, but you
need to check whether the space is suitable. Cramped conditions,

children or dogs running around, telephones ringing or babies crying while you are trying to perform a soothing, relaxing Reiki treatment would be awful! Another alternative is to hire a room, perhaps in a nearby complementary health clinic, but you would need plenty of clients to make this financially worthwhile. One of the most important considerations for locating your treatment room, though, is how it feels energetically. Even when they have been cleansed with Reiki some places just don't feel right, so let yourself be guided by your intuition on this matter. If you really want to work full-time as a Practitioner, you will need to do some market research in the locality where you want to set up to find out if there is a large enough market there for you to make a worthwhile profit.

Setting-up costs and legal responsibilities

For a Reiki Practitioner there are relatively few things you need, but it obviously looks more professional if you have a proper therapy couch; a portable couch is more adaptable for giving treatments at your own venue, or at a client's home, and you can fold it up and store it away when you're not using it. You will also need pillows, pillowcases, stretch-towelling sheets and one or two soft blankets, which you may already have.

You will need to be adequately insured to practise, so you must have public liability insurance, public indemnity insurance and, if you employ anyone else, employee liability insurance as well. It is good practice to have these certificates available or even discreetly displayed somewhere in your therapy room. Insurance can usually be obtained at a reasonable cost through an umbrella organisation such as the UK Reiki Federation or The Reiki Association, and it is possible to get reduced rates when you are still training. (Check with your initiating Master for similar organisations if you live and practise in other countries.) Another cost to bear in mind is anything you may decide to do to market your business, such as newspaper advertising or leaflets.

Don't forget that when you are in business you are legally responsible for keeping adequate records, because you will have to calculate how much tax to pay. Accounts don't have to be difficult. A simple two-column system of income and expenditure will suffice, where you write down everything you receive on one side and all the money you have spent in running the business on the other. Keep all your receipts and other paperwork regarding your business, such as bank statements, cheque stubs, credit- and debit-card statements, invoices, gift vouchers and so on – you are legally required to keep these for seven years in the UK; you will need to check the requirements if practising in another country.

What to Charge

You need to find out what other therapists charge in your area – not just for Reiki but for other therapies like reflexology and massage – because this will give you an idea about what price you can ask. This will also depend upon whether you have to pay for the hire of a room, or whether you are treating people in your own home or theirs – but in the latter case, remember it should cover your transport costs, too. But don't fall into the trap of thinking that if you undercut all the other local therapists, you will start to attract their clients. Firstly that is unfair (and will probably make you unpopular in a community which might otherwise be a good support for you); secondly it indicates that you do not value Reiki – or yourself – enough to charge a sensible price; and thirdly people may assume that as you charge less you might not be as good as the others.

Some people get very bothered by charging for Reiki treatments, but money is simply a convenient form of exchange, and if all you do is give and give and give you are putting other people under some form of obligation. Most of us have a well-developed sense of what is fair, and it can make us feel uncomfortable if we are always on the receiving end of someone's altruism. Another side of this question is that sometimes when healing is given freely people will take advantage of the healer, calling on their services constantly and expecting to be treated at almost any time regardless of any other commitments the healer may have. Essentially, this means they have 'dumped' the problem on the healer, so they don't have to take any responsibility for their own healing. This is one of the reasons why paying money for a treatment, even if it is only a small amount, actually gets them involved and builds a sense of commit-ment to taking part in their own healing.

Healing, intrinsically, is freely given. Reiki energy flows regard-less of any financial reward. But you deserve to be paid for your time – you would be in any other job – and to be recompensed adequately for the time, effort and money you have put into training and practising and setting up your equipment and premises. The principle is really that we should value ourselves, and learning to accept money in exchange for Reiki is a part of that valuing. Lots of people find it much easier to give than to receive, so there is a meaningful lesson to learn in setting charges for Reiki treatments. The first time you ask for money can feel a bit strange, but it can be a very important step in establishing self-worth. If you still feel awkward about this, then by all means give some of your time for 'free' treatments – perhaps helping out in a hospice or a nursing home for the elderly – but to be professional about your business you must set proper charges and stick to them.

MARKETING YOUR BUSINESS

To get your business off to a good start – and to keep it going – you will need to do at least a small amount of marketing, to make sure that people know where you are and what you do. There are lots of ways of bringing your services to the attention of other people.

Advertising

Placing advertising in local newspapers or other publications is quite expensive and rarely worthwhile unless it is a specialist publication designed to publicise green issues and alternative health. Yellow Pages is now free for a basic advertisement, which also appears on its website (www.yell.com). There are a growing number of opportunities to advertise in other directories on the internet so this is well worth looking into. You might even decide to have your own website – it can be easier and cheaper than you think to set one up. It doesn't cost much to register a domain name (that is, a website address), and there are plenty of websites that offer easy-to-use programs so that you can design and regularly update the site yourself, so there's no need to use professional website designers unless you particularly want to. There are some addresses and sites listed in Resources at the back of this book that you might find helpful. You might also consider getting involved in social networking on the internet, such as Facebook or Twitter, or Linked-in, or having an online blog, or taking part in online Reiki forums.

Publicity materials

It is certainly worth producing a good, professional leaflet – an A4 (21 × 29cm/8¼ × 11½in) piece of paper, folded into thirds, is the most popular size. This should tell people about Reiki, about you and your background, how long treatments last and how much you charge – but you mustn't make any claims about curing people. Doing so is illegal and unethical! If you don't have much experience at producing such materials yourself, get one done by a local printing firm, because a poorly designed and produced leaflet with grammatical and spelling mistakes can really put people off. Gift vouchers can be a good idea, so that people can buy a treatment as a present for someone, and it is sensible to have a few letterheads (they are easy to produce on a computer) so that you can send out occasional promotional letters. Business cards can be useful too, because you can hand them out to groups if you give a talk or write the next appointment time on the back before people leave.

Other publicity

There are other ways to publicise your business, such as giving short talks to groups or taking a stand at holistic health fairs, but you need plenty of confidence for those. The best publicity, however, is always by 'word of mouth' – building up a good reputation so that your clients come back for more and recommend you to other people. Also, remember that Reiki is not about competition – you need to trust in your potential for success, knowing that you will attract the right clients for you. The energy you put out will draw to you those people for whom you are the right person to help, so even if there are other Reiki Practitioners nearby, they will attract whoever is right for them, too. Just send Reiki to the situation, and visualise nice, friendly people coming to you, and that's what you will get! Another possibility is to set up reciprocal deals with other local therapists offering different kinds of treatment, so that you can refer clients to each other whenever that is appropriate.

GETTING YOUR TREATMENT SPACE READY

You will no doubt want to create the right atmosphere in your treatment space – an attractive blend of comfort and professionalism – so please put into practice all the suggestions in Chapter 7.

Also, you might like to adopt the principles of feng shui, and I have suggested a few books in Further Reading. The purpose of using feng shui is to help the occupants of any building (or room) to achieve success and prosperity, so you can use the principles to create a calm, relaxing atmosphere in your therapy room. The most important principle, though, is to clear away your clutter and always keep everything clean and tidy, so ensure that you clear your therapy room of all non-essential items.

WHAT DOES IT TAKE TO BE A GOOD PRACTITIONER?

If you go to a therapist of any kind, what sort of experience do you hope you will have and how do you want to be treated? Whatever your answer is, that is what it takes to be a good Practitioner. It means you need to be a good listener, have an understanding and caring nature, be empathetic and sympathetic with people, treat them with respect, but also be knowledgeable, confident and firm enough to command their respect. And, of course, you also need to be thoroughly experienced, well organised, and good at what you do.

So, being experienced in the practice of Reiki is not all it takes. You also need to be competent in a wide range of other abilities, especially those which help you to deal with people, for example coping with any emotional release which can be one of the effects of a Reiki treatment. You may therefore wish to acquire some knowledge, experience and qualifications in related skills, such as counselling or NLP (neurolinguistic programming), to help with this side of your practice. Another aspect of being a good Practitioner is your organisational skills. You could be a wonderfully empathetic therapist who channels Reiki beautifully, but if you are never ready when a client arrives or, worse, you are not even there because you had forgotten to write the appointment in your diary, then you will not be seen as a good Practitioner.

THE THERAPIST–CLIENT RELATIONSHIP

Naturally, it is important to be professional at all times and that includes having set boundaries; for example, it would be unacceptable to exploit your clients either financially or emotionally by insisting on regular appointments or by making them feel dependent upon you. It is also absolutely unacceptable to interfere with or exploit a client in a sexual manner and you should never ask a client to remove any clothing other than their coat and shoes.

Because many different types of people may come to you for treatment, it is very important that you are non-judgemental and do not show any preferences or prejudices, regardless of a person's race, colour, creed, gender or sexual orientation. Your non-judgementalism should also extend to accepting your clients' rights to make their own choices in respect of their health and lifestyles. Whatever opinions you might have on subjects such as smoking, heavy drinking or eating unhealthily, your clients have the right to live their lives in their own way, without being made to feel uncomfortable because of their habits.

You do have the right to ask that people do not smoke or drink alcohol on your premises and to suggest that they should be sober when coming for a treatment. Of course, you also have the right to refuse to treat someone if their behaviour is unacceptable; for example, if they are drunk, abusive, intimidating or if they make you feel physically or sexually unsafe. However, it is important that you should deal with such a situation sensitively and in an uncritical way, perhaps by suggesting that another therapy or therapist might be better for the person for the time being.

Codes of conduct

As a Reiki Practitioner, the most important ethical considerations are integrity, respect and confidentiality. The 'status' of being a therapist puts you in a privileged position when you are treating members of the public, because you will be regarded by many as a health professional – which you are not, unless you are medically trained. Whatever you say will be regarded as 'the truth' so this is a considerable responsibility. Needless to say, a Practitioner must never give the impression that they have medical qualifications if they do not.

You must keep all information (medical details and appointment records) relating to each client entirely confidential, even from members of their own family, unless you have the client's consent or unless legally obliged to do so by a court of law. A possible exception to this is if you believe there is a threat of suicide, which you are legally bound to report to an appropriate health professional such as a doctor or psychiatrist. (If you are practising outside the UK, please check what regulations apply in your country.)

To act with integrity you should make clear to your client what is involved in a Reiki treatment, how long it will last and how much it costs before starting a treatment, and explain what type of client records you keep. It may not be possible initially to estimate how many treatments will be needed, but it is the client's choice whether to take your advice to have further treatments or not. It is absolutely vital, however, that you do not offer any diagnoses, and do not claim or promise a cure.

If at any time you feel that a client should consult a doctor, you can suggest this but please do so in as calm and tactful a manner as possible; for example, if you felt a lump or unexpected mass when you placed your hands on some part of the client's body, you would naturally treat the area with Reiki, but afterwards you could check whether the client had detected anything there themselves. You could then calmly suggest that they see a doctor to reassure themselves, saying that it is always sensible to have such things checked out. Do not, under any circumstances, be drawn into saying what you think it might be. The best answer is always, 'I'm sorry, I'm not a doctor, so I have no idea. The best thing to do is to get it checked' – unless, of course, you are a doctor of medicine. It is not illegal for someone to refuse to consult medical advice, but you must write in the client's notes that you have advised them to do so.

Another thing to remember is that clients may be nervous when coming for a treatment, so it is important to treat them with gentleness and respect, and to invite them to ask any questions or discuss anything about the treatment that may be worrying them. You will then be able to reassure them so that they can relax and enjoy the treatment.

Record keeping

All client records are confidential, so they should be kept where other people do not have access to them, and in the UK you are legally required to keep such records safely for seven years from the time of the last consultation (please check the regulations if you live elsewhere). This also means that you should make some provision in your will for the proper disposal of your client records after your death. Your client records – and any lists you keep of the names, addresses and telephone numbers of people who have made enquiries about treatments – are also subject to the Data Protection Act in the UK (please check the position if you practise in other countries). Even if you do not keep these lists on a computer, you may still be required to register with the Data Protection Agency, although if your records are kept only for your own use this probably won't be necessary.

Your initial client records should include their name, address, telephone number and a brief case history including any medical problems they have had in the past (and present), any surgical procedures they have undergone, any medication they are taking now and any previous medication which might be important. You should also include any alternative remedies they are taking and other complementary therapies they have received or are currently receiving. You will also need the name, address and telephone number of their doctor (for emergency use only). Each time the client attends an appointment you should make a note of the date, time, a brief outline of the treatment and any particular results and/or experiences and any advice given. Your records should be clear and comprehensive but purely factual – no comments or opinions which, even if made in a jocular way, could be misinterpreted. Remember, your client has a right to see these records if they so request, and they could also be required as part of your defence in the unfortunate (although unlikely) event of any legal action being taken against you for negligence or injury. (That, of course, is why you need public liability insurance.)

COMBINING REIKI WITH OTHER THERAPIES

Reiki works well with virtually all complementary and alternative therapies, but particularly well with any 'hands-on' therapy, such as aromatherapy, reflexology, shiatsu, metamorphic technique, acupressure, cranio-sacral therapy, chiropractic, osteopathy and any others where massage or manipulation are involved. If the therapist is attuned to Reiki, then the energy will automatically flow from the therapist's hands during the complementary therapy session if the client needs it. For therapies that entail taking some form of preparation internally, such as homoeopathy, Bach flower remedies or herbal medicine, the bottle or container can be held in the hands to allow Reiki to flow into the medication.

If Reiki is the only therapy you practise, you might consider continuing your personal development by training in one or two others, to extend the service you can offer to your clients. I think Reiki is absolutely wonderful, but it is not the only thing that can help people. Sometimes an experience of a different therapy can give someone the 'kick-start' they need to continue with their healing. Also, it is important to realise that all these complementary and alternative therapies have particular benefits and to recognise and respect the contribution of other therapies, including allopathic medicine.

THE BALANCE BETWEEN REIKI AND CONVENTIONAL (ALLOPATHIC) MEDICINE

Some people seem to think that complementary and conventional medicine do not mix, but this is not the case. Many health professionals are taking an increasing interest in complementary and alternative therapies, and indeed, I have trained lots of doctors, nurses, physiotherapists and occupational therapists in Reiki. Many hospitals, hospices, clinics and doctors' surgeries now include healing and other forms of complementary therapies in their range of services on offer, and the number is growing each year.

If you do wish to carry out Reiki healing in any of these environments, however, they often require you to have qualifications in anatomy and physiology, even though an in-depth knowledge of such things is actually unnecessary for the practice of Reiki – some basic knowledge is needed, however, in order to comply with the National Occupational Standards. I would suggest that it is far better to gain the extra knowledge and then put your abilities to good use, if this is something you really want to do. You will also need to carry public liability insurance, which is normal for therapists anyway.

In terms of using Reiki with someone receiving conventional medical treatment, there are some general guidelines that are important for you to follow:

- *Never* advise anyone to stop taking any medicines or to stop seeing their doctor or other health professional.

- *Never* try to diagnose what is wrong with anyone (unless you are medically qualified).

- *Always* advise clients to check with their doctor, if they wish, that receiving Reiki healing is OK, and suggest to them that when they talk to their doctor about it they refer to it as a type of spiritual healing, as many doctors will not have heard of Reiki.

- Also, *always* advise them to see a doctor if their health problem does not respond to treatment or if you intuitively feel there may be some underlying serious problem. (This must only be done in a very tactful and sensitive manner, as you don't wish to frighten them in any way and, as already indicated above, it is not your place to diagnose.)

As with complementary therapies, any prescribed medication can be held in the hands and given Reiki to enhance its beneficial effects and decrease any side effects. Simply hold it and draw the Power Symbol over it, silently saying its mantra three times and *intending* that Reiki should work with the medication for the highest possible good.

MEDICAL RESTRICTIONS AND NOTIFIABLE DISEASES

There are a surprising number of rules and regulations regarding what you can or cannot do as a health practitioner, and it is essential that you get up-to-date information about any legal requirements or regulations for any country in which you wish to practise. Ignorance of the law is no defence. Your professional association should be able to help you with this, but to give you some examples, in the UK these are just some of the current instances where by treating someone with Reiki you might be going against the law:

- It is illegal to charge for the treatment of certain venereal diseases.

- Except in emergencies it is illegal to attend a woman in childbirth without qualified medical supervision.

- You cannot prescribe or sell remedies, herbs, supplements, oils, and so on, unless you have appropriate qualifications.

- It is illegal to diagnose or prescribe unless medically qualified.

- Although hands-on healing of animals is permitted in an emergency, or if it is your own animal, an owner must be advised to have a sick animal examined by a vet for diagnosis and treatment.

- It is an offence to advertise treatments or remedies purporting cures for the following diseases: Bright's disease, cancer, cataracts, diabetes, epilepsy, glaucoma, locomotor ataxia, paralysis and tuberculosis.

- Any of the following infectious diseases must be reported to the Medical Officer of Health in your local area, and if you suspect any client is suffering from anything on this list, you should also insist that they see a doctor: acute encephalitis, acute poliomyelitis, anthrax, cholera, diphtheria, dysentery (amoebic or bacillary), food poisoning, leprosy, leptospirosis, malaria, measles, meningitis, meningococcal septicaemia (without meningitis), mumps, opthalmia neonatorum, paratyphoid fever, plague, rabies, relapsing fever, rubella, scarlet fever, smallpox, tetanus, tuberculosis, typhoid fever, typhus, viral haemorrhagic fever, viral hepatitis, whooping cough and yellow fever.

- In addition, the WHO (World Health Organization) requires countries to report other disease outbreaks or public health events which might become international threats to health, so clearly if you come across any of these, inform your doctor immediately: influenza, severe acute respiratory syndrome (SARS), vector borne viral infections (that is, transmitted to humans by insects such as mosquitoes and ticks), anti-microbial resistance (that is, resistance to antibiotics), chemical* safety (such as toxic substances), dengue fever, HIV/AIDS, and zoonoses (infectious diseases transferred from animals to humans).

Do take the above information in context, however – it is highly unlikely that someone suffering from dangerous or infectious diseases would contact a Reiki Practitioner before calling a doctor!

RED FLAG SYMPTOMS

A 'red flag' symptom is something that indicates your client should be referred immediately to a doctor. Obviously, it is important not to frighten your client, so please act sensitively and tactfully. You might consider taking a course in first aid so that you will have a better idea of what to do, and in the UK these are offered by St John Ambulance, the Red Cross, and some other organisations.

There are six major sets of red flag symptoms:

1   Paralysis in the arms or legs, tingling, numbness, confusion, dizziness, double vision, slurred speech, trouble finding words or weakness, especially on one side of the face or body – these are potentially signs of a stroke.

2   Chest pain or discomfort, pain in the arm, jaw or neck, breaking out in a cold sweat, extreme weakness, nausea, vomiting, feeling faint or dizzy, or being very short of breath – these are all potentially signs of heart attack.

3   Tenderness and pain in the lower leg, chest pain, shortness of breath, or coughing up blood – these are symptoms of a potentially dangerous blood clot.

4   Blood in the urine, even without accompanying pain – this could potentially be symptomatic of kidney stones, or bladder or prostate infection.

5   Asthma attacks – severe wheezing or difficulties in breathing – if symptoms get worse these could be potentially fatal.

6   Depression and suicidal thoughts – symptoms could include sadness, fatigue, apathy, anxiety, changes in sleep habits and loss of appetite.

Apart from the six mentioned above, there are other symptoms which could also be classified as 'red flag', including abnormal bleeding from the rectum or vagina, sudden changes in bowel habit, severe constipation, unexplained vomiting, persistent coughing, or breathing difficulties, severe headache, sudden weight loss, unexplained exhaustion or loss of appetite.

LOOKING AFTER YOURSELF

Remember the old adage 'Healer, heal thyself'. Running a successful Reiki practice can be hard work, so you really need to look after yourself first – and always. You will not be much help to other people if you let yourself get run down or become ill, so it is vital to set in motion those things that can help you to remain healthy, whole and energetic. That means concentrating on your physical well-being with good nutrition and sensible exercise, but also on your mental, emotional and spiritual well-being. You work with a wonderful holistic healing energy, so please don't neglect yourself. A daily self-treatment of a minimum of 30–40 minutes is important – preferably an hour, when you can – and having a regular Reiki treatment from another Practitioner is also excellent. Monthly would be fine, but if you are going through a particularly busy or stressful time, try to make it once a week. Also, make sure you have a good self-cleansing routine, using the techniques recommended in Chapters 15 and 20, especially before, between and after doing treatments, as this will help to keep your energies clear and balanced.

Whether you are just starting out or have been running a busy practice for some time, one of your priorities should be to manage your time effectively to prevent burn-out. If you always find you are rushing around 'chasing your tail', then you need to take stock of your life and see how you can reorganise things to make your life easier. Many of us tend to take on too much, so we run ourselves ragged or begin to let other people down; the first thing to do is to start being assertive and say 'no' to everything you don't really want to do (and probably to some of the things you would like to do but simply don't have the time). You will also need to build up your strength and stamina, as standing up doing treatments can be quite tiring otherwise. Taking up yoga, t'ai chi, qigong or martial arts is a good way to strengthen yourself and to get your energies flowing well.

Your Personal Support System

When you spend a lot of time helping others, it is vital to have your own personal support system – people you can turn to for advice and assistance if you have problems or need encouragement. Your support group should include your Reiki Master and perhaps other Practitioners or the members of a Reiki sharing group and the other students you met when you did your Reiki training, as well as family and friends. One way that would undoubtedly help is if you could encourage some family members or friends to train in Reiki, as then you could swap treatments regularly.

Your Further Development as a Practitioner

You might choose to further your development as a Practitioner by studying other forms of Reiki, such as Karuna Reiki (see the Appendix), or by taking courses in advanced Reiki techniques. Some Reiki Masters offer a course for Personal Mastery, sometimes called Master Practitioner or Reiki 3A (see Chapter 18), where you are taught and attuned to the Usui Master Symbol; however, you are not taught how to carry out the attunement processes, so you cannot call yourself a Reiki Master, but having the Master attunement and using the Master Symbol will enhance your capabilities. (Please read the next chapter to decide whether you are ready to take on the commitment the Master attunement brings with it.) You might want to study other forms of healing or other therapies, or learn meditation or other relaxation methods, or simply read extensively about such techniques to help you improve your practice.

Continuing professional development (CPD)

As a registered Reiki Practitioner you will be required to undertake a minimum of 12 hours additional training each year as CPD (continuing professional development) in order to remain on the register, of which at least six hours must be Reiki-specific, such as attending Reiki Shares or learning Japanese Reiki techniques. The other hours could be on other subjects that will help you in your professional development, such as first aid, counselling or meditation. This doesn't just mean attending additional courses, although sometimes that would be appropriate. Alternatively you might shadow another Practitioner in their work, or take part in Reiki sharing groups or attend conferences, or it could be self-directed learning such as reading and reviewing books, journals or articles relevant to your practice; however, it isn't sufficient to just 'do' something, you also have to reflect on that activity and see how it can improve your practice, and you have to provide evidence of what you have done, such as certificates, testimonials, evaluation notes, project reports, articles you've written, and so on. This evidence may have to be sent to your professional association (for example, the UK Reiki Federation) in support of your renewal of membership.

Continuing your personal and spiritual development

One of the imperatives when you start to use Reiki professionally is to work with it on your personal and spiritual development, allowing Reiki to teach you who you really are. It has the power to transform you and change your life, increasing your self-awareness and your intuition, and bringing a greater happiness and contentment. It is therefore necessary to prioritise Reiki, giving it time in your life so that you gradually develop a deeper and more meaningful relationship with it. Hopefully, the last chapter will give you some ideas for your spiritual practice, and you will find more suggestions in Part 5 on the Japanese traditions, especially in Chapters 20 and 21.

One of the areas to be aware of, however, is attracting clients who mirror your own issues. If you get a stream of people with the same problem, whether they are headaches, bad backs, sore throats or frozen shoulders etc., then maybe you need to start looking at the metaphysical causes behind those conditions, too. Perhaps you have been unwilling to look at certain areas of your life, so Reiki conveniently brings you people who can, metaphorically, push the problem under your nose so that it is hard not to look at it!

Another area that you might give some attention to is working on your abundance/money issues with Reiki and visualisations: visualising yourself attracting plenty of clients; seeing yourself as a successful Reiki Practitioner; having a good lifestyle, with a lovely home, beautiful things around you and relaxing holidays; with happy, satisfying relationships, and seeing yourself fulfilling your dreams. And remember, you can use Reiki on all aspects of setting up a business, from attracting the right number of clients to attracting the appropriate funding, and even manifesting a therapy couch. (I did that, and within two days someone offered me a deluxe adjustable one as an exchange for teaching them Second Degree!)

The key to much of this, as well as working on these issues with Reiki, is to feel gratitude for what you already have and to turn that feeling into something tangible. Perhaps you could tithe a proportion of the money you receive for treatments to a favourite charity or you could give some of your time to do voluntary work in hospices or nursing homes where Reiki would be so beneficial.

In the next chapter, we look at progressing further in Reiki by becoming either a Reiki Master/Practitioner – advancing your knowledge of techniques for treating clients – or a Reiki Master/ Teacher, where you learn the skills necessary to train others in Reiki.

Chapter 18

Third Degree Reiki (Master Level)

Do you *really* want to be a Reiki Master? Being a Reiki Master can be interesting, rewarding and usually great fun too, but it is not an easy path to follow and, like any journey, you need to be well prepared and have a good map. That is why I have put an emphasis on the word *really* in the question above, because it is not a decision to be made lightly on a whim; it definitely deserves a lot of thought. Becoming a Reiki Master is not just about getting another, higher qualification. It is not even about being able to teach other people. It is much, much more than either of those. Perhaps the question should read, 'Do you *really* want to *commit your life* to Reiki?', because that is what it actually entails. It is a commitment for life to mastering Reiki – a commitment to a healing practice and a spiritual discipline which will inevitably change you and in all probability will change your whole life too. This is a lifetime decision, and you cannot change your mind once you have received the Master attunement.

Being a Reiki Master can be like a rollercoaster ride, and how you experience it depends very much upon your point of view. You can see it as exciting, exhilarating, enjoyable, fun, challenging and full of adventure, or you can see it as frightening, full of too many responsibilities and you may have an overwhelming urge to shout, '*I want to get off!*' but, of course, you can't. Just as when you ride a rollercoaster, unless you go with it, bending and turning as it does, it can be very uncomfortable; if you fight to stay upright, rigidly holding on to what you have always known, then you make the ride difficult; however, surrender to the experience, move as it moves, adapt to its speed and angles, just let it be, and you go with the flow. That is when it becomes fun. And that is when being a Reiki Master becomes fun – when you go with the flow. That is when you are *being* a Reiki Master instead of *doing* Reiki Master. Reiki Master is not a job. It is you, *being* you. It is you *being* Reiki. It is you living what you love. And that is special. Rise to the challenge, and it can be the best kind of life you could imagine.

So, if you really like the life you are living now, *don't* become a Reiki Master – at least, not yet – because change is inevitable; however, nothing stays the same forever, no matter how much we like it or dislike it. So, if you love Reiki and you are curious, interested and keen enough to explore a life that is filled with Reiki – then go ahead.

THE ROLE OF A REIKI MASTER

By now you will have gathered that the role of a Reiki Master is an important one. It is a sacred responsibility where you not only need knowledge and experience but you also need wisdom, understanding, compassion and a genuine interest in people – and you need to live a life that is a good example to your students. But being a good example does *not* mean being 'holier than thou' and living an ascetic life just for the sake of it. Reiki Masters are human beings with the same foibles and failings as everyone else, so some of them smoke, some of them drink and most of them are aware that they could be looking after their bodies in better ways. But any changes they make in that direction tend to be slow and easy, and because they *want* to, not because they feel *obliged* to. It is actually more important to show an understanding of the Reiki Principles and to use Reiki regularly, especially on yourself, than to force yourself to give up meat or caffeine-laden drinks (although that might be a direction you will be happy to follow later on in your development), because you will just end up feeling deprived. Demonstrating a balanced life, one that shows you are trying to look after yourself and care for others, is more 'real' and honest than trying to achieve some unrealistic idea of 'perfection'.

The role of Reiki Master is that of a respected teacher, someone who knows Reiki 'inside out'. By that I mean someone who lives with Reiki as an essential part of their daily lives as well as someone who has plenty of knowledge and experience of using Reiki in different ways. Please realise, however, that no Reiki Master knows *everything* about Reiki. Reiki is itself a teacher, so the longer a Master uses and teaches it, the further along the path *towards* mastery they go. And for each Master that is a very personal journey, because each comes from a different starting point. Each of us has a unique set of life experiences and it is inevitable that these will influence how, when and why we came to Reiki. Reiki Masters come from all walks of life, and this diversity means that there is bound to be a Reiki Master somewhere whose approach will appeal to you, and who will therefore be just the right person to guide you through your own personal Reiki path.

Being a Master is not just about knowing how to attune someone, or how to carry out a Reiki class. It is essentially about empowering others, knowing how to lead someone towards their own personal and spiritual fulfilment – without judgement, without censure, but with love and compassion. As a Master's self-awareness, knowledge and understanding of Reiki grows, so they are even better able to carry out their role.

That is what I meant when I chose the title for this book, *Reiki for Life*. When you become attuned to Reiki, you have Reiki for life; when you become a Master, Reiki gradually becomes more and more important to you, until it is your life.

WHAT DOES A REIKI MASTER NEED TO KNOW?

It might seem common sense, but in order to teach as a Reiki Master you need to know as much as possible about Reiki so that you can pass on your knowledge and experience to your future students. This should include:

- A basic understanding of energy theory.

- A thorough knowledge and understanding of what Reiki is, the four Usui Reiki symbols and how to use them.

- The hand positions and how to carry out self-treatments and treatments on other people lying on a therapy couch or seated on a chair.

- How Reiki can be used as an emergency treatment.

- How Reiki can be used on animals, plants and inanimate objects.

- How to prepare for and carry out attunements at each level.

- How to prepare your students if they wish to practise professionally.

You also need to know:

- How to run a small business, including relevant UK and European legislation, ethics and codes of practice.

- How to communicate effectively and appropriately to create professional relationships.

- The importance of confidentiality.

- How to reflect on your practice and identify development needs.

- How to look after your own physical, mental, emotional and spiritual health and well-being to support yourself and your work.

That might look like a pretty long list, but even when you know all of that (and much of the theory is included in this book, with further guidance in *The Reiki Manual*) it is important to continue to learn so that you continue to improve what you can offer to students. You might consider attending courses with other Reiki Masters, perhaps to gain practical experience in the techniques from the Japanese tradition, or joining a meditation group, or doing voluntary work in a hospice, or broadening your knowledge by training in other therapies such as EFT (emotional freedom technique). Remember, being a Reiki Master is a journey, not a destination, so you might as well make it as interesting as possible!

HOW TO PREPARE FOR MASTER TRAINING

Before Reiki Master training it is especially important to raise the vibrations of your energy bodies – physical, mental, emotional and spiritual – so that you will be better prepared for the power of the Master energy coming through you. Your preparations could include daily meditation, self-treatments and practice of *Hatsurei-ho* (see pages 354–5) plus weekly Reiki treatment 'swaps' whenever possible, either with another Practitioner or preferably with the Master who will be training you. This enables you to get to know each other more, and if they have trained in the Japanese traditional techniques this would also give you the chance to receive regular *Reiju* attunements to increase the flow of Reiki.

In addition, you could meditate on the Reiki Principles and the Reiki symbols, and perhaps carry out a visualisation to meet your Reiki Master spirit guides, asking them to help you with your preparation. You might also look at other possibilities for self-improvement and growth, perhaps by reading spiritually inspired books, or attending personal growth groups or workshops, plus of course thinking about the ethics, responsibilities and commitment of being a Reiki Master. Also, it would be useful to look at what experience you already have and to thoroughly practise all the techniques detailed in this book. If you have practised Reiki professionally for several years, this would obviously be of greater benefit to your future students than if you had done only an occasional Reiki treatment on family or friends, because you would then have a wealth of experience to share with them. Equally, if you confidently and regularly use the Reiki symbols this will enable you to teach them more effectively. I would also recommend that you get some qualifications and/or experience in teaching or training. Not only will this help your own confidence but it will also, hopefully, lead to an even better experience for your future students.

CHOOSING YOUR TYPE OF TRAINING AND INITIATING MASTER

Reiki Master training in the West can be minimal and take a very short time or very comprehensive and take a long time – or anywhere in between those two points; for example, some Masters, like me, insist that you should have at least three years' experience of Reiki, preferably part of that time as a professional Practitioner, before they will accept you for Master training, while others have no minimum time requirements and some even actively encourage every student to become a Reiki Master as soon as possible.

You therefore have several options – you can take the fast track, which could mean taking all levels of Reiki (1, 2 and 3) within a matter of a few months, weeks or even days, or you can take the slow and easy route, taking as much time as you feel you need between initiations. Whichever you choose is always at the right speed for you at a soul level, because at that level it is not possible to make mistakes – all experience is valid; however, that is not always the case at the human level, where the fast track can have some rather unpleasant consequences, because your physical body has to adapt very quickly to huge changes in vibrational frequencies. This can lead to a rapid (and uncomfortable) cleansing period, not only of your physical body but also of all areas of your life. Changes are an inevitable consequence of becoming a Reiki Master – it is just the speed at which they happen that tends to be different because, in general, growth needs time.

The system for Master training that was most prevalent until the early 1990s was that of Reiki Alliance Masters, who usually train by the apprenticeship system where a student Master works alongside a fully trained and experienced Master for at least a year, gradually learning how to organise and teach classes for Reiki 1 and 2 by observing, and then taking over certain parts of the class as they gain knowledge and confidence. When their initiating Master considers them ready, they are taught the Master Symbol and receive the Master attunement. They are also taught (and practise at Reiki classes alongside their initiating Master) the attunement processes for the first two levels, but the attunement process for the Third Degree is often not taught until several years later, when the newly qualified Reiki Master has acquired plenty of experience.

Clearly, this system limits the number of Masters who can be trained, as it would be unwieldy to have more than a couple of 'trainees' working with a Master on each Reiki course, so unless they are members of The Reiki Alliance, few Masters use this type of training today. It is much more common now to learn how to be a Reiki Master in the same way as you learn the skills required in Reiki First and Second Degrees – by attending a short course. Obviously, what can be taught will be limited by the amount of time the course takes, and since this varies between one day and 10–14 days, with most probably taking an average of between three days and a week, there is considerable variation in content, style and quality of training.

Because the vast majority of Reiki Masters work independently, they can set their own training guidelines and prices, so the cost of training as a Master varies enormously from less than £100 (US$160) up to £6,000 ($10,000), which is the price charged by members of The Reiki Alliance; however, you cannot necessarily assume that a Master charging a high price is a good teacher offering high-quality tuition, or that one charging a low price is an ineffective teacher offering poor tuition. There are as many variations in Reiki Masters as there are in any other profession. There are some excellent, dedicated and highly experienced Reiki teachers who charge moderate prices, whereas there are others who have little experience and offer inadequate information and poor support, yet who charge high prices. I am afraid it is very much up to you to decide which is which, and probably the best way is to meditate on it and ask your Higher Self – after all, Reiki is a spiritual discipline as well as a healing modality, so this is an appropriate way to make your decision, especially at this level!

WHAT MIGHT BE INCLUDED IN REIKI MASTER TRAINING?

Some Masters divide the training into several parts, so that on the first course (usually one or two days) students are taught and attuned to the Usui Master Symbol, and receive instruction in a few advanced techniques, thereafter they can call themselves 'Master Practitioners'. This is sometimes called Reiki 3A, Advanced Reiki Training, or ART, and usually precedes a further two-day Reiki Master training course where students are taught and given some time to practise the attunement processes for all three Reiki levels. This final stage, often called 'Master/Teacher' also frequently includes a further two symbols – another Master Symbol with a four-syllable Japanese mantra and an Energy Symbol which has a three-syllable mantra in English (although both are apparently from a Tibetan source) to which the students are attuned. Many Masters refer to this as the 'Reiki Master attunement', although these symbols were never a part of the original Usui Reiki Ryoho, but were introduced by the American Reiki Master William Lee

Rand as part of his Usui/Tibetan Reiki system. These short courses generally contain only very brief instructions (but no practice) on how to teach the three levels of Reiki.

Other Masters offer longer courses, some of which give you an opportunity to practise the teaching skills required, and which may also include preparatory material either as written manuals, or as CDs or DVDs. A few Masters offer courses which extend the students' knowledge to other types of Reiki (at Master level) in addition to the Usui Reiki and Usui/Tibetan Reiki referred to above, such as Tera-Mai Seichem, Sekhem, Karuna Reiki and Reiki Jin Kei Do (all of these are described in the Appendix), including any extra symbols those systems use. There would also be some instruction in the attunement processes (normally quite different) for each system, so these are very intensive and energetically challenging courses.

There are obviously some basics that *must* be included in Reiki Master training and other aspects that would be an advantage but which are not essential. I have put together a checklist, which you might find useful when making your decision on where to go for training, but I don't believe it is appropriate to include any of the following Master level techniques or processes in this book, as they should really be taught in person:

Essential training	Possible advantageous additions
How to draw the Usui Reiki Master Symbol	How to draw the Tibetan Master Symbol and Energy (Fire Serpent) Symbol
Mantra for the Usui Reiki Master Symbol	Mantras for the Tibetan symbols
Attunement to the Usui Reiki Master Symbol	Attunement to the Tibetan Master Symbol and Energy (Fire Serpent) Symbol
Ways of using the Usui Master Symbol including Master Practitioner techniques for treatments	Methods for using the Tibetan Reiki symbols (e.g. balancing chakras, meditation)
Learning and practice of *Hui Yin* (muscular contraction to hold energy)	The single (integrated) attunement method for Usui Reiki First Degree

Essential training	Possible advantageous additions
What to include in teaching Reiki at First Degree (for individuals and groups)	The single (integrated) attunement method for Usui/Tibetan Reiki First Degree, using Tibetan symbols
Learning and practising the four attunement methods for Usui Reiki First Degree	The single attunement method for Usui/Tibetan Reiki Second Degree using Tibetan symbols
What to include in teaching Reiki at Usui Reiki Second Degree (for individuals and groups)	The Japanese tradition two- and three-attunement methods for Usui Reiki Second Degree (*Okuden*)
Learning and practising the single attunement method for Usui Reiki Second Degree	Hiroshi Doi's Japanese *Reiju* empowerment (in the Usui tradition)
The spiritual and business responsibilities of being a Reiki Master	Learning and practising the Violet Breath technique
Learning and practising the single attunement method for Usui Reiki Third Degree (does not have to be learned at the same time as First and Second Degree attunement methods)	Learning the Antahkarana Symbol and its uses (this is an ancient healing and meditation symbol from China and Tibet, not a Reiki symbol)
What to include in teaching Reiki at Third Degree (Master) level for individuals and groups	Learning and practice of a Psychic Surgery technique (aura clearing/ removal of negative energies using Reiki)
Developing the Master–Student relationship	Learning and practising a technique called a Healing Attunement
The ongoing responsibility for personal and spiritual development	

Other opportunities may also be offered, such as observation and co-teaching of Reiki 1 and Reiki 2 courses. Something to be aware of, however, is that a significant proportion of Reiki Masters in the West do not actually use – or teach – the original Usui system for attunements, and some don't even teach the Usui Master Symbol or attune you to it. Since so many Reiki Masters have been taught in the 'modern' way on short courses lasting between one and three days, they use the Tibetan Reiki symbols (pioneered by William Lee Rand), which bring through a different healing energy that is somewhat 'fiercer' than the very gentle, flowing Usui Reiki energy. These symbols seem to stimulate and raise the *Kundalini*, (a very strong spiritual and sexual energy stored in the base chakra, sometimes called 'serpent power') which is wonderful, powerful and life enhancing, and which can create the most profound spiritual connections; however, because it can also activate and break through the blockages in a person's sexual energy, it can occasionally have slightly unpleasant side effects on some people – mostly nausea or uncontrollable shaking for a short time. This is not entirely surprising because in the Buddhist tradition it would normally take many years of meditation and other practices to prepare for it.

THE MASTER SYMBOL

This symbol is the fourth in the Usui system of Reiki, and it comes from the Japanese *kanji*. There are a number of variations, the one probably used by most Masters consists of 22 strokes, but in recent years a slightly different Japanese version consisting of 17 strokes, called *Reisho*, has become popular. They both work, however, as I mentioned above, becoming a Master is a sacred responsibility, so although I have included the Second Degree symbols in this book, I don't feel comfortable doing the same with the Master Symbol. The Master Symbol is described as 'a Zen expression for one's own true nature or Buddha-nature of which one becomes aware during the experience of enlightenment or satori'. One translation of its four-syllable mantra is 'treasure house of the great beaming light'. These definitions indicate how profound this symbol is, as its use gives us direct and immediate connection to the Light, the Source, the Master within – the essence of 'enlightenment'. In fact, it represents that part of the self that is already completely enlightened, so when we use the Master Symbol we are actually connecting with our Higher Selves – that enlightened part of our being which has total wisdom and understanding. The Master Symbol brings in even higher and purer dimensions of light and healing – Reiki – to assist with self-awareness, personal growth, spiritual development, intuition and a deep understanding of 'being', and is therefore connected with the crown chakra.

The Master Symbol can be used to bring Light into any situation, and it is an essential part of each Master's development to use this symbol to surround themselves with higher and finer vibrations as often as possible to help with self-cleansing and self-purification (on spiritual levels) to help to create a more harmonious and balanced life. Meditating on this symbol can bring enormous benefits, as it directly enters the consciousness to allow Light to enter even the darkest and most deeply buried blockages, whether those blockages are on a physical, mental, emotional or spiritual plane. It can also be used in combination with the other Reiki symbols when it will increase their effectiveness and allow them to act from only the very purest and highest motivations.

There are various ways of using the Master Symbol, once you have been attuned to it. It can be drawn in the same way as the other symbols – with the whole hand, the fingers or the eyes, or visualised. It is multi-dimensional energy having height, width and depth but also operating in time, space and light. It can appear to be any colour, but the most usual are white, gold, purple, violet, turquoise, pink or rainbow-coloured. You can draw it and 'step into it', you can visualise it filling your whole being, you can imagine breathing it in with each breath, and you can draw the symbol and chant its mantra (when you are alone) to purify and fill your body and the space where you are with light, love and peace before and after any activity. It also plays a part in the attunement process for all levels of Reiki, as well as helping the Reiki Master to create a unique sacred space in which to carry out the sacred ceremony of initiation.

AFTER A REIKI MASTER COURSE

The first and most important thing to remember is that receiving a Master attunement does not make you a Reiki Master. It is just the beginning of a long journey *towards* the mastery of Reiki – a journey without end, because this amazing, Divinely guided energy is beyond mastery by humans. But we can do our best to live up to it, to 'walk our talk', to gradually 'become' Reiki so that it forms a vital and inexorable part of our lives.

At Master level, personal and spiritual development is no longer an option – it is a necessity. Reiki will lead you towards a more spiritual way of being, through experiences that will give you a greater level of wisdom and understanding about yourself and about other people. To become a Reiki Master is to become the *embodiment* of Reiki – the embodiment of love, light, healing, harmony and balance. That might seem pretty daunting, especially at first, but at a soul level you always make the right decisions, so whenever you decide to become a Reiki Master is always the right time.

Like the other Reiki courses, after being attuned as a Reiki Master you will go through another 21-day clearing process, but it does tend to be a bit deeper in its effects, as one might expect, since the Master energy has a very high vibration. I would suggest that you don't attune anyone else for a month at the very least, and preferably six months or longer from the time of your attunement. Of course, you might not choose to attune anyone for many years, preferring to use the higher energies and the Master Symbol for your own personal and spiritual development and in your Reiki treatments on yourself and others, and that is fine. That is still working with the energy. So, let yourself go at a pace that suits you, and don't feel pressurised by family or friends, who might be looking forward to you attuning them. Only do it when you feel it is right, and trust your inner instincts, your intuition, to let you know when that is.

EXPLORING REIKI AS A SPIRITUAL DISCIPLINE

Part of a Master's personal responsibility is to explore Reiki more deeply as a spiritual discipline, and the tools for this are meditation, the Reiki Principles and the four Reiki symbols and their mantras, but particularly the Master Symbol.

Because the Master Symbol works at very high and fine vibrational frequencies, it can connect you in a deep way with aspects of your Higher Self/Higher Consciousness which usually reside in higher dimensions, and this can result in a very profound personal connection to the Source/God/All That Is, leading to intense and wonderful experiences of enlightenment. These periods of illumination can last for brief seconds or for several hours, but their effects are more long lasting and, not surprisingly, can be life changing.

They can lead to amazing insights into your life path and life purpose, so that you can confidently step out on the next phase of your spiritual journey. To begin with you may need to draw the Master Symbol on a piece of paper (to be burned later) so that you can focus on it for your meditation, but after a while you will be able to visualise its image easily and to hold the image in your mind to meditate upon. You can also chant its mantra, either silently in your mind or aloud if you are alone, which can provide a deeply relaxing meditation. You might also like to try an alternative meditation technique, which is to 'walk' the symbol. Imagine the Master Symbol drawn on the ground, and walk the shape of each stroke, chanting the sacred mantra as you walk. This can be done inside but seems to be even more powerful if done outside, perhaps in a private area of a garden or in a clearing in a wood where you can be sure of being alone.

You can also meditate on the Master Symbol to entrust to Reiki any problems or difficulties you have not yet been able to solve, and the solutions will come to you intuitively. Because it connects to even higher dimensions, it is also especially useful to infuse any worldwide disasters with peace and healing. (The Master Symbol can eventually be used in place of the other three symbols, but it is better to leave this until much later in your development, when you have sufficient experience and practice with using all four symbols and have absorbed and embodied their energy fully.)

Other aspects of Reiki as a spiritual discipline are: daily self-treatment (preferably for at least an hour); thinking about and putting into practice the Reiki principles on a daily basis; performing at least one *Hatsurei-ho* each day, plus self-cleansing (with Reiki – and remember the cold showers too!); and using Reiki as a normal part of your everyday life so that it becomes your automatic response to anything and everything. You can start and end each day by first placing your hands in the *Gassho* position for a few moments, and then drawing in the air (or visualising) the Master Symbol and chanting its mantra with the intention that Reiki should fill your being and your day (or night). This is a really powerful way of enhancing your spiritual growth, especially if you combine it with some suitable affirmation(s) for your personal and spiritual healing, guidance and well-being.

Reiki, the more your energy channels will
and expanded so that you can receive increas-
nergy. Eventually you integrate Reiki into the
d energy fields that make up your whole self,
and physical, and when that happens your total
being es Reiki so that everything and everyone within your
expanded energy field will be touched by the vibration of Reiki.
You will be spreading healing, harmony and balance wherever you
go. To quote Sensei Hiroshi Doi, 'When everything and everyone
is vibrating to its/their maximum potential, then life will cease to be
a struggle, and we will experience the fullness of Who We Truly
Are – Spirit having a physical experience'.

In Part 5 we look at the Japanese traditions for teaching and practising Reiki, including the three training levels *Shoden*, *Okuden* and
Shinpiden, and many spiritual and practical techniques that can add
an interesting dimension to your practice of Reiki.

Part 5

The Japanese Tradition

Chapter 19

Reiki Training in Japan

Japanese culture and language can be difficult to understand, because it is so different from what we are used to in the West. This is why it has taken so long for us to become aware of the Japanese traditions of Reiki, because information is not easily or readily made available, especially to outsiders. In this and the following three chapters, when mentioning Japanese people I will be using the Japanese form of names, where the surname comes first, and the term Sensei instead of Master, as well as using a number of Japanese words. At this stage you might want to be reminded of some of the relevant names:

- Usui Mikao, the founder of the system (Usui Sensei)

- Hayashi Chujiro (Hayashi Sensei), one of Usui's *Shinpiden* students who passed his knowledge on to Takata Hawayo, who brought Reiki to the West

- Doi Hiroshi (Doi Sensei), a Japanese Reiki Master who has trained in both Western and Japanese Reiki

- Taketomi Kan'ichi and Koyama Kimiko, former Presidents of the Usui Reiki Ryoho Gakkai

Of course, it isn't necessary for you to learn Japanese in order to practise Reiki, even when you're practising techniques from the Japanese tradition! However, you might like to know how to pronounce the words, so here is a quick guide to Japanese pronunciation:

VOWELS

Japanese vowels can be either short or long, and making this distinction can be important, as vowel length can change the meaning of a word.

Vowel	Short	Long
A	usually *u* as in fun	like *ah* in father
	Or like *a* in fan	
E	like *e* in bed	like *ai* in pain
I	like *i* in pin	like *ee* in feed
O	like *o* in got	like *aw* in law
U	like *u* in but	like *oo* in shoot

Some vowels are used together, like the diphthongs in the English language, either just two vowels, or vowels followed by particular consonants:

AI	like *ai* in aisle
AIR	like *ai* in stair
EI	like *ay* in may
OW	like *ow* in cow
OY	like *oy* in soya

CONSONANTS

Most Japanese consonants are very close in sound to those in English, although double consonants should have a slight pause between the letters.

Consonant	English	Consonant	English
B	as in bin	P	as in pin
CH	as in church	R	half way between L and R
D	as in dig		as in run (a 'rolled' r)
F	as in football	S	as in sew
G	as in goal	SH	as in show
H	as in hip	T	as in tip
J	as in jump	TS	as in hits

K	as in kitchen	W	as in win
M	as in move	Y	as in yes
N	as in no	Z	s/z sound as in is

REIKI TECHNIQUES

Thanks to research conducted in Japan (see Chapter 1) we now know that Dr Usui left a rich heritage of healing techniques that has been passed down from his *Shinpiden* students in Japan (a *Shinpiden* is the equivalent of a Western Reiki Master). It is believed that most of the techniques I will be describing in these four chapters were part of Dr Usui's original system, the Usui Reiki Ryoho, or Usui Teate, meaning 'hand touch' or 'palm healing', and some of them use one hand only, which seems to have been quite usual for Dr Usui, according to his original manual, the *Usui Reiki Hikkei*. I have tried to ensure that the information included is as thorough and accurate as possible, but details do vary quite a lot depending upon the source, and as I've mentioned before, some material has been withheld, but hopefully you will find this and the following more detailed chapters on the training levels both interesting and useful.

INFORMATION SOURCES

In Chapter 1, I explained that most of the information we have gained about the Japanese traditions, and about Usui Sensei's original system, has been the result of research by some Western Reiki Masters, especially a German Reiki Master, Frank Arjava Petter, who lived in Japan with his Japanese wife Chetna Kobayashi; however, the majority of the detail has come from Doi Sensei (Doi Hiroshi), a Japanese Reiki Master whose first visit to the West in 1999 was at the invitation of two of my Reiki Masters, Andrew Bowling and Richard Rivard. They organised a workshop in Canada for Reiki Masters from all over the world where Doi Sensei taught a range of techniques from the Usui Reiki Ryoho, Usui's original system, and he has run further training sessions in Japan for Reiki Masters from many countries.

Doi Sensei's Reiki training began in 1982, and he has studied with both Japanese and Western-style Reiki Masters, include Ohta Hiroshi, Mieko Mitsui, Manaso Swami, Koyama Kimiko (Mrs), the late President of the Usui Reiki Ryoho Gakkai who had trained with Taketomi Kan'ichi, one of Usui's students, and finally with Mrs Yamaguchi, who had herself trained with Hayashi Sensei in 1938. Doi Hiroshi is now a member of the Usui Reiki Ryoho Gakkai (Usui Spiritual Energy Healing Method Society), the organisation set up to continue Usui Sensei's teachings, and he and some other Japanese *Shihan* (Japanese Reiki Masters who teach) who are sympathetic to sharing information with the West have helped us to understand much more about Usui's teachings, and the workings of the Gakkai. Other information has come from contact made by Chris Marsh and a few other Western Masters with a number of Usui Sensei's original students, including Suzuki-san, a Buddhist nun. It is unlikely that any of them will still be alive by the time this book is published, as they were all more than 100 years old in 2005, one apparently being 112 at that time! However, we should be very grateful that they were willing to share some information about Usui and his original teachings, although, as I said previously, they still held back some details as they felt they were too sacred to be passed to Western 'outsiders', so we will probably never know the whole story.

THE TRAINING BASICS

The system taught by Mikao Usui emphasised spiritual development and self-healing practice based on a number of main aspects:

1   Receiving *Reiju* empowerments regularly

2   Focusing on and living the *Gokai* (the five Reiki Principles or Precepts)

3   Practising meditation and mindfulness

4   Carrying out *Kokyu-ho* – breathing and energy exercises

5   Practising *Tenohira* – the practice of palm healing for self and others

6   At *Okuden* level and above, learning *Jumon* (chants) and *Shirushi* (symbols) and *Kotodama* (mantras), if required

The Usui Reiki Ryoho Gakkai has continued to teach Usui Sensei's system in a similar way since his death in 1926, as it does have in its possession Usui's original *Hikkei*, or manuals, although it is likely that some changes have been made. It has always been a closed learning society and, like Usui, they do not advertise. Although Japan passed a law in the early 1980s requiring a hands-on healer to have training in massage therapy, the Gakkai were able to continue to use this method because of their private membership. In recent years, however, they have apparently taken a more cautious approach and no longer teach any 'hands-on' positions.

We now know that the Gakkai used an energy-ranking system to determine the level of ability of a student, and as a means to determine if a student was ready to be taught new techniques and receive new energies. A teacher within the Gakkai would be assigned students, and the students would meet with their teacher (*Shihan*) on a regular basis to receive instruction and *Reiju*, the Japanese empowerment (attunement) ritual, to assist the student to strengthen their connection to Reiki and the amount of Reiki their body could hold, and they would be expected to practise regularly between meetings.

The training levels

Students were assigned grading levels in reverse order when they were training, in a similar way to martial arts, so they would start at level 6, rather than at level 1.

- When the student received the *Shoden* initiation (equivalent to Reiki 1) they would be assigned an energy rating of 6, called *Roku-to* (sometimes called *Rokyu*), and as they practised with Reiki, their energy abilities would grow, and the teacher would show them *Byosen Reikan-ho*, a scanning technique. The student would then be given an energy ranking of 5, called *Go-to* (*Gokyu*).

- As they grew skilled in this technique, the teacher would then show them an advanced method called *Reiji-ho*, which involved using Reiki to guide their hands to wherever it was needed on the body. This brought the student to energy rating 4, called *Yon-to* (*Yonkyu*).

- When they excelled at this, the teacher would notice the improvement in their energy and rate them as a 3, *San-to* (*Sankyu*), and at this point, the student would be offered *Okuden* training. (Therefore the levels 6, 5, 4 and 3 would all be equivalent to Reiki 1 in the West, although 3 would be transitional, taking them into the next level, *Okuden*.)

- *Okuden* level (equivalent to Reiki 2) would be taught in two stages; *Zenki* or first step, and *Koki* or latter step, over a lengthy period of time. They would receive three separate energy transformations (attunements) over a period of time to each of the energies: Focus (Power), Harmony (Mental–Emotional) and Connection (Distant). Hayashi Chujiro in his training gave these along with *Shirushi* (symbols) and *Kotodama* (mantras), but in the Gakkai, these are not taught.

- *Shinpiden* or 'mystery training' (equivalent to Reiki 3/Master in the West) involves yet another empowerment (to the Empowerment or Master energy) and training in giving the *Reiju* empowerments (attunements).

- After the *Shinpiden* student demonstrated proficiency with techniques and dedication to meditation and energy practices, the student would become first an assistant teacher (*Shihan-Kaku*) and eventually would be allowed to have their own students as a qualified *Shihan*.

The *Reiju* attunement ceremony is very simple compared to modern Western ceremonies and, according to Doi Hiroshi, it has changed a few times. Even Usui apparently modified this from the very simple process that he taught his earliest *Shinpiden* student, Eguchi Toshihiro, a well-known natural healer of the time. Eguchi's fame eventually outgrew that of Usui in Japan, as he is believed to have taught about 500,000 students in his lifetime.

Originally, Usui Sensei, as a highly spiritual man, would simply be able to sit in meditation with the student and pass on an attunement by transferring the Reiki energy connection across the room with his powerful thought energy. But he obviously found that a small ceremony was more useful to assist the focus of some of his *Shinpiden* students, and also when there was a large group involved (empowerments were given on a one-to-one basis). The process

Dr Hayashi taught Tatsumi Sensei was indeed very simple, and reportedly that used in the Gakkai was even more so. Doi Sensei is not permitted to demonstrate the current Gakkai process (*Reiju*) in public, although evidently he did give it to one of my Reiki Masters, Andrew Bowling. Instead he has developed his own version of *Reiju* – something that closely reproduces the process of the Gakkai empowerment. He uses this in all his Reiki gatherings and, just as in the Gakkai meetings, each teacher goes around the room giving *Reiju* to others.

Usui saw the purpose of Reiki as a way to put us in touch with our spiritual path, to encourage enlightenment in this life, so he developed definite spiritual techniques, which form 'the way', techniques that were designed to allow us to connect fully with ourselves. Healing was simply a by-product. Doi Sensei explained that Usui taught and made use of techniques and energies he learned long before his Reiki experience on the mountain (Kurama-yama), including the Reiki Principles, meditations and energy techniques from his martial arts training, such as *Kenyoku-ho* (dry bathing), which unblocks the *Ki*, allowing it to flow, so that we 'become' Reiki.

He also shared four specific energies with his experienced students, without the use of any physical representations such as *Shirushi* (symbols) or *Kotodama* (mantras), although he may have instructed his students to use *Jumon* (chants) to help develop their acquisition of these energies. Apparently, since the *Okuden* student would be very sensitive to energy, having developed their connection through the *Shoden* levels, such things were usually not required, but at some point he is believed to have made allowances for some of his students – notably the three naval officers including Dr Hayashi – who had difficulty with such things because they did not have a very spiritual background, and were seemingly unwilling to put in the time to practise *Jumon* regularly. These people were given what Doi Sensei calls 'training wheels' – the *Shirushi* (symbol shapes) and *Kotodama* (mantras) – to assist in their focus.

In *Shoden* training, the Gakkai has apparently always taught Usui's simple five hand positions for the head and given out his *Shoden* class booklet, the *Usui Reiki Hikkei*. This contained a reference table of hand positions for various body parts, as well as for common illnesses and conditions that could be followed if the student could not naturally sense where to place his or her hands.

These hand positions originated from traditional Chinese medicine, but they appear to have only survived in the Eguchi style of healing, although they are reportedly in Tatsumi's notes. Usui seemed to rely more on *Byosen Reikan-ho* (a form of scanning) and *Reiji-ho* (letting Reiki guide you to the area of need). According to Tatsumi Sensei's information, originally Dr Hayashi did not have formal hand positions, but after 1931 he evolved a complex system that involved two Practitioners, with the patient lying on their back, including new hand placements for the lower half of the body. These may have been the basis for the series of 12 hand positions Mrs Takata taught using the front and back of the body, for one Practitioner – it is not known if Hayashi had a one-Practitioner formula as well.

THE THREE LEVELS OF USUI REIKI RYOHO TRAINING

As I have indicated, traditional Japanese Reiki training is in three levels, *Shoden* (the opening) *Okuden* (the deep inside) and *Shinpiden* (mystery teachings). According to Doi Sensei, the student would receive *Reiju* (empowerment) at each training session, and the techniques taught at each of the levels would be over a significant period of time. There is a separate chapter for each of the levels, but briefly the following would be included:

Shoden

The purpose of this level was to learn to sense *Ki*, cultivate *Ki*, and use this knowledge to ground and heal the self. During their *Shoden* training, students would receive copies of the *Usui Reiki Hikkei* (Usui Sensei's teaching manual) and the *Reiki Ryoho Shishin* (Usui's healing guide), they would learn the five Reiki Precepts as well as Usui's selection of *Gyosei*, 125 examples of the Meiji Emperor's poetry, and a number of energy, breathing and meditation techniques (*Kenyoku-ho*, *Joshin Kokyu-ho* and *Seishin Toitsu*). In addition they would be taught *Byosen Reikan-ho*, a method for sensing imbalances by scanning the body, and Usui's original five hand positions on the head, and they would be expected to practise *Teate* (hands-on healing) for themselves and others. They would take part in some healing methods in groups (*Reiki Mawashi*, *Shuchu Reiki* and

Renzoku Reiki) and would learn *Nentatsu-ho*, a deprogramming technique, and *Jakikiri Joka-ho*, a method for purifying negative energy from objects. At a later stage in their training they would be taught *Reiji-ho*, a technique for allowing Reiki to guide you to wherever on the body needs healing. When they were seen to be proficient in all aspects of *Shoden* training, they would be invited to progress to the *Okuden* level.

Okuden

This is divided into two parts: *Okuden-Zenki* and *Okuden-Koki*, and the student would progress to the second part only when their teacher felt they were ready. This level was about strengthening their ability as a channel, learning to use specific energies and receiving more spiritual teachings.

Okuden-Zenki

At this level, students would be taught *Hatsurei-ho*, a combined meditation and cleansing technique, and a number of ways of using the hands differently for performing treatments (*Uchite Chiryo-ho*, *Oshite Chiryo-ho* and *Nadete Chiryo-ho*), *Tanden Chiryo-ho*, a method of releasing toxins, *Heso Chiryo-ho*, a navel healing technique, plus ways of using Reiki through breathing (*Koki-ho*) and with the eyes (*Gyoshi-ho*).

Okuden-Koki

When a student had shown proficiency in all of the above techniques, they could then progress to the second part of *Okuden* training. They would receive three separate empowerments over a period of time, one to each of the Focus, Harmony and Connection energies, and receive the relevant *Shirushi* and *Kotodama* and training in the use of each energy if required – this would be dependent upon the student's spiritual development and level of understanding. Other techniques at this level would include *Seiheki Chiryo-ho* (natural habits healing technique), *Hanshin Chiryo-ho* (half-body treatment) and *Zenshin Koketsu-ho* (full-body blood cleansing), as well as *Enkaku Chiryo-ho*, a technique for distant healing, *Genetsu-ho*, for bringing down fever or inflammation, and *Byogen Chiryo*, for getting to the root cause of a disease.

Shinpiden

The purpose of this level was to focus on furthering personal and spiritual development, and learning how to pass on the system of Reiki to others, but it would only be offered to very few highly experienced and committed students. They would receive further spiritual teachings and would receive attunement to the Empowerment (Master) energy, and its corresponding *Jumon*, *Shirushi* and *Kotodama*, as well as training in its use. At this level they might be taught the process for carrying out *Reiju*, although this may have been a further level called *Shihan*, meaning teacher, and they would be expected to make a commitment to the life-long Reiki journey.

THE WESTERN WAY

It is becoming quite popular now for Western Reiki Masters to call their Reiki training by the Japanese names, *Shoden* (Reiki 1), *Okuden* (Reiki 2) and *Shinpiden* (Reiki Master); however, there is huge variation between the training offered, some of which is quite close to the original way in which Usui Sensei taught, whereas others are basically Western-style Reiki courses with some Japanese techniques added. (Some courses using the usual Western names of Reiki 1, Reiki 2 and Reiki Master also include some Japanese techniques.) That's not a bad thing, indeed it adds to a student's experience and can be very enjoyable, but if you do find yourself attracted to the Japanese way, then those courses wouldn't fulfil your expectations.

It is almost unknown for any supposedly Japanese-style training to take more time than a typical Western-type course, so most are offered over one or two days, whereas in Japan each level would take many months, and possibly even years, to complete; for example, if a Japanese student was taught the *Shirushi* (symbols) and *Kotodama* (mantras) they would not all be taught in one day, as is typical in a Western Reiki 2 course or Western *Okuden* course. They would be introduced first to the Focus (Power) *Shirushi*, and be expected to work with that, including meditating on it and chanting the *Kotodama* (or *Jumon*), for many weeks or months before being introduced to the Harmony (Mental–Emotional) *Shirushi* and *Kotodama*, and there would be a similar time lapse before the Connection (Distant) *Shirushi* and *Kotodama* were offered.

Some Western Reiki Masters do teach a range of practical techniques appropriate to each level; others might include them in their manuals but don't demonstrate or practise them on their courses, preferring to concentrate on the more spiritual, meditative aspects of Reiki. Also, some offer monthly Reiki Share meetings where their students can receive regular *Reiju*, and a few offer ongoing study on a one-to-one basis, especially at *Shinpiden* level.

Therefore, if you decide to take a *Shoden* course, for example, instead of a Reiki First Degree, do find out first exactly what will be included. You can ask the Reiki Master to provide you with the course programme, and check it against what you find in Chapter 20, and you can also ask them about their lineage; if their lineage includes Mrs Takata, then unless they also have an additional Japanese lineage, as I do, it is unlikely that the course they offer will be authentically Japanese in style. The most likely Japanese lineages to look out for will include Doi Hiroshi (Usui Mikao – Taketomi Kan'ichi – Koyama Kimiko – Doi Hiroshi) or Yamaguchi Chiyoko (either Usui Mikao – Hayashi Chujiro – Yamaguchi Chiyoko – Hyakuten Inamoto; or Usui Mikao – Hayashi Chujiro – Yamaguchi Chiyoko – Yamaguchi Tadao).

THE JAPANESE REIKI TECHNIQUES

In the following three chapters I have tried hard to make all of the described Japanese techniques as easy to understand as possible so that you can try them out; however, you would undoubtedly still find it beneficial to attend a workshop with a Reiki Master who has a good understanding of these methods so you would then be able to practise them, under supervision, with other Reiki students. Whatever level of Reiki you have now – 1, 2 or 3 – these techniques are a tremendous addition to an already excellent healing practice, so I hope you will enjoy discovering their potential.

Chapter 20

Shoden Techniques
(First Level)

The emphasis at this level, as with all the levels, is spiritual development and self-healing to create health in mind and body (healing
by *Ki*) and spiritual growth (healing by *Rei*), and to understand the
journey you are taking.

GASSHO

First, an explanation about *Gassho*, which you will have seen mentioned briefly before in this book. The word itself literally means
'to place the two palms together' and it is probably the most fun-
damental of all the *mudras* (symbolic hand gestures or positions)
that we use. It is a gesture of respect, humility and reverence and
is used to concentrate the mind and to express the total unity of
Being. It is seen as a connection between body and mind, bringing
together the *in* and *yo*, the Japanese words meaning the same as the
more familiar Chinese *yin* and *yang*. In Reiki, it is used during the
Japanese 'blessing' ritual or empowerment called *Reiju*, and during
the Western-tradition attunement process. It can also be used to
begin and end any of the techniques in this or the following two
chapters, as a sign of prayerful respect and honour of the system,
the energy, the client and all creation.

To make a *Gassho*, place both hands together with their palms
touching and the fingers and thumbs close together and extended
upwards in a prayer position, and hold them so that the thumbs are

held close to the centre of the chest. At the end of any meditation or other technique, keeping your hands together, bow slightly to show respect.

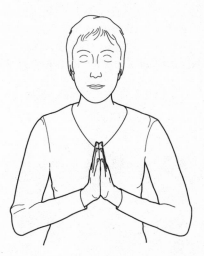

THE REIKI PRECEPTS

One of the first things students would learn would be the Reiki Precepts, known perhaps better in the West as the Reiki Principles. The Principles, which have been taught in the West through Mrs Takata's lineage, are slightly different from those now available from Japan, and you will find those in Chapter 16.

Usui is thought to have adapted his precepts from a similar teaching used in the Tendai Buddhist sect of Shugendo from the 9th century:

> *Do not bear anger,*
> *For anger is illusion.*
> *Do not be worried,*
> *Because fear is distraction.*
> *Be true to your way and your being,*
> *Show compassion to yourself and others,*
> *Because this is the centre of Buddhahood.*

He instructed his students to sit with their hands in the *Gassho* position and repeat his precepts aloud twice a day as part of their responsibility to improve both body and soul with Reiki, which he described as 'the secret method to invite happiness' and 'the spiritual medicine for all diseases of body and mind'. The Japanese version is given below, together with the principles originally thought to have been written in Usui's own handwriting (read from right to left), but we now believe these were probably written by Ushida Sensei, the second President of the Usui Reiki Ryoho Gakkai:

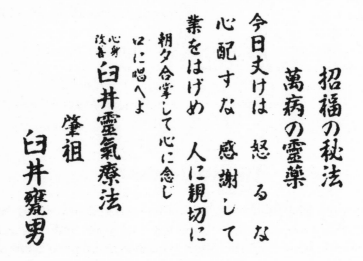

The secret art of inviting happiness
The miraculous medicine of all diseases
Just for today, do not anger
Do not worry and be filled with gratitude
Devote yourself to your work and be kind to people
Every morning and evening join your hands in prayer,
Pray these words to your heart
And chant these words with your mouth
Usui Reiki treatment for the improvement of body and mind.

The founder, Usui Mikao

Another slightly different translation, with its phonetic pronunciation in Japanese, is:

Japanese	English
Kyo dake wa	Just for today
(Kee oh dah kay wah)	
Okuru-na	Do not get angry
(Oh koh roo nah)	
Shinpai suna	Do not worry
(Shin pie soo nah)	
Kansha shite	Show appreciation/be grateful
(Kan shah she tay)	
Goo hage me	Work hard (on yourself)
(Gyo oh hah gay may)	
Hito ni shinsetsu ni	Be kind to others/show
(Hee toe nee shin set tzoo nee)	compassion to yourself and others

WAKA POETRY

Usui also recommended that his students should read aloud some of the *waka* poetry as part of their spiritual work, and he selected 125 poems by the Emperor Mutsuhito and the Empress Shoken in the Meiji period, 1868–1912. *Waka*, also called *tanka*, are very short, fixed forms of poetry containing 31 syllables – five lines of 5, 7, 5, 7 and 7 syllables – and are said to be very expressive of the feelings of the Japanese people. Here is an example:

Nami	The Wave
Aruruka to	One moment stormy
Mireba nagiyuku	The next moment it is calm
Unabara no	The wave in the ocean
Nami koso hito no	Is actually
Yo ni nitarikere	Just like human existence

(There is a list of all 125 *waka* poems in *Spirit of Reiki* by Walter Lubeck, Frank Arjava Petter and William Lee Rand.)

CLEANSING AND MEDITATION TECHNIQUES

Students would be expected to follow a daily practice including *Kenyoku-ho*, and either (or both) *Joshin Kokyu-ho* and *Seishin Toitsu*. The techniques could be carried out when standing or, more usually, when sitting, either on a chair, or in *seiza*, which is a kneeling position, sitting back on your ankles, with your back straight.

Kenyoku-ho – dry bathing or brushing off

(*Kenyoku*: dry bathing; *ho*: method.)

This technique can be practised on its own, or before other techniques, and the physical actions combined with the breath stimulates the clearing of energy through the body and arms. This is therefore an ideal technique to use before using Reiki in treatments, as clearing the arms and hands allows the Reiki to flow more freely through them.

1　First, place the fingers of your right hand near the top of your left shoulder, with the palm of your hand facing the floor, fingers and thumb close together, and draw your hand diagonally down, quickly and positively, across your chest down to your right hip. At the same time, expel your breath quickly and loudly, making a sound throughout the movement, such as 'Haaah'.

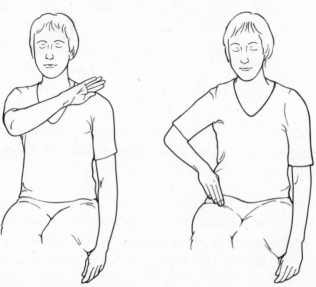

2 Now do the same thing on the other side, placing your left hand on your right shoulder, and brush down from the right shoulder to the left hip, again exhaling loudly.

3 Repeat the action, with your right hand on your left shoulder, brushing diagonally from your left shoulder to your right hip and exhaling loudly.

4 Next, hold your left arm out, parallel to the ground with the palm facing upwards, and place your right hand on your left shoulder again, but this time, draw your right hand quickly and positively down your left arm, all the way across and then off the palm and fingertips of your left hand, while expelling your breath noisily, as before.

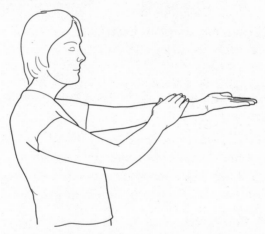

5 Repeat this process on the other side, with your left hand on your right shoulder, brushing down quickly and positively to the fingertips of your right hand, expelling your breath loudly as before.

6 Complete this process by once more sweeping your right hand down your left arm from shoulder to fingertips, again exhaling loudly.

(It may seem strange that each action is made three times, rather than four, but the reason is that in Japan there is superstition about doing things four times, at least among the older generation, as the word for the number four is apparently the same as the word for death!)

Joshin Kokyu-ho – the cleansing breath

(*Joshin*: focus, pure mind; *kokyu*: breath; *ho*: method.)

This is a meditation technique that cleanses and clears your energies with Reiki.

1   Begin by sitting in *seiza* (or on a chair) with your back straight, your eyes gazing with soft focus at the floor, then breathe deeply to release all the tension from your body, and bring your mental focus to your *hara* (just below your navel). Place your hands in *Gassho*.

2   When you are ready, lower your arms and put your hands on your lap with your palms facing upwards, and let yourself breathe naturally and steadily through your nose.

3   As you breathe in, *intend* to breathe in Reiki for your cleansing, and allow the breath to flow all the way down to your *hara*, filling it with Reiki.

4   Then, as you breathe out, *intend* that the Reiki flows through to fill your whole body, and eventually through your skin into the area surrounding you, as if you are filling a big balloon with air.

5   Continue to breathe in Reiki through your nose down to the *hara*, and breathe out Reiki to fill your whole body and the area around you (your big balloon), for about five minutes.

6   When you finish, place your hands in *Gassho* again.

With experience, you can carry out this technique for up to an hour, but if at any time you feel a bit faint, stop; this is just a possible reaction to the energy clearing, but you can continue with this practice the next day.

Seishin Toitsu – concentration or meditation

(*Seishin*: spirit, soul, mind, intention; *toitsu*: unite, unify, make one.)

This technique would probably not be taught until you had several months of experience with the previous technique as it is a much more concentrated and potentially powerful meditation.

1   Begin by sitting in *seiza* (or on a chair) with your back straight, your eyes gazing with soft focus at the floor. Breathe deeply to release all tension from your body, and bring your mental focus to your *hara* (just below your navel), and place your hands in *Gassho*.

2   Keeping your hands in *Gassho*, focus your mind on your *hara*, and as you breathe in Reiki, take your focus away from breathing through your nose, and imagine that you are breathing into your hands. As you breathe in, visualise the light of Reiki flowing up your arms to your shoulders and then down through your body to your *hara*.

3   As you breathe out, sense the energy flowing from your *hara*, up through your body, down your arms and out of your hands.

4   Continue breathing in and out, moving the Reiki from your hands down to your *hara* and back to your hands.

5   Carry on with this process for about five minutes, but with experience you can extend this to about an hour, letting your mind settle into a peaceful, meditative state.

The Reiki Shower technique

This technique from the Japanese tradition may have been taught by Usui, although the description below is the one I use which is probably a bit more Westernised. The technique consists of activating and cleansing your whole energy body by absorbing Reiki energy throughout the body like a shower. You can use this technique almost anywhere for cleansing yourself, and it can also help to centre yourself, raising your consciousness and bringing you into a meditative state.

1   Stand or sit and make yourself comfortable. Close or half-close your eyes and begin to slow down and deepen your breathing until you can maintain a naturally slow and steady pace.

2   Place your hands in the *Gassho* position. Stay like this for a few moments, and *intend* to use Reiki to cleanse and activate your energy body.

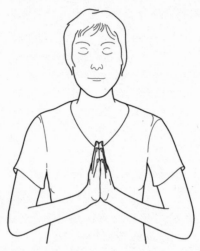

3   Then separate your hands and lift them above your head, as high as possible, keeping them about 20–30cm (8–12in) apart.

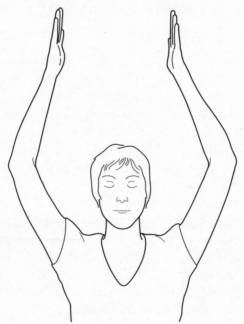

4　Wait for a few moments until you begin to feel the Reiki building up between your hands, and then turn your palms downwards so that they are facing the top of your head.

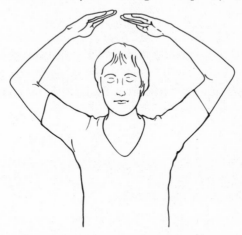

5　Visualise and *intend* that you are receiving a shower of Reiki energy from the palms of your hands which flows over and through your whole physical and energy body, cleansing you and removing any negative energy.

6　When you feel the vibration of the Reiki energy flowing over and through you, move your hands, palms still facing towards you, and begin to draw them slowly down over your face and in front of your body, keeping your hands about 20–30cm (8–12in) away from the body. *Intend* that Reiki is flowing from your hands and continuing to cleanse and revitalise you as you draw your hands all the way down your body and then down your legs to your feet. Eventually, turn your palms to face the floor and gently throw the energy off your hands so that any negative energy flows out of your feet and into the earth below, where it can be transformed and used by the planet.

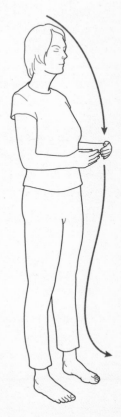

7   Repeat this exercise a few times – I find three times to be ideal –
    and you should feel cleansed, revitalised and more alive as Reiki
    healing and light flows into all of your cells and fills every part
    of your body.

8   Place your hands together again in the *Gassho* position and
    spend a few moments experiencing gratitude for the Reiki, and
    then finish. You may find it helpful to clap your hands once or
    twice to help you to return to a more wakeful state, if this exer-
    cise leaves you feeling a bit 'spaced'.

BALANCING AND SENSING ENERGIES

Connecting the three diamonds

As I mentioned in Chapter 2, Reiki is not traditionally linked with
the chakra system, as this was essentially an Indian concept, and
was not used in Japan; however, Usui was well versed in energy
techniques from his martial arts training, so this technique would
have been taught to students to help them to expand and balance
their energies. It is similar to a qigong technique called *Dao Chi*,
and the idea is to connect the three energy centres known as *hara*,
tanden, *tandien* or in Reiki practice as the three diamonds: Earth *Ki*,
Heaven *Ki* and Heart *Ki*.

* **The lower *tanden*, or Earth *Ki*,** is in the abdomen, at the
  hara (just below your navel). Earth *Ki* is heavy, powerful
  and grounding, helping you to feel strong and secure, and
  physically connected to the environment.

* **The middle *tanden*, or Heart *Ki*,** is located in the middle of the
  chest, in the heart area. Heart *Ki* is seen as the point of perfect
  balance that comes from merging Earth *Ki* and Heaven *Ki* to
  connect body, mind and spirit, and it helps to bring peace, love
  and compassion into your life.

* **The upper *tanden*, or Heaven *Ki*,** is located within the upper
  brain, in the brow area. Heaven *Ki* is light and expansive, and
  it helps your intuition and mental acuity.

A student would first be taught to sense each of the three diamonds individually by spending some time breathing slowly and deeply and *intending* to draw energy into each of them, one at a time. When they had mastered that, they would then be taught the following technique to connect all three, to balance the energies of Heaven and Earth and bring them into the Heart, the centre of your being. You can do this on yourself, or on a client, and it is an especially nice way to end a treatment – the following instructions assume you are doing this with a client who is lying down, but if you are doing this on yourself, your palm would be facing towards you.

1   Place your hands in *Gassho*, breathe slowly and deeply, and state your intent that you are going to connect the three diamonds.

2   Put your dominant hand with the palm downwards over the brow about 10cm (4in) off the body, and wait for a few moments until you feel the energy connection. (The non-dominant hand remains relaxed next to your body throughout the exercise.)

3   Move your dominant hand to above the heart area and stay until you feel a connection again.

4   Now move your dominant hand to above the *hara* (just below your navel) and again stay until you feel the connection.

5   Now, slowly repeat this in the reverse direction, moving the energy up from the *hara* to the heart area, pausing briefly, and then to the brow area.

6   Then, repeat the original process, moving the energy slowly from the brow, pausing briefly, then to the heart, pausing briefly, and finishing at the *hara*, leaving your hand there for a minute or two to enjoy the connection with the energy.

7   Place your hands in *Gassho* once more, and give thanks.

A technique for developing sensitivity

When a student first begins their *Shoden* training they may find it difficult to sense subtle energies when carrying out the next technique, the *Byosen Reikan-ho*, so this is a method taught by Doi Sensei to encourage sensitivity in the hands.

1   Begin to rub your palms together until they feel hot, then the backs of your hands, then each thumb and each finger, and finally rub the palms together again.

2   Move your hands apart and hold them with the palms facing each other about 20cm (8in) apart and feel the tingling sensations of the energy between your hands.

3   Bring your attention to your breathing, and each time you breathe out, expel the air with a 'haaah' sound. Look at the space between your hands and, as you continue this deep breathing (called *Hado*), for a while, imagine that you are breathing in and out through your hands.

4   Finally, clench your hands tightly into fists and then release them.

5   Hold your hands at chest height about 20cm (8in) apart and visualise or imagine that you are holding an empty balloon. With your eyes half closed, keep looking at the space between your hands, imagining the balloon there. Continue with the *Hado* breathing, breathing out with a 'haaah' sound, and as you do so, feel and *intend* that the energy from your palms is going into the balloon. As you breathe out Reiki into this imaginary balloon your hands move wider apart as it fills with energy and gets larger, and as you breathe in again the balloon shrinks and your hands come closer together.

6   Continue this visualisation for a while and gradually the sensation of moving energy into and out of the space between your hands will become more and more real. When this happens you can change back to natural breathing. Experiment with the energy between your hands, moving your hands together then apart, always with the palms facing each other, to sense the tingling and warmth of the energy.

7   Finally, clench your hands tightly into fists and then release them.

8   Bring your hands down towards your abdomen, and place both hands with their palms facing towards the *hara* (just below your navel), keeping them about 10cm (4in) away from your body. Feel the energy flowing from your hands into your *hara*, and

keep them there until you can feel the energy quite strongly, which will mean you have built up enough sensitivity to be able to sense energy differences in different parts of your body.

9 Now, slowly move your hands to other parts of your body, keeping your palms facing your body as you slowly scan over each area – give yourself time to sense the energy. (If you find your sensitivity becoming weaker, go back to steps 1 to 3 until the energy returns.)

Practise all of the above from time to time until you are fully confident that you can sense energy easily and clearly.

My quick version!

The above method for intensifying the sensitivity in your hands might seem a bit complex, so I developed a quick-and-easy technique that seems to work reasonably well. Simply rub your hands together vigorously – palms, backs of hands, fingers and sides of hands – for about 30 seconds, then separate your hands and sense the tingling energy between them. You are then ready to begin sensing your own or a client's energies.

Byosen Reikan-ho

(*Byo*: disease, sickness, imbalance; *sen*: before, ahead, previous, future; *rei*: energy, soul, spirit; *kan*: emotion, feeling, sensation; *ho*: treatment, method, way.)

This is a method for sensing imbalances with your hands, and it can be used on yourself or with others. The type and amount of sensation will vary from person to person, depending upon the severity and condition of any imbalance or 'dis-ease' (physical or energetic), and can include tingling, tickling, pulsating, piercing, stinging, pain, numbness, heat, cold and so on. In Japanese, these sensations are called *Hibiki*. They normally occur only in the hands, but can occasionally be felt in the arms or even up to the shoulders in extreme cases.

Whenever dis-ease is present, there will be a *Byosen*, even if the client is unaware of any physical condition, as the imbalance is usually presented first in the energy body. If you sense a *Byosen* in someone's body and work on it until it disappears, the related disease/symptom (or potential disease) should either completely heal or never manifest on the physical level (unless there is a higher reason for it to do so, such as needing the lesson that illness will teach that person). Sometimes, however, the *Byosen* may appear in a different part of the body from any physical symptom, as the energetic imbalance may be linked through the meridians of the energy system. The ability to sense a *Byosen* will vary from person to person, so practise on yourself and friends or family until you feel reasonably confident.

1   Sit or stand comfortably next to the recipient.

2   Sensitise your hands with one of the two methods above (and repeat that method whenever you find it more difficult to feel sensations in your hands).

3   Spend a few moments centring yourself with your hands in the *Gassho* position, and allow your mind to become calm. Then *intend* to activate your intuitive ability to detect *Byosen* by saying silently to yourself, 'I begin *Byosen Reikan-ho* now.'

4   Place your hands, palms downwards, slightly above (5–15cm/2–6in) the recipient's body, starting at either the head or the feet, and begin to move them slowly down (or up) the body. Sometimes, it is helpful initially to close your eyes, so that you can 'tune in' more easily to any sensations in your hands. You will probably find that there is a general 'background' sensation of gentle warmth or tingling or even a cool breeze when you pass your hands over one of the major energy centres (such as one of the three diamonds, or if you are more familiar with them, the chakras); however, some areas will feel different, and these are the areas of *Byosen*. The more you practise, the easier it will become to identify the subtle differences, but pay attention to changes in heat or tingling, or any of the other sensations detailed above.

5   When you sense a *Hibiki* (the sensation of *Byosen*), hold your hands on or over that area. The sensations will ebb and flow in natural cycles, increasing and then decreasing. Don't automatically assume that when the sensation reduces it is time to move your hands, as these cycles will continue for as long as your hands are on the body. The longer you hold your hands over a particular place the more energy cycles you will feel, but with

each cycle the intensity diminishes. Keep your hands over the *Hibiki* for at least one cycle, and if you have time, keep your hands in the same place until there is virtually no discernible difference in sensation (that is, more of a continuous sensation than an ebb and flow).

6   When you are ready, move your hands gently and slowly to the next area of *Byosen* and repeat step 4.

7   When you have completed *Byosen Reikan-ho* on the entire body, remove your hands from the recipient and place them at mid-chest height in the *Gassho* position. Mentally give thanks for the Reiki, bowing slightly as a mark of respect.

Reiji or *Reiji-ho*

(*Rei*: energy, spirit, soul; *ji*: show, indicate, express, display; *ho*: treatment, method, way.)

This technique would not usually be taught until a student was fully competent at *Byosen Reikan-ho*. *Reiji-ho* encourages relaxation, enhances your intuition and allows Reiki to guide your hands to places on the body that are in need of treatment. (As I have previously mentioned, in Japan they do not use the pattern of 12 or more hand positions taught in the West, as students are encouraged to develop their sensitivity, perception and intuition by using this and the previous two techniques, so that they can place their hands wherever they intuitively sense is most in need of Reiki.) Practising this technique will help you to expand and enhance your awareness of subtle energies.

1   Sit or stand comfortably next to the recipient, and spend a few moments centring yourself (hands in *Gassho*). Focus your attention on your *hara* (just below your navel) to connect with Earth *Ki*, allowing your breathing to become deep and even, and then *intend* to activate your intuitive ability, saying to yourself, 'I begin *Reiji-ho* now' or 'Reiki guides me now to where it is needed.'

2   Next, with your hands either palm upwards on your lap if you are sitting, or loosely by your side if you are standing, allow your body to completely relax, releasing any tensions and anxieties, and gently encourage your client to do the same. Silently

call upon Reiki to fill you and your client with healing energy, and imagine Reiki flowing into you as you breathe in, filling your whole body with healing energy, and sense it flowing out of your hands into your client's energy field, healing all levels of your being for both of you. Let yourself experience this feeling for a while and then move to step 3.

3   Move your hands (still in the *Gassho* position) upwards until your thumbs are resting on your brow (Heaven *Ki*) and silently ask Reiki to guide your hands to the places in need of energy. Let your hands remain in that position until you feel you need to move them, and then your hands will be guided or drawn like magnets to areas of imbalance in the body, and you can either place your hands directly on the body or hold them 5–10cm (2–4in) above or in front of your client, palms facing towards their body, and allow Reiki to flow. When you feel that part has been balanced by the Reiki, your hands will be guided to the next place, and this process will continue until all parts of the body in need of energy are balanced. The more you practise this technique, the more you will find that Reiki automatically tells you what to treat and for how long, and this intuition can be received either kinaesthetically (in feelings or sensations) or mentally (as thoughts/words, images, insights or intuitions).

4   When all parts of your client's body have been balanced, or when there is no need for more Reiki at this particular time, your hands will be naturally guided to your knees if you are sitting or to the sides of your body if you are standing.

5   *Gassho*, give thanks for the Reiki and end with a bow of respect.

Usui's Reiki Manual

The original Reiki manual, the *Usui Reiki Hikkei*, has a section called Ryoho Shishon: 'Guide to a Method of Healing'. The purpose of the guide was to assist the Reiki Practitioner who had not yet developed *Byosen* or *Reiji-ho* (the ability to feel where Reiki is required). This included the specific hand positions for all the major body parts, as well as major illnesses that were common in Usui Sensei's time. Depending on the size of the treatment area, the Practitioner could lay one or two hands on the area, or simply place the index and middle fingers on the area. (Reiki also flows out of the fingertips.) Most of these hand positions (there were 68 in total), and which of them should be used to treat various illnesses or specific parts of the body, are shown in Frank Arjava Petter's book, *The Original Reiki Handbook of Dr Mikao Usui*.

What we should remember is that the ultimate aim of Usui's system was not to heal others but to heal oneself, because by healing the Self you affect others, so all his Reiki students were encouraged to practise *Tenohira* – the practice of palm healing – for themselves and others. Also, the only thing that was kept secret was the *Reiju* empowerment. Usui simply gave people the tools to heal themselves.

USUI'S ORIGINAL HAND POSITIONS

Despite having the 68 potential hand positions referred to above for treating various ailments, it seems that Usui mainly concentrated on hand positions on the head, unless areas on the torso appeared to be out of balance energetically, apparently because the belief in the East at the time was that most ailments arise in the brain. A number of different hand positions are in use today as Reiki has developed, although the 12 hand positions taught by Mrs Takata do include four or five on the head, with seven or eight on the trunk of the body. These positions correspond to Eastern traditional teachings (such as Chinese medicine) where the 'body' is the head and torso, whereas the limbs are considered 'external' and are therefore not normally treated. It is considered that applying healing energy to the head and thorax is sufficient to treat the whole body–mind.

The person receiving healing was usually seated, not lying down, and the healing began at the head. For a self-treatment there were five hand positions as shown overleaf.

1 *Zento-bu*: Place your hand on top of your forehead, between your eyebrows and the line where your hair starts to grow.

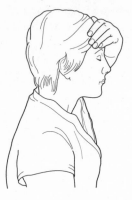

2 *Koutou-bu*: Place your hand at the back of your head, roughly at the middle point between the top of your head and the top of your spine.

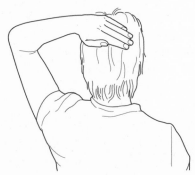

3 *Enzui-bu*: Place your hand at the base of the skull, where the brain and spine meet.

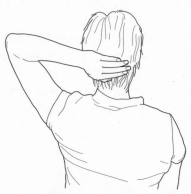

4 ***Sokuto-bu***: Place one hand on each of your temples.

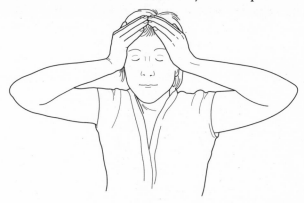

5 ***Toucho-bu***: Place your hand right at the top of your head, on your crown.

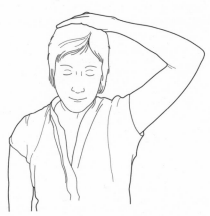

The same individual hand positions can be used when treating someone else, or they can be combined into three hand positions. The Practitioner's hands would either be placed on the head, or could be held 5–10cm (2–4in) away from the head. These would be held for as long as necessary, but the total time would be about 30 minutes, after which other positions on the body would be treated; that is, wherever showed an imbalance when the patient's energy field was scanned by the Practitioner's hand(s).

1   Combine *Zento-bu* and *Enzui-bu*, the forehead and back of neck.

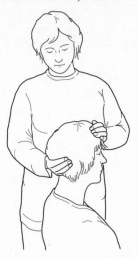

2   Combine *Koutou-bu* and *Toucho-bu*, the back of the head and the crown.

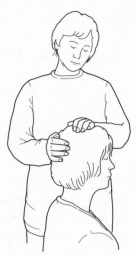

3   *Sokuto-bu* – treat both temples.

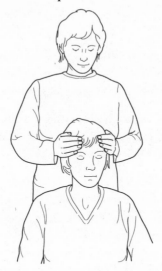

ADDITIONAL *SHODEN* TECHNIQUES

At a later stage in their training, *Shoden*-level students would be taught some additional techniques to use for self-healing and, if they were drawn to do so, for helping others.

Nentatsu-ho

(**Nen**: sense, idea, thought, concern; **tatsu**: discontinue, sever, abstain; **ho**: treatment, method, way.)

This was a technique for working on your own or a client's subconscious mind to use Reiki to reprogramme the mind, for instance to overcome bad habits, remove negativity, achieve goals, help with learning or even prevail over an illness. A literal translation of *Nentatsu-ho* is 'method for discontinuing a concern'.

1   Decide what it is you wish to work on. Create a simple, clear affirmation in the present tense as if you were already there. Some examples are: I am healthy, energised and full of vitality; I am confident and successful; I am my ideal weight and I look good and feel great; my job is fulfilling and rewarding; my life is joyful and abundant; my relationships are happy and loving.

2   Get into a comfortable position, either sitting or lying down, close your eyes and allow your breathing to become slow and steady.

3   Spend a few moments centring yourself with your hands in the *Gassho* position, allowing your mind to become calm, and then say silently to yourself, 'I begin *Nentatsu-ho* now.'

4   Place one hand on your forehead, over your brow (Heaven *Ki*/ brow chakra) and the other hand on the back of your head over the indentation at the base of your skull.

5   Then *intend* that Reiki should flow into the issue you want to work on – to be rid of a habit or a physical condition, to achieve your goal or improve your memory, and so on, always remembering to add 'for my highest and greatest good'. Repeat your affirmation(s) as you hold this position and feel the Reiki flowing into you and into your wishes and intention, for about five minutes.

6   Then remove your hand from your forehead, but keep your other hand in place at the back of your head. (You can now have both hands behind your head if you wish.) Then spend about five minutes in meditation, visualising yourself as you would be if you were rid of the habit, or as if you had achieved your goal, and so on.

7   *Gassho*, give thanks for the Reiki and end with a bow of respect.

Jakikiri Joka-ho

(*Jaki*: bad, negative energy; *kiri*: cut; *joka*: purification, cleansing; *ho*: treatment, method, way.)

   This is a technique from Doi Sensei, the purpose of which is for energy purification, or cleansing and energy-boosting of *an object*, to remove strong negative energy within an object (such as a crystal) by purifying it with Reiki energy and putting in positive energy. Please note that this technique should NOT be used on a person or animal.

1   Place your hands in *Gassho*, and centre yourself, ready to use Reiki.

2   Say silently to yourself, 'I begin *Jakikiri Joka-ho* now.'

3   Pick up the object you wish to clear in your non-dominant hand.

4   Using your dominant hand, 'chop' the space about 5cm (2in) above the object with your hand horizontally and make a sudden stop of your hand movement. When you do this chopping action, focus your attention on your *hara* (just below your navel) while holding your breath, and chop the length of your hand.

5   Repeat this three times. This means you are doing three abrupt chops. This apparently turns the vibration into a good one.

6   Give Reiki for purification and to boost the object's energy, by holding your hand over it and letting the Reiki flow for a short time (30 seconds–one minute should be enough).

7   You can repeat from step 4 again in order to keep the negative vibration away, and do this as often as you feel necessary.

8   When finished, lay the object down, *Gassho*, then clap your hands and shake your wrists well, to remove any negative energy which may be present.

This technique can be applied to crystals, charms or any object, regardless of size. If it is a large object, do the actions to selected points, or visualise a miniature version of the object in the palm of your hand, and then treat it as above.

GROUP TECHNIQUES

Shoden students would take part in group healing sessions as well as using the individual Reiki techniques above. Dr Hayashi apparently taught these techniques, and they were believed to help students to develop more confidence.

Reiki Mawashi

(***Rei***: spirit, soul; ***ki***: energy; ***mawasu***: pass on.)

This is the traditional method of a Reiki Circle or Reiki Group, which can help to sensitise a gathering of Reiki Practitioners to feel energy flow.

1   All the Reiki Practitioners form a circle, either sitting or stand-
    ing. (Ensure that your feet are shoulder-width apart, to balance
    you effectively.)

2   Everyone joins hands and, in order to ensure the correct flow
    of Reiki, it is usual to ensure that each person first has their left
    hand palm up (to receive), and their right hand palm down (to
    send). In other words, your left hand is under the right hand
    of the person on your left, and your right hand is over the
    person's hand on your right. (It is easier to do than it sounds!)

3   Next, keeping your hands in the same (under or over) position,
    gently loosen hands but continue to hold your hands 2.5–5cm
    (1–2in) apart from your partners on each side, so that the circle
    is still complete energetically, but no one is touching each other.

4   Someone in the circle (usually the *Shinpiden*/Reiki Master, if it
    is a class) begins by *intending* to send Reiki flowing down their
    right arm, so that it flows anti-clockwise around the circle. As
    each person joins in, the Reiki moves from one hand to another,
    resulting in a strong flow or current of energy around the circle,
    through each Practitioner, and this should continue for several
    minutes, or longer if you wish. (To increase the intensity of the
    current, you might like to try vibrating whichever hand is palm
    down, which is a qigong technique to increase energy.)

5   Now, switch your hands, so that your left hand is over your
    partner's hand on your left, and your right hand is under your
    partner's hand on your right, and let the current flow in a
    clockwise direction for several minutes, or longer if you prefer.

6   You may find that the current can be quite strong at times, and
    often the whole group can feel the need to move (or sway) anti-
    clockwise or clockwise like a big spiralling whirlpool.

Shuchu Reiki

(**Shuchu**: concentrated; **rei**: spiritual, soul; **ki**: energy.)

This is a traditional method for giving a group treatment or concentrated Reiki to someone, often used during a Reiki course, at
Reiki meetings or healing circles, and it ideally follows the *Mawashi*
(above), so that the group of Practitioners are channelling Reiki as
effectively and strongly as possible. The idea is that two or more

Practitioners work on one client (as Hayashi had in his clinic), and this concentrates the Reiki energy exponentially, so that the Reiki is intensified with each additional Practitioner who joins the treatment. As usual, while the group channels Reiki, every Practitioner *intends* that the Reiki flows into the recipient for their highest and greatest good.

1   Ideally, the client/recipient should be lying (face up) on a massage table/therapy couch, made comfortable with pillows under their head and knees, and a blanket to cover them, but if you don't have a massage table then please improvise appropriately.

2   Everyone who is about to carry out the treatment performs a cleansing technique first, such as the *Kenyoku-ho* or the Reiki Shower, and then they place their hands in *Gassho*, *intending* that Reiki should flow.

3   Two or more Reiki Practitioners carry out a hands-on treatment, covering all the usual hand positions, and the more Practitioners work together, the more hand positions can be covered at the same time, so the stronger the flow of energy will be; for example, four people on each side can cover all the classic hand positions, and if more Practitioners are available, then the arms, legs and feet can also be covered.

4   Generally, the head and the front of the body would be treated first, and then the client could be asked to turn over so that the back of the body could be covered; however, if ten or more Practitioners are working on the same person, there is no need to ask the person to turn over, as treating the whole of the front of the head, body and legs is sufficient.

5   One person would then perform the Three Diamonds technique over the body of the person who had just received the treatment, to balance their energies and end the treatment.

6   At the end of a treatment, each Practitioner finishes by placing their hands at mid-chest height in the *Gassho* position and mentally giving thanks for the Reiki, bowing slightly as a mark of respect.

7   Then each person performs another cleansing technique before
     treating the next person in the group; that is, they all take it in
     turns to lie on the therapy couch to receive a group treatment.

Renzoku Reiki

(**Renzoku**: continuous; **rei**: spiritual, soul; **ki**: energy.)

This is the traditional method of the Reiki Marathon, or Relay
Treatment, a practice where several Practitioners take turns (one
or two at a time) to provide Reiki in a continuous treatment session
– often over many hours or even days – to a single client. Another
version of this is for eight Practitioners to give Reiki continuously
for eight hours to a single client.

DAILY PRACTICE AT SHODEN LEVEL

All Usui Reiki Ryoho students at every level would be expected to
commit to carrying out a daily practice to enhance their physical,
mental and spiritual health, and at *Shoden* level this would be:

1   To prepare by deciding which techniques they would do that
     day.

2   Then they would either stand, or sit with their back straight on
     a chair, or more usually in *seiza* (correct sitting), meaning to be
     in a kneeling position, sitting back on their ankles, with their
     legs folded underneath and their back straight.

3   They would then gaze softly down towards the floor, release all
     tension from their body, bring the focus of their mind to their
     hara (just below their navel), and place their hands in *Gassho*.

4   Then they would chant the Reiki Principles in Japanese, but
     you can do so in your own language. (This would be done three
     times in the morning, and repeated again three times in the
     evening.)

5   Next, they would clear their energies with *Kenyoku-ho*, and
     follow this with either (or both) the *Joshin Kokyu-ho* and when
     they were more experienced, the *Seishin Toitsu* technique.

6   They would follow this by giving themselves either a head treat-
    ment or a full-body self-treatment, either sitting or lying down,
    for about half an hour.

7   For their final practice, they would be encouraged to keep a
    journal or diary, writing at least one page each day.

Remember, the *Shoden* training would probably take many months
or even years, and each student would be expected to attend
regular meetings with their *Shihan* where they would receive a *Reiju*
empowerment and additional training, plus they would be required
to practise every day, as shown above. It could therefore be a long
time before they were assessed by their *Shihan* as being ready for
the next level, *Okuden*, which is covered in the next chapter.

Chapter 21

Okuden Techniques (Second Level)

The purpose of *Okuden* training was to introduce additional tools to strengthen a student's connection with the Reiki energy, as well as enhancing their knowledge and experience. It included breathing and meditation techniques, alternative ways of using the hands when healing, as well as, at a later stage, connecting the student to the Focus, Harmony and Connection energies. It was divided into two parts, *Okuden-Zenki* and *Okuden-Koki*; however, students were still expected to undergo personal practice, similar to that at *Shoden* level, but with a few additions, as you will see at the end of this chapter.

STAGE 1 (FIRST STEP): *OKUDEN-ZENKI*

Hatsurei-ho

(**Hatsu**: to generate; **rei**: spiritual, soul; **ho**: method.)

Probably one of the first things the *Okuden* student would learn would be to combine some of their *Shoden* techniques into *Hatsurei-ho* to generate greater amounts of spiritual energy. You can follow the instructions for *Kenyoku-ho*, *Joshin Kokyu-ho* and *Seishin Toitsu* from Chapter 20, or you might like to try my slightly adapted version below, which is also available on CD from my website. It is an ideal way to start the day, or to begin your practice of Reiki, whether treating yourself or other people.

It is split into three main parts, and its basic functions are:

1   To cleanse the outer part of your physical and energy bodies with dry bathing or brushing (*Kenyoku-ho*) so that your energies can flow freely.

2   To cleanse the inner part of your energies with the cleansing breath (*Joshin Kokyu-ho*).

3   And finally, when you are cleansed internally and externally, to allow you to bring more Reiki into yourself for your own personal healing, and to fulfil part of your spiritual purpose by sending Reiki out to wherever it is needed (*Seishin Toitsu*).

It can take as little as ten minutes, or you can stretch out the more meditative parts of it (*Joshin Kokyu-ho* and *Seishin Toitsu*) to half an hour or more – it is up to you. (Some of the hand positions are illustrated on pages 330–3 in Chapter 20.)

1 *Kihon Shisei* – Standard Posture

Sit on a chair or in *seiza* and make yourself comfortable, then allow yourself to relax and close your eyes. Focus your attention on your *hara* (Earth *Ki*), which is just below your navel, and with your hands in *Gassho* spend a few moments bringing your breathing into a slow, steady rhythm as you centre yourself and intend to begin the *Hatsurei-ho*.

2 *Kenyoku-ho* – dry bathing or brushing off

1   First, place the fingers of your right hand near to the top of your left shoulder, with the palm of your hand facing the floor, fingers and thumb close together, and draw your hand diagonally down quickly and positively across your chest to your right hip. At the same time, expel your breath rapidly, making a loud sound throughout the movement, such as 'Haaah'.

2   Now do the same thing on the other side, placing your left hand on your right shoulder, and quickly brush down diagonally from the right shoulder to the left hip, again exhaling noisily.

3   Repeat the action, with your right hand on your left shoulder, brushing diagonally from your left shoulder to your right hip and exhaling loudly.

4   Next you put your left arm out parallel to the ground with the palm facing upwards, and place your right hand on your left shoulder again, but this time, draw your right hand quickly and positively down your left arm, over your palm and fingertips of your left hand, while expelling your breath noisily, as before.

5   Repeat this process on the other side, with your left hand on your right shoulder, brushing quickly and positively down your arm and over the palm and fingertips of your right hand, expelling your breath loudly as before.

6   Complete this process by once more sweeping your right hand down your left arm from shoulder to fingertips, again exhaling loudly.

3 Connect to Reiki

Now, raise both your hands high up in the air above your head, with your palms facing each other about 12–15in (30–40cm) apart, and visualise and feel the light and vibration of Reiki flowing into and between your hands and running through your whole body.

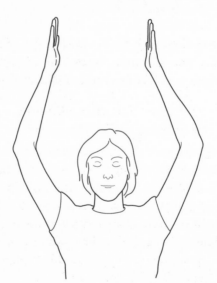

4 *Joshin Kokyu-ho* – the cleansing breath

Next, lower your arms and put your hands on your lap, with your palms facing upwards, and let yourself breathe naturally and steadily through your nose. Then say to yourself:

'I now breathe in Reiki for my cleansing, so that as the Reiki flows around my body and energy field, it breaks through any blockages and picks up any negativity, so that as I breathe out, the Reiki takes the blockages and negativity away, to beyond my energies where they can be safely healed and transformed.'

As you breathe in, visualise Reiki as white light pouring into you through your nostrils and through your crown chakra, filling your head, neck, shoulders, arms and hands with Reiki, and then flowing down your back, chest, waist, hips, abdomen and down into each leg, all the way down to the tips of your toes. Then imagine the Reiki spreading out, expanding to fill the whole of your aura, and *intend* that as the Reiki flows through the whole of your physical body and energy field, it is cleansing you.

Continue this process for two or three minutes, or up to 20 minutes or more if you wish, breathing in Reiki to cleanse you, and breathing out Reiki so that it takes away any negativity. Finally, when you feel ready, take a really deep breath and blow out the rest of the negativity, and then move on to the next section.

5 *Gassho*

Put your hands together with palms and fingers flat against each other in the *Gassho* position (see pages 326–7) and hold them in front of the centre of your chest, at about the level of your heart.

6 *Seishin Toitsu* – concentration or meditation

Say to yourself:

'Now I breathe in Reiki for my own healing – healing on all levels, physical, emotional, psychological and spiritual, wher-ever I need Reiki at this time – and as I breathe out I can share the wonderful gift of Reiki, allowing it to flow in all directions to heal the planet, the people, the animals, birds, fish and other creatures, the trees, crops and other plants, and any-thing else that needs Reiki at this time.'

1 Keeping your hands in the *Gassho* position, take your focus away from breathing through your nose, and imagine that you are breathing through your hands and, as you breathe in, visu-alise the light of Reiki flowing in through your hands and then

flowing up your arms into your heart chakra (Heart *Ki*) and down into your *hara* (Earth *Ki*) (just below your navel). Imagine it filling your heart chakra and *hara*, and then sense it flowing into your *hara* line, the energy line that connects all of your energy field from the base up to the crown. Visualise it flowing up and down your *hara* line, so that your *hara* line is filled with light, and see or sense the Reiki spreading out to fill the whole of your physical body and your energy field with its healing, balancing and harmonising energy.

2 Then imagine that, as you breathe out, Reiki flows from your *hara* to your heart, and then down your arms to your hands, where it then flows beyond your energy field in all directions, to heal anything on this beautiful planet Earth that needs Reiki at this time.

3 Continue this process for two or three minutes, or up to 20 minutes or more if you wish, and let your mind settle into a peaceful, meditative state.

7 *Gokai Sansho* – five principles, three times

In the traditional way, Japanese Reiki students would at this point say the Reiki Principles aloud three times, as instructed by Dr Usui – obviously in Japanese. This is an important part of your spiritual practice, so you may feel that you would like to do this in Japanese or in English – whichever English version of the Principles you prefer.

Japanese	**English**
Kyo dake wa	Just for today
(Kee oh dah kay wah)	
Okuru-na	Do not get angry
(Oh koh roo nah)	
Shinpai suna	Do not worry
(Shin pie soo nah)	
Kansha shite	Show appreciation/be grateful
(Kan shah she tay)	
Goo hage me	Work hard (on yourself)
(Gyo oh hah gay may)	
Hito ni shinsetsu ni	Be kind to others/show
(Hee toe nee shin set tzoo nee)	compassion to yourself and others

8 *Mokunen* – setting the intent

Place your hands back onto your lap with palms facing downwards, and *intend* that the *Hatsurei-ho* is now complete. When you feel ready, open your eyes and rub or gently clap your hands together for a few seconds, to bring you back to a greater state of physical awareness.

You are now ready to get on with your day; however, to continue your spiritual practice, this is an ideal time to carry out a self-treatment, placing your hands in each position on your head and body for between three and five minutes, or longer if you prefer, depending upon how much time you have available.

REIKI UNDO

(**Rei**: spiritual; **ki**: energy; **undo**: movement.)

This is another cleansing technique that uses physical movement to get rid of negative energy, allowing the body to move involuntarily (for example, rotating the head and neck from side to side, or moving the legs or arms) to release negative energy, sometimes performed on its own, or before or after *Hatsurei-ho*.

1   Stand or sit and make yourself comfortable, and place your hands in *Gassho*. Raise your hands up as high as possible, and *intend* to connect to Reiki, and sense the vibrations of the Reiki showering into your whole body.

2   Slowly move your hands down and place them on your lap, palms facing up, and keep them relaxed, and say to yourself, 'I begin *Reiki Undo* now.'

3   Focus on your breathing, allowing it to be deep and even, and *intend* to release as much as you can while exhaling.

4   After several breaths you may find that your body begins to move, guided by the flow of energy pulsing through you – and if it does, allow this to happen. It may be slow and rhythmic, or it might become more vigorous, but just allow Reiki to guide your body, don't try to consciously control it.

5   When you sense that the time is right to finish this technique, place your hands in *Gassho*, bow as a form of respect to Reiki, and continue with your day.

6   If performed regularly, some people find that there is a 'natural' detoxification of the physical body over a period of about three months.

ALTERNATIVE WAYS OF USING THE HANDS WITH REIKI

The methods below can all be used during a Reiki treatment as an occasional alternative to holding your hands flat and still on or just above the body, perhaps to provide additional stimulation with Reiki on the physical body in the areas where you have found energetic disturbances when scanning (*Byosen Reikan-ho* – see Chapter 20). As always while carrying out these techniques, you *intend* that the Reiki will continue to flow through your hands (palms and fingertips), for the highest and greatest good of the client. Also, it is advisable to tell your client what you are intending to do, as they may not expect anything other than hands being held still, if they have had a traditional Reiki treatment before.

Another point to remember is that it would not normally be necessary or sensible to use any of these methods on physically or socially sensitive areas of the body, so do not treat near or on the breasts on a woman, or the genital area on either men or women. Naturally, there is no need for the client to remove any clothes for these techniques (or for any Reiki techniques), as the Reiki flows through clothing in the same way as when you keep your hands still. In the *Usui Reiki Hikkei*, Usui's teaching manual, it states that Reiki emanates from all body parts, but strongest from the hands, the eyes and the breath. You may have noticed this already; for example, I often feel Reiki flowing from my feet as well as my hands, and from my brow, heart and solar plexus chakras.

Uchi-te Chiryo-ho

(*Uchi*: slap, hit, pat; *te*: hand; *chiryo*: treatment, remedy; *ho*: method.)

This is a technique for patting with the hands, and it can be used for areas of numbness or where energy feels stagnant and blocked, as well as to encourage greater energy flow and movement. It can be used at any stage during a treatment, but may be best towards the end, as it will help the client to come out of a deeply relaxed state. Clients usually find it especially pleasant to have this done on their shoulders and upper back.

1   Using a firm but gentle motion (not hard enough to hurt), use the flat of the hand (palm and fingers flat) to pat and stimulate the area, starting with very soft patting and gradually getting a bit stronger, so that the motion becomes a soft slapping. Continue until you sense it is time to move to another position (probably between 30 seconds and a minute).

2   This will stimulate the surface of the physical body and enable Reiki to penetrate into the body quickly, waking up the cells and breaking up any energy blockages.

3   *Gassho*, give thanks for the Reiki and end with a bow of respect.

Nade-te Chiryo-ho

(**Nade**: stroke, smooth down; *te*: hand; *chiryo*: treatment, remedy; *ho*: method.)

This method of stroking with the hands encourages the body's own natural energy flow, and also promotes a greater flow of Reiki so that it quickly and easily penetrates the body. Clients often find this technique very comforting and soothing, especially on their shoulders, back, arms and legs.

1   Place your hands flat on the body. Gently, but with an acceptably firm pressure to avoid tickling, stroke your hands in a downwards direction in short movements of about 5–10cm (2–4in), encouraging the energy flow with Reiki, giving gentle stimulation with the friction of the hands.

2   You can also use the same stroking motion from the left side to the right side, and then back again on the shoulders and back, again making sure you do not touch any sensitive or intimate areas.

3   *Gassho*, give thanks for the Reiki and end with a bow of respect.

Oshi-te Chiryo-ho

(**Oshi**: push, pressure; *te*: hand; *chiryo*: treatment, remedy; **ho**: method.)

This is a method of using slight pressure with the fingertips, pushing them gently but firmly into areas such as stiff or aching muscles, or places where there is some numbness or a feeling of energy blockage or stagnation. Care must be taken not to press too hard, of course, and also please be aware of the necessity for reasonably short nails! This technique can be used at any stage of a treatment, but is probably best either at the beginning or the end, so that the client is not disturbed during the more relaxing phases, and again, clients seem to like this technique best on their shoulders, back, upper arms and thighs.

1   Place your fingertips – usually only two on each hand, (or on one hand only), so use either the index and middle fingers or the middle and ring fingers or the tips of both thumbs on the area that is stiff or where you detect a blockage. Gently apply a little pressure, *intending* that Reiki should flow through the fingers to treat that area and/or to break up energy blockages.

2   To loosen particularly stubborn stiff shoulders or aching muscles, start to gently vibrate or rotate your fingers/thumbs back and forth slightly, sending Reiki through the fingertips.

3   *Gassho*, give thanks for the Reiki, and end with a bow of respect.

OTHER *OKUDEN-ZENKI* HANDS-ON TECHNIQUES

Tanden Chiryo-ho

(**Tanden**: energy vessel; **chiryo**: treatment, remedy; **ho**: method.)

This is a particularly useful traditional technique for removing poisons or toxins from the body, whether physical (such as germs, poisons, fumes or chemicals), or mental (such as toxic thoughts, depression, old patterns/habits or negativity), or emotional (such as sadness, anger or grief). It can be used on yourself or on clients; the instructions below are for when using it on yourself, but the hand positions are the same when using it on others.

1   Perform a Reiki Shower or *Kenyoku-ho* on yourself before and after this technique if you are using it on someone else.

2   Sit or stand comfortably, and spend a few moments breathing deeply to help you to become centred with your hands in the *Gassho* position, and allow your mind to become calm. Then *intend* that the Reiki should flow to remove poisons or toxins from the body, and say silently to yourself, 'I begin *Tanden Chiryo-ho* now' or 'let Reiki remove poisons or toxins now.'

3   Place one hand on your *hara* (just below your navel), and the other hand on your forehead, over the brow, and wait. Sense the energy in your hands and hold this position for about five minutes, or until the energy balances in both hands (sometimes it is better to hold the hands slightly away from the body).

4   Remove your hand from your forehead and place it on top of the other hand on the *tanden*, and say silently 'Reiki, please remove all poisons and toxins from my/the body, mind, emotions and spirit.' Then, keeping both hands in place, let Reiki flow to your *tanden* for as long as you feel is necessary – between 10 and 20 minutes.

5   When complete, finish by placing your hands at mid-chest height in the *Gassho* position and mentally give thanks for the Reiki, bowing slightly as a mark of respect.

Heso Chiryo-ho

(*Heso*: navel; *chiryo*: treatment, remedy; *ho*: method.)

This technique works on what is considered in Eastern medicine to be the most important point to heal all diseases – the navel – because it is seen as the energy centre of the body (that is, location of the *hara/tanden/*sacral chakra). This method allows the Reiki to flow directly into the *hara* to balance and harmonise the flow of *Ki* in the body. It requires you to sense the body's energetic pulse – the ebb and flow of *Ki* – which may take a bit of practice, but note that it is not necessary to press hard enough to feel the aortic pulse (blood flow), which can also be detected deep within the body at this point. The instructions below are for self-healing, but the process is the same for working with clients (although it could be seen as a bit intrusive!).

1   Sit or stand comfortably, and spend a few moments breathing deeply to centre yourself with your hands in the *Gassho* position, and allow your mind to become calm. Then *intend* that the Reiki should flow into you to promote deep healing for your greatest and highest good. Say silently to yourself, 'I begin *Heso Chiryo-ho* now' or 'I begin the navel healing technique now.'

2   Place one hand (usually your dominant hand) against your body, with your middle finger inserted into your navel, ensuring that you can feel your own energetic (not blood flow) pulse. (You can place your other hand elsewhere on the body if you wish.) Sense that your energetic pulse is harmonising and balancing with Reiki, as it begins to resonate in harmony with it.

3   Hold this position until you feel relaxed and balanced, which will probably take about five to ten minutes, and then remove your finger from your navel.

4   Place your hands in *Gassho*, give thanks for the Reiki and end with a bow of respect.

USING THE BREATH AND THE EYES WITH REIKI

Koki-ho

(**Koki**: exhalation, breath; **ho**: method.)

This is a method for sending healing energy with your breath, which can be particularly helpful if you are working with clients who have injuries such as burns that are painful to touch or whom you cannot touch for some other reason. You can do this technique at any time during a regular Western-style Reiki treatment, although if you are blowing onto someone's face (not recommended), please ensure that your breath is sweet! It is also suitable for use in general 'first aid' or at many other times when you wish to let Reiki flow to a person, place, object, animal or plant, and so on.

1   Perform a Reiki Shower or *Kenyoku-ho* on yourself before and after carrying out this technique.

2   Spend a few moments breathing in through your nose and out through your mouth, pursing your lips so that they form an O-shape. *Intend* that you are drawing in Reiki with every breath,

and that every exhalation is filled with Reiki. When you gradually feel your chest, throat, nose and mouth become warm, or possibly slightly tingly, you are ready to perform *Koki-ho*.

3   Continue to breathe in Reiki through your nose, and breathe gently and steadily out through your mouth, with your lips still forming an O-shape, directing your breath to the area you wish to receive Reiki.

4   Do this for one or two minutes to each area which needs this form of treatment. To finish, place your hands in *Gassho*, give thanks for the Reiki and end with a bow of respect.

Gyoshi-ho

(*Gyoshi*: gaze, stare; *ho*: method.)

This method for sending healing with the eyes is another one that can be used at almost any time during a Reiki treatment, or for first aid or any other general purpose, as well as for treating burns or injuries that cannot be touched, because it is so easy to do. Gazing with unfocused eyes is soft and gentle, and combined with love, compassion and Reiki it can be very healing; however, it is important not to stare or look aggressively while doing *Gyoshi-ho*. A soft, gentle gaze at the area with unfocused eyes is all that is required.

1   Perform a Reiki Shower or *Kenyoku-ho* on yourself before and after carrying out this technique.

2   Spend a few moments becoming centred by breathing slowly and deeply, and then begin to look at the place to which you wish to send Reiki, let your eyes defocus and soften your gaze. *Intend* and feel that loving Reiki energy is pouring out through your eyes into the recipient, and 'see' them perfect, whole and balanced. You may notice that this technique often creates a particularly compassionate connection between you and your client.

3   Continue for one or two minutes, until you feel guided to move your gaze to the next position, or until you feel that this part of the treatment is complete.

4   Place your hands in *Gassho*, give thanks for the Reiki and end with a bow of respect.

Stage 2 (latter step): *Okuden-Koki*

The Reiki *Shirushi* (symbols)

When a student has demonstrated proficiency at all of the above techniques, they would be allowed to move on to *Okuden-Koki*, or second step. This would include some additional practical techniques, plus three separate empowerments to the Focus, Harmony and Connection energies, plus the *Shirushi* (symbols) and *Kotodama* (mantras) associated with each energy, if required. This would depend on each individual student's spiritual development and level of understanding, as some students would naturally develop the ability to draw upon those energies. In Japan these *Shirushi* would be identified as numbers 1, 2, and 3 (and eventually 4, if a student progressed to *Shinpiden* level) rather than by the names we are more familiar with in the West. The students would be taught how to use the energies after each of the individual empowerments, but these would be introduced slowly over a period of time, with the student practising and meditating on one symbol before being allowed to move on to the next. The interpretation of the symbols in Japan is somewhat different from the Western understanding of their meanings.

- **Symbol 1** is about re-establishing your personal power and connection with Earth *Ki*, so this is the necessary foundation for the other symbols.

- **Symbol 2** is about exploring your mental and intuitive abilities and connection with Heaven *Ki*. The grounding work of Symbol 1 supports this so that any psychic development can be carried out safely.

- **Symbol 3** is about experiencing the concept of Oneness, and your connectedness with everything, where distance does not exist. This therefore links with Heart *Ki*, the balance between Heaven and Earth, so working with Symbols 1 (Earth) and 2 (Heaven) is necessary before introducing Symbol 3 (Heart).

The Reiki *Kotodama* and *Jumon*

The Reiki *Kotodama* are the mantras we are fairly familiar with in the West, but the *Jumon* are vowel sound phrases – the word in

Japanese means 'spell', or 'incantation'. They are based on the ancient idea of the sacred power of sound and speech – that the intonation of special sounds can bring about a mystical or spiritual state, or even achieve a particular outcome in the physical world. Such sounds are used in Shintoism as invocations, in Buddhism as mantras, and in martial arts, such as Aikido as a way of focusing *Ki*.

According to Doi Sensei, the *Kotodama* (mantras) are taught alongside the *Shirushi* (symbols), but other sources say that *Jumon* were used by Usui to help students to resonate with the corresponding energies, and these predated the physical shapes of the *Shirushi* and the *Kotodama*, which he introduced specifically to help the three naval officers to connect to the energies, as mentioned previously.

There are four *Jumon* taught in Reiki, three at *Okuden* level, and one at *Shinpiden* level, and they can be used as an alternative to, or to complement, the *Shirushi*, and they are a wonderful focus for meditation. The three *Jumon* introduced at *Okuden* level are:

1   **The Focus *Jumon***, representing the energy of Earth *Ki*.

2   **The Harmony *Jumon***, representing the energy of Heavenly *Ki*.

3   **The Connection *Jumon***, representing a state of Oneness.

The *Jumon* are considered to be especially sacred, so it is inappropriate to reproduce them in this book, but obviously they can be learned on an *Okuden* or *Shinpiden* course, and some Masters do teach them on the more Westernised Reiki 2 or Master courses. Also, because they are so sound based, it is much easier to learn them if you can hear them being demonstrated!

DEPROGRAMMING AND DISTANT TECHNIQUES

Seiheki Chiryo-ho

(*Seiheki*: habit; *chiryo*: treatment, remedy; *ho*: method.)

This is a technique for releasing bad habits, or 'deprogramming' negative thinking. It requires you to formulate an affirmation, (a short, precise, positive and personal statement), to work on whichever issue you wish at a particular time. (Or you can use the Reiki Principles instead, but making them personal and positive; for example, 'Just for today, I will remain calm' (rather than 'I will not anger').

1   Place your non-dominant hand on your forehead, and your dominant hand on the back of your head, and *intend* that Reiki should flow into your thinking.

2   Repeat your affirmation over and over for several minutes, keeping your hands in place as you do so.

3   Stop repeating your affirmation, and remove your hand from your forehead, placing it with the other behind your head, and continue to give yourself Reiki for a few minutes.

4   *Gassho*, give thanks for the Reiki, and end with a bow of respect.

Enkaku Chiryo-ho

(**Enkaku**: distant, remote; **chiryo**: treatment, remedy; **ho**: method.)

This is a technique from Doi Sensei to send energy from a distance. It may be that Usui Sensei would not teach distant healing, and the necessity of 'connecting' to another person, because he believed in the 'Oneness' and connectedness of all things. In Buddhist teachings, the idea that 'I' is separate from 'you' is an illusion, as we are all One; however, this method is similar to the Western-style Reiki 2 distant healing techniques, and is taught by Doi Sensei.

1   Acquire a photograph of the intended healing subject (person or animal).

2   Place your hands in *Gassho*, and then extend your hands upwards, *intending* to bring in the Reiki energy.

3   Focus on the combined *Okuden*-level Reiki energies, from Connection, to Harmony, to Focus.

4   *Intend* that Reiki flows to the recipient.

5   When you sense that enough Reiki has flowed, place your hands in *Gassho* and give thanks to the Reiki, ending with a small bow of respect.

PRACTICAL *OKUDEN-KOKI* TECHNIQUES

Hanshin Chiryo-ho

(***Hanshin***: half body; ***chiryo***: treatment, remedy; ***ho***: method.)

This is a very soothing, relaxing treatment using very gentle stimulation of both sides of the spinal column, which Dr Usui apparently used to help with nervous conditions, and for metabolic or blood problems.

1   Perform a Reiki Shower or *Kenyoku-ho* on yourself before and after this technique when using it on someone else.

2   Sit or stand comfortably, and spend a few moments breathing deeply to help you to become centred with your hands in the *Gassho* position, and allow your mind to become calm.

3   With the client either seated or lying face down, place one hand flat on each side of the spinal column, starting at the top of the spine (shoulder level) and sweep each hand sideways across the back from the spine (centre) to the sides (either left or right, as appropriate), and gradually work your way down the spine (making about 10–15 outward sweeps).

4   Then hold your index and middle fingers together on both hands and place them one on each side of the spine. Sweep firmly (but not too hard) down each side of the spine from the neck to the bottom. Repeat this action about 10 or 15 times.

5   Take your hands away, *Gassho*, and give thanks for the Reiki, ending with a bow of respect.

Zenshin Koketsu-ho

(***Zenshin***: whole body; ***koketsu***: blood exchange; ***ho***: method.)

This technique is an excellent way of 'grounding' a client after a treatment, and is apparently calming when used with mentally disturbed clients, as well as being useful for blood disorders or metabolism problems. It can be done with the client standing, sitting or lying down.

1   Perform a Reiki Shower or *Kenyoku-ho* on yourself before and after carrying out this technique.

2   Sit or stand comfortably, and spend a few moments breathing deeply to help you to become centred with your hands in the *Gassho* position, and allow your mind to become calm.

3   Place your hands on each of the head positions (front and back, both sides, forehead and base of the skull, as on pages 346–7) and *intend* that Reiki should flow for a few minutes in each position for the client's highest and greatest good.

4   Then give Reiki by placing your hands for a few minutes on first both lungs (either side of the chest), then the heart (centre of chest), then the stomach (solar plexus), and finally the intestines (belly).

5   Sweep your hands gently but firmly down both of the client's arms from the shoulder to the tips of the fingers several times.

6   Then sweep your hands down each of their legs from the thighs to the tips of the toes.

7   Take your hands away, *Gassho*, and give thanks for the Reiki, ending with a bow of respect.

Gedoku-ho

(**Ge**: bring down, lower; **doku**: poison, toxin; **ho**: method.)

This technique is similar to *Tanden Chiryo-ho*, and works to detoxify yourself or a client. It is believed to be especially useful to help to counteract any side effects from medication or chemotherapy.

1   Perform a Reiki Shower or *Kenyoku-ho* on yourself before and after this technique, if you are using it on someone else.

2   Sit or stand comfortably, and spend a few moments breathing deeply to help you to become centred with your hands in the *Gassho* position, and allow your mind to become calm.

3   Place both hands on the body, one in front and one behind, at the level of the *hara* (just below the navel). *Intend* that Reiki should flow into the body of the recipient (yourself or a client).

4   Think or imagine that all toxins and poisons within the body are draining away (you can imagine them draining into the earth, where they can be transformed and used). You might

find it helpful to 'see' with your inner eye the toxins as a thick, dark liquid, which gets lighter and lighter the more Reiki flows into the body. When the thick liquid is replaced by bright white light (this may take 10 to 15 minutes or more), you have finished.

5   Take your hands away, and finish by placing your hands at mid-chest height in the *Gassho* position and mentally give thanks for the Reiki, bowing slightly as a mark of respect.

Genetsu-ho

(**Ge**: bring down, lower; **netsu**: fever; **ho**: method.)

This was apparently one of Dr Usui's main treatments for most diseases, but particularly those involving fever or inflammation. It involves treating the forehead, temples, back of the head, neck and throat, crown of the head, stomach and intestines.

1   Perform a Reiki Shower or *Kenyoku-ho* on yourself before and after carrying out this technique.

2   Sit or stand comfortably, and spend a few moments breathing deeply to help you to become centred with your hands in the *Gassho* position, and allow your mind to become calm.

3   With the client sitting or lying comfortably, place one or both hands on their forehead and *intend* that Reiki should flow for their greatest and highest good. Leave the hand(s) there for several minutes.

4   Move your hands to the client's temples, and let Reiki flow for several minutes.

5   Place your hands at the back of the client's head, letting Reiki flow for several minutes.

6   Place one hand at the back of the client's neck, and the other on their throat (perhaps a few inches above the throat, so that they don't feel threatened) for several minutes.

7   Place one (or both) hands on the client's crown for a few minutes.

8   Place one hand on the client's stomach (midriff area) and the other hand over their intestines (belly area) for several minutes.

9   Remove your hands, *Gassho*, give thanks for the Reiki, and end
     with a bow of respect.

Byogen Chiryo-ho

(**Byo**: disease; **gen**: origin, root; **chiryo**: treatment, remedy; **ho**:
method.)

This is very similar to the *Genetsu-ho* above, and was apparently used by Dr Usui to help to get to the root of a physical
problem, regardless of where in the body the symptoms appeared.
Sometimes, when using this technique, you will receive intuition or
insight (as words, pictures or feelings) about the physical and metaphysical causes behind the illness or disease, and so will the client,
so this is one of my favourite techniques! Ask the client to think
about their condition while you carry out their treatment – they
don't have to tell you what it is – and while your hands are in each
position, see what comes to your mind, and mentally make a note
of it so that you can discuss it with your client afterwards.

1   Perform a Reiki Shower or *Kenyoku-ho* on yourself before and
     after carrying out this technique.

2   Sit or stand comfortably, and spend a few moments breathing
     deeply to help you to become centred with your hands in the
     Gassho position, and allow your mind to become calm.

3   With your client either sitting or lying down, place one hand
     behind the client's neck, and the other in front of their throat
     (perhaps a few inches away, so that they don't feel threatened),
     and let Reiki flow for their greatest and highest good for about
     five minutes, or longer if you feel this is necessary.

4   Then place one (or both) hands on the client's crown, letting
     Reiki flow for five minutes or more.

5   Finally, place one hand on their stomach (midriff area) and
     the other over their intestines (belly area), again holding your
     hands there for five minutes or more.

6   Remove your hands, *Gassho*, give thanks for the Reiki and end
     with a bow of respect.

DAILY PRACTICE AT *OKUDEN* LEVEL

Much of the daily practice students are required to undertake would be the same as at *Shoden* level, with some additions.

1   Begin by preparing yourself for your daily practice by deciding which techniques you will do that day, then sit (in *seiza* or on a chair) or stand, gaze softly downwards towards the floor, release all tension from your body, bringing the focus of your mind to your *hara*, and place your hands in *Gassho*.

2   Chant the Reiki precepts (in Japanese, or in your own language) three times in the morning, and again in the evening.

3   Clear your energies with *Kenyoku-ho*, and follow this with the rest of the *Hatsurei-ho* technique.

4   At *Okuden-Koki* level, follow this with *Jumon* and *Shirushi* techniques (for example, chanting the *Jumon* or meditating on the *Shirushi*).

5   Give yourself a head treatment and/or *Gedoku-ho* (or one of the other *Okuden* techniques) for about half an hour, either sitting or lying down.

6   Keep a journal or diary, writing at least one page each day.

Chapter 22

Shinpiden Techniques (Third Level)

Shinpiden is the Japanese word for 'mystery teachings', and a student would not be accepted for *Shinpiden* training unless they had been practising, and had shown excellence, at *Shoden* and *Okuden* level techniques. The purpose of this level was to focus on furthering personal development and the passing of the system of Reiki on to others. They would receive further spiritual teachings and review and practice in *Shoden* and *Okuden* techniques, as well as another *Shirushi, Kotodama* and *Jumon*; however, being taught *Shinpiden* level would be seen as a beginning, not an end, as the *Shinpiden* student would be expected to make a commitment to Reiki as a life-long practice and learning journey, and as a vital part of their everyday lives.

THE EMPOWERMENT ENERGY

The *Shinpiden* student would receive an empowerment to the last of the four energies used by Usui – the Empowerment energy – and would be taught the Empowerment (Master) *Shirushi, Kotodama* and *Jumon*, and would be instructed in its meaning and usage. The *Kotodama* for this final *Shirushi* means 'great bright light', and becoming this light is to acknowledge the Oneness of everything. This is the task of the *Shinpiden* student – to recognise that there is no duality, no separateness, that everything is connected, and a part of the whole, that we all come from the same Source, and that this is the true nature of existence. The *Shinpiden* teachings are therefore to support the student on their journey of spiritual discovery and development.

MEDITATION AND MINDFULNESS

At *Shinpiden* level the student would be expected to be skilled at meditation, and to be able to reach advanced levels of mindfulness, the Buddhist principle of 'living in the present', having your mind right here, right now, not allowing your thoughts to wander into the past or the future. This engenders a state of tranquillity and relaxation, and enables you to be fully engaged in what you are doing.

Meditation is a really holistic discipline. It creates change at all levels of being, including the physical, emotional and psychological. It also has the power to awaken us to the spiritual levels of our being, and it enables us to discover who we really are and what we might achieve. It brings us to a state of self-realisation, which is the highest expression of human nature.

Meditation is an umbrella word that encompasses a multitude of techniques (see Chapter 16) aimed at achieving an altered state of consciousness which results in a deeply relaxed state that can eventually bring about a state of enlightenment or ecstasy, or both, and there are two major types of meditation.

Most Christian, Sufi and yoga meditation techniques are based on heightened concentration, where you give your undivided attention to a single idea or perception, seeking the total absorption, which leads to understanding. If this is successful, it leads to a trance-like state where external awareness dims and the effects of competing external stimuli fade away. This is probably the oldest type of meditation, and it is found in most cultures in some form.

The other type of meditation is Buddhist, which is itself divided into two strands – *samatha*, which means 'calm', and *vipassana*, which means 'insight'. Both involve the passive examination and then letting go of whatever content drifts into the individual's awareness. *Samatha* is designed to bring peaceful awareness and acceptance, and *vipassana* to bring mindfulness and understanding.

✳

My personal view is that meditation simply allows you to experience and enjoy a feeling of being at one with yourself and with the Universe. It brings an acceptance of yourself and your part in 'the grand scheme of things', and leads to a deepening of 'inner knowing', as opposed to simply having acquired knowledge. Meditation is a mental and spiritual discipline that is open to anyone who is willing to try it (not just to *Shinpiden* students!), although it does require some practice and self-discipline.

Part of what Dr Usui asked us to do was to be mindful and live in the present (just today) and to work hard on ourselves, by which I believe he meant to work on our personal growth and spiritual development through meditation. There have been examples of traditional Japanese meditations in Chapters 20 and 21. But the ideal of meditation practice is to be aware in every moment of your waking life, not just those moments when you are sitting quietly, deliberately meditating. There is no more joyful place in the world than exactly where you are, right now – because you cannot experience real joy when your mind is elsewhere, thinking of what has happened in the past, or what might happen in the future.

Expanding awareness Meditation

Here is a Reiki meditation that is useful at any level of Reiki, not just at *Shinpiden*, as it helps to expand your awareness, and at the same time expand your energies – Earth *Ki*, Heart *Ki* and Heaven *Ki*.

1 Begin by sitting in *seiza* (or on a chair) with your back straight and your eyes gazing with soft focus at the floor. Breathe deeply to release all tension from your body, and bring your mental focus to your *hara* (just below your navel), and place your hands in *Gassho*.

2 Breathe in and place your hands on your *hara* and, as you breathe out, move your hands and arms upwards and outwards, so that your arms are parallel to the ground and your hands are 60–90cm (2–3ft) apart, whichever feels comfortable.

3 Then as you breathe in, move your hands and arms back downwards and together again, and place both your hands on your *hara* again.

4 Repeat this nine more times (ten times in all).

5 Next, as you breathe in, place both hands on your middle *tanden*, in the centre of your chest, and as you breathe out, move your hands and arms outwards in front of you so that your arms are parallel to the ground and your hands are 60–90cm (2–3ft) apart.

6 Then as you breathe in, move your hands and arms back towards your body and place both hands together on your middle *tanden* again.

7 Repeat this nine more times (ten times in all).

8 Next, as you breathe in, place your hands in *Gassho*, and move them upwards until your thumbs are resting on your forehead, the top *tanden*.

9 This time as you breathe out, leave your hands in *Gassho*, still resting against your forehead.

10 Repeat this nine more times (ten times in all).

11 When you have finished, place your hands on your lap and spend a few minutes resting peacefully in your expanded energy.

LEARNING *REIJU*

One important aspect of training at *Shinpiden* level is learning the physical process of *Reiju*, as well as its esoteric (secret and spiritual) meanings, so that you can perform this with your *Shoden* and *Okuden* students; however, *Shinpiden* level does not automatically mean you have to teach – it can be taken as a means to your own spiritual development. The teaching level is described as 'Shihan' and in the Japanese tradition would have required additional training, firstly as a *Shihan-kaku*, or assistant teacher, only progressing to *Shihan* and able to have their own students after gaining considerable practice and experience.

At the workshop in Canada in 1999, Doi Hiroshi taught the Masters gathered there how to carry out a *Reiju* empowerment, although, as I have mentioned before, this was a version of *Reiju* that he developed which is very similar to, but not exactly the same, as the one used by the Usui Reiki Ryoho Gakkai. At a further workshop for Reiki Masters from all over the world held in Kyoto, Japan in November 2000, he held a special *Reiju* class where he again taught *Reiju*, as well as an additional process, which he called Power *Reiju*, which is his way of giving a more intense attunement. He also taught a process of Self *Reiju*, as a method of giving *Reiju* to yourself to help your spiritual development at *Shinpiden* level. Just as with the Western-style attunements, however, it is not appropriate to describe the *Reiju* processes in this book.

To receive *Reiju*, a student would normally sit on a chair in a relaxed but upright posture, with their eyes closed and their hands held in *Gassho*, and this would usually be received during meditation, especially during the *Seishin Toitsu*.

DAILY PRACTICE AT *SHINPIDEN* LEVEL

Much of your daily practice is the same as at *Okuden* level, with some additions, and would be for no less than, and probably considerably more than, one hour per day.

1　Begin by preparing yourself for your daily practice by deciding which techniques you will do that day, then sit (in *seiza* or on a chair) or stand, and gaze softly downwards towards the floor. Release all tension from your body, bringing the focus of your mind to your *hara* (just below your navel), and place your hands in *Gassho*.

2　Chant the Reiki Principles (in Japanese, or in your own language) three times in the morning, and again in the evening.

3　Clear your energies with *Kenyoku-ho*, and follow this with either or both the *Joshin Kokyu-ho* and the *Seishin Toitsu* techniques, or the full *Hatsurei-ho*. Follow this with *Jumon* and *Shirushi* techniques (for example, chanting the *Jumon*), and then with *Reiju* preparation and practice.

4　Give yourself a head treatment and/or *Gedoku-ho*, or a full-body treatment, for at least half an hour, either sitting or lying down.

5   Other meditations and techniques can also be included.

6   Keep a journal or diary, writing at least one page each day.

TEACHING *SHODEN*, *OKUDEN* AND *SHINPIDEN*

Realistically, it is very difficult to combine many of the Japanese techniques into a traditional Western Reiki 1 or Reiki 2 course, so my suggestion would be to include the Reiki Shower and *Hatsurei-ho* in both Reiki 1 and Reiki 2, and perhaps *Byosen* in Reiki 2; however, for many of the other techniques, quite a lot of experience of using Reiki is required before a student can attain the levels of intuition, or trust in the guidance of Reiki, in order to use them. I did start teaching *Reiji-ho* in my Reiki 2 classes, but I found that all I was doing was building in failure (not a good thing to do!), as almost all of the students found it too difficult because, as I soon realised, they hadn't had enough experience with the Second Degree-level energy to develop their perception. This is fairly obvious when you understand that in Japan they would take many months, or possibly even years, to progress their intuitive abilities.

If you want to teach in the traditional Japanese way, then it is important to realise that it is much more about spiritual development than healing techniques, and such growth takes time. Just as with Western Reiki, you need to develop confidence that you have a thorough knowledge of all the meditations and techniques in each of the levels, as well as the origins of Reiki, the four *Shirushi*, *Kotodama* and *Jumon*, and the *Reiju* process. Ideally, you would then teach *Shoden* over a period of about six months or a year, meeting up with your students on a regular basis, perhaps with a foundation weekend, and then one day per month, teaching them one or two new techniques each time, performing *Reiju* on them, and supervising their practice.

When you felt they had made sufficient progress, *Okuden* could then be taught in two parts, with *Okuden-Zenki* techniques in one weekend, followed perhaps six months or a year later by *Okuden-Koki*, but making sure the students practise the techniques in between. One way of doing this would be to hold regular Reiki Share evenings where the students could practise the techniques under your supervision, and receive a *Reiju* empowerment each time. They could then continue meeting regularly after the *Okuden-Koki*, so that you could ensure that they had learned all the techniques effectively.

Shinpiden would not normally be taught for several years after *Okuden*, and could be added to a traditional Western Reiki Master/ Teacher course, teaching the students how to do the *Reiju*, Power *Reiju* and Self *Reiju*. (Some Masters teach only the basic *Reiju* process.) However, doing that would not really be in the spirit of the traditional Usui Reiki Ryoho, so you might consider teaching the *Reiju* processes over a weekend with the students, and then supporting them over the following 12 months with regular meetings to practise meditations and techniques until they – and you – felt confident in their abilities, before giving them a certificate entitling them to teach.

Appendix

Other Forms of Reiki

There has been a considerable increase in interest in healing over the past 25 years, and this has been part of the reason for the spread of Reiki worldwide; however, over that period of time – and particularly since the mid-1990s – there have been many changes in, and an evolution of, the original Reiki system in the West. When, in the late 1990s, information finally came out of Japan about the real history of Dr Usui and the healing system he started and the techniques that we did not know, this caused great upheaval in some Reiki communities, as it challenged their assumption that what they were offering was 'traditional Reiki'.

The situation now is probably even more confused, because 'new' Reiki healing systems are being developed all the time, mostly based on the original Usui Reiki but incorporating new symbols, different attunement methods and lots of new ideas. Add to this the claims that one system is supposedly 'better' than another and counter-claims that other systems 'just do not work', and it is very difficult to cut through the dross and find out what each system offers.

As I explained in Chapter 1, because the word Reiki in Japanese can refer to any healing energy, most of these new healing systems are using that word to identify themselves – and also, presumably, to benefit from the reputation of the original Usui Reiki, which is well known now in almost all countries. I have direct experience of only a few of these new systems – I am a Karuna Reiki Master and a Usui/ Tibetan Reiki Master, as well as a Master in the Usui Shiki Ryoho system from a Western lineage, and in the Japanese Usui Reiki Ryoho system through the lineage of Sensei Hiroshi Doi; however, I have tried to summarise very briefly the main points of those 'off-shoot' Reiki systems that exist at the time of writing this book, most of which seem to have developed in the US. I hope the information I give below will help you to identify any that you might find interesting, because there are many healing paths, and one of these might be right for you. Reiki is a dynamic energy, so it is bound to develop, and we will probably see even more 'versions' of Reiki in the future.

The following is an alphabetical list of the main Reiki styles that exist today, or have existed in the recent past, with some brief details about each. It is designed for information purposes only and is not intended to be a list of recommended styles. I would suggest that if you would like more detail on any particular form of Reiki you carry out some internet research – my own searches have revealed that some of them have generic websites which give more detail, whereas others seem only to have one or two Masters or Practitioners with individual websites.

Amanohuna Reiki

Amanohuna means the 'Abundance of the Right Way of Life'. This system, which claims to have ten levels, was channelled by Arthur Cataldo in Hawaii.

Angelic Reiki

A modern style of Reiki, combining the Usui and Shamballa lineages with what is described as an angelic vibration through Archangel Metatron. (Shamballa Reiki is supposed to originate from the ancient land of Atlantis.)

Ascension Reiki

This is a system taught in nine levels, which claims to have nine additional symbols, and its founder appears to be Jayson Suttkus, from the US.

Blue Star Reiki

This was originally called Blue Star Celestial Energy. It is a channelled energy supposedly originating from an Ancient Egyptian Mystery School and brought through by channelling Makuan, the spirit guide of John Williams, a Reiki Master from South Africa. This system has been modified by Gary Jirauch, who changed the name to Blue Star Reiki. It has 14 symbols (added by Gary) and two levels, both available only to Reiki Masters.

Brahma Satya Reiki

This system was channelled by Deepak Hardiker and claims to be based upon shiva-shakti energy (presumably linked to Hinduism), and is only taught in India and the Philippines. Little else is known about it.

Buddho-Enersense

Sometimes called EnerSense-Buddho, this system claims to be from Buddhist Lamas in Nepal, Tibet and Northern India. It was inaugurated by the Venerable Seiji Takamori, a Buddhist monk. It is a system of spiritual discipline related to healing involving meditation practice and empowerments, using ancient symbology, mantras, yantras (lines, shapes, figures and designs used to impart hidden or concealed meaning) and other aspects of Buddhist teachings and philosophy. (See also Reiki Jin Kei Do.)

Eastern Reiki

A modern term, indicating any Reiki lineages that do not include Chujiro Hayashi or Hawayo Takata.

Gendai Reiki-ho

A system founded in Japan by Hiroshi Doi who trained with Mieko Mitsui, Kimiko Koyama, Hiroshi Ohta and Chiyoko Yamaguchi. Gendai Reiki-ho techniques are based on both traditional Japanese Usui Reiki Ryoho and Western-style Reiki techniques. Its goal is to achieve a state of great spiritual peace.

Golden Age Reiki

This is a system in three levels developed by Maggie Larson (who is also called Shimara) that is similar to Tera-Mai, but with additional channelled symbols and an apparently different type of elemental energy.

Hayashi Reiki Kenkyukai

Hayashi Reiki Kenkyukai means the 'Hayashi Reiki Research Society', and is a term used by Chujiro Hayashi for what he taught.

Ichi Sekai Reiki

This system of four levels was started by Andrea Mikaha-Pinkham, who calls herself a Reiki Grand Master. It is based on Usui Reiki and Johrei Reiki, but with different forms of attunement and an additional Heart Attunement developed by Andrea.

Japanese Reiki

A modern term, usually indicating that the Practitioner or Master is practising or teaching Western Reiki with the addition of specific techniques from Japan that were brought into the West in the late 1990s, mostly by the author Frank Arjava Petter and the Japanese Reiki Master Hiroshi Doi.

Jikiden Reiki

A style of Reiki whose title means 'directly taught Reiki', with the lineage coming through Chujiro Hayashi, Wasaburo Sugano, Chiyoko Yamaguchi and Tadao Yamaguchi. It concentrates on treatment, although it also encourages the broadening of spiritual awareness.

Jinlap Maitri Reiki

This five-level system is also known as Tibetan Reiki, and was developed by Gary Jirauch to follow on from Karuna Reiki Mastership. It claims to be 'Tibetan Reiki in the Medicine Buddha Tradition'. It has 25 symbols and includes techniques such as Meridian Therapy and trauma release.

Johrei or Jo Reiki

This system seems to have been developed from a combination of Raku Kei Reiki and the Johrei religion by a man named Jim Davis in the US, who taught it as one level, but it was the equivalent of going from First Degree to Master in a weekend. The Johrei Fellowship (a non-profit religious fellowship) does not recognise it, and they have trademarked the name Johrei so that any unauthorised usage is forbidden. It is therefore probable that this system is no longer being taught.

Karuna Reiki®

Karuna means compassion, and this healing system was developed by William Lee Rand at the International Center for Reiki Training in the US. It is based on two levels and nine new symbols, plus one Usui symbol and two Tibetan symbols, and the attunement system is different to that of Usui Reiki. William Lee Rand specifies that this system should only be available to Reiki Masters as he wishes it to be an addition to, not an alternative to, Usui Reiki. It seems to activate a different type of healing energy to that brought in by Usui Reiki – powerful and more intense than the gentle flow of Reiki – and it has an interesting spiritual dimension.

Komyo Reiki

In Japan, the word *komyo* means 'enlightenment', so the name Komyo Reiki can be translated as 'Enlightenment Reiki'. Its lineage comes through Chujiro Hayashi, Wasaburo Sugano, Chiyoko Yamaguchi and Hyakuten Inamoto, so it has a very similar origin to Jikiden Reiki, but is closer in content to some other Western/ Japanese-style Reiki lineages.

Mari-el®

This system of one degree (plus advanced techniques) and three symbols was developed by Ethel Lombardi, one of Mrs Takata's original 22 Reiki Masters in the US, apparently in preference to siding with either Phyllis Furumoto or Dr Barbara Weber Ray after Mrs Takata's death. The name comes from Mari, meaning Mary, Mother of Christ, and El, which is said to be one of the names of God. It is not certain whether this system is still being taught.

Men Chhos Reiki® or Medicine Dharma Rei Kei

This system of three levels is supposed to be based on reconstructed teachings from Dr Usui's notes, letters to his students and some of the rare and secret Buddhist teachings which he studied, including 'The Path of the Thunderbolt of Transcendent Light that Heals the Body and Illumines the Mind'. The translations have been carried out by Lama Yeshe Drugpa Thrinley Odzer, a former Shingon Buddhist priest and the Spiritual Advisor of the Men Chhos Rei Kei Institute.

New Life Reiki

This form of Reiki has four levels, and possibly as many as 150 symbols. It seems to have been started by Dr V. Sukumaran of the International Institute of Reiki (an Indian foundation).

Raku Kei Reiki

Raku Kei Reiki has been called 'The Way of the Fire Dragon', and supposedly encompasses the energies of the Fire Dragon. This style of Reiki was developed by Iris Ishikuro, Mrs Takata's sister, and Arthur Robertson, and it is supposed to be an advanced Reiki originating in Tibet. The name Raku apparently means the vertical flow of energy, and Kei is the horizontal flow of energy in the body. It is taught in four levels, with the use of Master Frequency plates, which are supposed to switch the polarity of the body. Aspects of it are also included in Usui/Tibetan Reiki developed by William Lee Rand. It is normally taught only to qualified Reiki Masters from other lineages.

Reido Reiki

A blend of traditional Japanese Reiki and Western Reiki which emphasises meditation and 'living a Reiki way of life'. It was developed by Fuminori Aoiki, whose lineage is Chujiro Hayashi, Hawayo Takata, Dr Barbara Weber Ray, and it consists of seven levels.

Reiki-ho

This is the name given to the system of Reiki healing, also known as Iyashi No Gendai Reiki-ho, meaning the Modern Reiki Method for Healing, developed by Hiroshi Doi, a Reiki Master in Japan who has trained in both the Japanese and Western Reiki traditions. It is taught in four levels; Level 1 is for opening the Reiki channel; Level 2 is for enhancing the Reiki power and extending the use of Reiki; Level 3 is for reaching a higher level of vibration of consciousness and being more creative; and Level 4 is becoming a Reiki teacher.

Reiki Jin Kei Do

Reiki Jin Kei Do is a spiritual lineage and system of Reiki that emphasises the development of compassion and wisdom within one's own life. Its lineage is through Chujiro Hayashi, Venerable Takeuchi, Seiji Takamori, Ranga Premaratna. (See also Buddho-

Enersense.) *Jin* is the Japanese word for 'compassion' and represents the Buddhist concept of universal compassion for all beings. *Kei* is the Japanese for 'wisdom' and represents the Buddhist understanding of universal wisdom, which is the product of deep spiritual practice. *Do* is the Japanese for 'way' or 'path'. It has been transmitted through Buddhist Reiki Masters and therefore has a greater content of Buddhist practices.

Reiki Plus®

This is a system developed by David Jarrell, the founder of the Reiki Plus® Institute (RPI), and is said to embody the philosophy of 'Freedom through Responsibility', the key teaching of Saint Germain. The lineage is through Chujiro Hayashi, Hawayo Takata and Virginia Samdahl, and it is based on Western Reiki with additional metaphysical elements. It is taught as four Practitioner levels and two Master levels in a total of 310 class hours, which include etheric body and soul-level healing techniques and counselling approaches

Saku Reiki

This is a comprehensive wellness programme built around Reiki, but also incorporating nutrition, exercise, herbs, crystals and other natural remedies. It was developed by Eric Bott originally from Germany, but now based in California, US. It is derived from Usui Reiki as well as Karuna Reiki and Tera-Mai, and is taught in six levels over a number of years.

Satya Japanese Reiki

This is another branch of Reiki which originated in Japan, with an Eastern lineage from Usui, Eguchi, Miyazuki, Mitsui, Takahashi, Mochizuki and Sakuma. Mitsui also studied The Radiance Technique with Dr Barbara Weber Ray, and the teaching is similar to that. It is taught in three levels and is found mostly in India.

Sekhem

This system, also known by the initials SKHM, was originated by Patrick Ziegler, a student of Dr Barbara Weber Ray in America, and is apparently based on a combination of Usui Reiki and his experiences in the Egyptian Great Pyramid. (*Sekhem* is an Egyptian word meaning 'power' or 'might' and is the Egyptian equivalent of *ki*.) It has some additional symbols and is taught in five main levels.

Sun Li Chung Reiki

This is a system from Israel that has been channelled by Yosef Sharon. It is taught in five levels and claims to use thousands of symbols (for example, 1,600 symbols at Reiki 2), but the symbols are not given to the students, because they are expected to 'channel' whatever they need, and undergo attunements with their spirit guides.

Tera-Mai® and Tera-Mai® Seichem

This system, taught in three levels, was originated by Kathleen Ann Milner in the US, and it seems to be based on the Raku Kei Reiki system but with different attunement methods and more symbols, some of which are the same as those used in Karuna Reiki®. It includes energy activations to three additional strands of energy called Sakara, Angeliclight and Sophi-el, and uses up to 31 symbols.

The Radiance Technique® (TRT)

Also referred to as Authentic Reiki® or Real Reiki®, this form of Reiki was originated by Dr Barbara Weber Ray, one of Mrs Takata's original 22 Masters in the US. She decided to call her system The Radiance Technique in the mid-1980s, because she described what others were teaching as 'polluted' – hence the other names. The system used to be taught in three levels, but now there are seven levels, still based on the original symbols, but with some additional ones.

Tibetan Reiki

This system, developed by Ralph White, claims a lineage to Tschen Li, further claiming that Tschen Li taught Dr Usui. There are several ways of teaching this system: one that has one level and 19 symbols and another that has 25 symbols. Although the symbols are said to be of Tibetan origin, they do not have Tibetan names. Another version of this system appears to be similar to Usui/Tibetan Reiki developed by William Lee Rand (shown on page 390).

Traditional Japanese Reiki

A school of Reiki developed by Dave King in Canada, incorporating information from the Hayashi line in Japan that does not include the Takata lineage. See Usui-do below.

Traditional Reiki

Traditional Reiki generally refers to the practices of The Reiki Alliance and those Masters who follow closely the Hawayo Takata/ Phyllis Lei Furumoto lineage (see Usui Shiki Ryoho below).

Usui-do (Traditional Japanese Reiki)

This system is from the Japanese lineage through Chujiro Hayashi (but not through Hawayo Takata) and was developed by Dave King and Melissa Riggall. It is very different from other Reiki styles, as it has no Masters, and the attunements are regarded simply as ceremonies. The whole system is driven solely by the intent of the Practitioner who has at his or her disposal a number of 'tools' that affect the way the energy is directed. There are seven levels in a similar ranking system to that used in Japanese martial arts.

Usui Reiki Ryoho

The 'Usui Spiritual Energy Healing Method' is the term used by people with lineages running through the Usui Reiki Ryoho Gakkai organisation in Japan, through the lineage of Kan'ichi Taketomi and Kimiko Koyama, as well as through Hiroshi Doi's Gendai Reiki-ho organisation.

Usui Reiki Ryoho Gakkai

This is a closed society in Japan that was set up to continue the teachings of Mikao Usui. Lineages come through the past and present Presidents of that society, Juzaburo Ushida, Kan'ichi Taketomi, Yoshiharu Watanabe, Hoichi Wanami, Kimiko Koyama, Masayoshi Kondo, and their students.

Usui Reiki/Traditional Usui Reiki

A term used by many Reiki Masters to indicate that they teach Reiki, but they may not confine themselves to any one system, so they may teach elements from a number of different Reiki styles.

Usui Shiki Ryoho

What is usually referred to as traditional Reiki in the West, with the lineage from Mikao Usui, Chujiro Hayashi and Hawayo Takata to Phyllis Lei Furumoto, Mrs Takata's granddaughter. Furumoto and another of Takata's Masters, Paul Mitchell, set up 'The Office of Grand Master' – a term meaning the recognised lineage bearer, which her followers use to describe Phyllis Furumoto – which has outlined what they call the four aspects (healing practice, personal growth, spiritual discipline, mystic order) and nine elements (oral tradition, spiritual lineage, history, principles, form of classes, money, initiation, symbols, treatment) of the Usui Reiki system, all of which they believe should be incorporated into Reiki training and practice. Masters who belong to The Reiki Alliance generally follow this system of teaching in three levels with four symbols. Some independent Reiki Masters also use this system with some minor adaptations.

Usui/Tibetan Reiki

This system, which includes two additional symbols, was developed by William Lee Rand, an American Reiki Master, and is a combination of traditional Usui Reiki, Raku Kei Reiki and his own understandings. It is taught in four levels – Reiki 1, 2, Advanced Reiki Training (ART), Reiki Master – incorporating the four Usui Reiki symbols and two additional symbols said to be from Tibet, but with a different attunement system to that of Usui Reiki, although details of the traditional Usui system are also given to Reiki Masters. Levels 1 and 2 are normally taught on consecutive days. Rand set up the International Center for Reiki Training, and training with Center-accredited Reiki Masters can be counted as part of the training through The National Certification Board of Therapeutic Massage and Bodywork (US) and the American Holistic Nurses Association.

Vajra Reiki®

This system originally came from Johrei Reiki, and was founded, named and trademarked by Wade Ryan who trained in India in the 1970s. He revised the Johrei Reiki system and created a 'new' energy that is claimed to be particularly effective with some of the new bacteria and viruses which have appeared in recent years. It is taught in three levels and includes mantras, meditation and energy polarity.

Resources

Useful Websites and Contact Addresses

Penelope Quest: For information about Reiki courses, retreats and other workshops with Reiki Master Penelope Quest, and for details of all her books and CDs, visit www.reiki-quest.co.uk and www.penelopequest.com. You can also email: info@reiki-quest.co.uk

For details of other Reiki Masters and Practitioners, and useful information about Reiki and other forms of healing, you might like to try the following organisations and websites (contact details correct when going to press):

UK

The UK Reiki Federation, PO Box 71, Andover, SP11 9WQ; website: www.reikifed.co.uk; email: enquiry@reikifed.co.uk

The Reiki Association, website: www.reikiassociation.org.uk; email: co-ordinator@reikiassociation.org.uk

The Reiki Council, website: www.reikicouncil.org.uk; email: info@reikicouncil.org.uk

The General Regulatory Council for Complementary Therapies (GRCCT), website: www.grcct.org; email: admin@grcct.org

The Reiki Alliance – UK and Ireland, website: www.reikialliance.org.uk; email: mail@reikialliance.org.uk

Reiki Healers and Teachers Society (RHATS), website: http@///www.reikihealersandteachers.net; email: info@reikihealersandteachers.net

Reiki Inspirations (Helen Galpin),
website: www.reikiinspirations.co.uk;
email: reikiinspirations@hotmail.co.uk

National Federation of Spiritual Healers (The Healing Trust),
websites: www.nfsh.org.uk; www.thehealingtrust.org.uk

British Complementary Medicine Association (BCMA),
website: www.bcma.co.uk; email: chair@bcma.co.uk

Institute for Complementary Medicine (ICM),
website: www.i-c-m.org.uk; email: infor@i-c-m.org.uk

Healthy Pages Reiki Forum,
www.healthypages.co.uk/forum/reiki-energy-healing

US and Canada

The Reiki Alliance – Worldwide, PO Box 41, Cataldo, ID 83810-1041;
website: www.reikialliance.com; email: info@reikialliance.com

Usui Shiki Ryoho (The Office of the Grand Master – Phyllis Furumoto
and Paul Mitchell), website: www.usuireiki-ogm.com

The International Center for Reiki Training (William Lee Rand),
21421 Hilltop St, #28, Southfield, MI 48034-1023;
website: www.reiki.org; email: center@reiki.org

International Association of Reiki Professionals (IARP), PO Box 481,
Winchester, MA 01890; website: www.iarp.org; email: info@iarp.org

Southwestern Usui Reiki Ryoho Association, PO Box 5162, Lake
Montezuma, Arizona 86342-5162; website: www.reiho.org;
email: adonea@msn.com

The Radiance Technique International Association Inc (TRTIA),
PO Box 40570, St Petersburg, FL 33743-0570; website: www.trtia.org;
email: TRTIA@aol.com

Canadian Reiki Association, Box 54570, 7155 Kingsway, Burnaby,
BC, V5E 4J6; website: www.reiki.ca; email: reiki@reiki.ca

Usui-Do (Traditional Japanese Reiki), The Usui-Do Foundation,
Toronto, Ontario, Canada; website: www.usui-do.org;
email: askme@usui-do.org

Worldwide

Reiki Dharma (Frank Arjava Petter) [Translations available in English,
Spanish and German], website: www.reikidharma.com;
email: Arjava@ReikiDharma.com

Australian Reiki Connection,
website: www.australianreikiconnection.com.au

Reiki Australia, website: www.reikiaustralia.com.au

International House of Reiki (Frans and Bronwen Stiene),
website: www.reiki.net.au; email: info@reiki.net.au

Shibumi International Reiki Association,
website: www.shibumireiki.org

Reiki New Zealand Inc., website: www.reiki.org.nz;
email: info@reiki.org.nz

The Wellness Directory, website: www.wellnessdirectory.co.nz

The Reiki Association of Southern Africa,
website: www.reikiassociation.co.za

Reiki Masters Association of South Africa,
website: www.reikihealing.co.za

World Reiki Association, website: www.worldreikiassociation.org

International Holistic Therapies Directories,
website: www.internationalholistictherapiesdirectories.com

SETTING UP A BUSINESS

There are a number of organisations that may provide help or useful
information when setting up your business, and if you practice outside
the UK an internet search should provide you with similar organisations in your country:

Business Link, website: www.businesslink.gov.uk
HM Revenue & Customs, website: www.hmrc.gov.uk/index.htm
Information Commissioner's Office (formerly the Data Protection
Agency), website: www.ico.gov.uk
Health and Safety Executive, website: www.hse.gov.uk
British Red Cross (first aid training), website:
www.redcrossfirstaidtraining.co.uk
St John Ambulance (first aid training), website: www.sja.org.uk

Website providers: There are many companies providing both website
hosting and easy-to-use programs to build your own website, both in
the UK and in other countries, such as:

www.oneandone.co.uk
www.fasthosts.co.uk

www.host-review.co.uk
www.webhosting.reviewitonline.net

Social networking sites: There are lots of social networking sites on the internet, but the best known and most popular are:

www.facebook.com
www.linkedin.com
twitter.com

Further Reading

The following books are my recommendations from the many available on each subject, and I have placed them under headings to make it easier to find the topics you want to pursue, but many of them cover several categories.

Reiki

Ellis, Richard, *Reiki and the Seven Chakras*, Vermilion, 2002
Hall, Mari, *Reiki for Common Ailments*, Piatkus, 1999
Lubeck, Walter, and Frank Arjava Petter, *Reiki Best Practices*, Lotus Press, 2003
Lubeck, Walter, Frank Arjava Petter and William Lee Rand, *The Spirit of Reiki*, Pilgrims Publishing, 2004
Petter, Frank Arjava, *The Original Reiki Handbook of Dr Mikao Usui*, Lotus Press, 1999
Quest, Penelope, *The Basics of Reiki*, Piatkus, 2007
Quest, Penelope, *Living the Reiki Way*, Piatkus, 2010
Quest, Penelope, *Self-Healing with Reiki*, Piatkus, 2009
Quest, Penelope, and Kathy Roberts, *The Reiki Manual*, Piatkus, 2010
Reiki Council, *The Reiki Council Resource Handbook*, Douglas Barry Publications, 2010 (available through the Reiki Council)
Steine, Bronwen and Frans, *The Japanese Art of Reiki*, O Books, 2005
Steine, Bronwen and Frans, *The Reiki Sourcebook*, O Books, 2003

Energy, auras and chakras

Braden, Gregg, *The Divine Matrix*, Hay House, 2007
Brennan, Barbara Ann, *Hands of Light: Guide to Healing Through the Human Energy Field*, Bantam Books Ltd, 1990
Chopra, Deepak, *Quantum Healing*, Bantam Books, 1990
Eden, Donna, *Energy Medicine: Balancing Your Body's Energy for Optimal Health, Joy and Vitality*, Piatkus, 2008

Edwards, Gill, *Conscious Medicine*, Piatkus, 2010

Emoto, Masaru, *The Hidden Messages in Water*, Pocket Books, 2005

Hunt, Valerie V., *Infinite Mind – Science of the Human Vibrations of Consciousness*, Malibu Publishing Co., 1996

Judith, Anodea, *Wheels of Life*, Llewellyn Publications, 1987

Kingston, Karen, *Clear Your Clutter with Feng Shui*, Piatkus, 2008

Lipton, Bruce, *The Biology of Belief*, Hay House, 2011

McTaggart, Lynne, *The Field: The Quest for the Secret Force of the Universe*, Element, 2003

Simpson, Liz, *The Book of Chakra Healing*, Gaia Books Ltd, 2005

General healing and self-help

Angelo, Jack, *Your Healing Power*, Piatkus, 2007

Chopra, Deepak, *Perfect Health*, Bantam Books, 2001

Chopra, Deepak, *Reinventing the Body, Resurrecting the Soul: How to Create a New Self*, Rider, 2010

Edwards, Gill, *Life is a Gift*, Piatkus, 2007

Edwards, Gill, *Living Magically*, Piatkus, 2006

Edwards, Gill, *Stepping into the Magic*, Piatkus, 2006

Gawain, Shakti, *Living in the Light*, New World Library, 1998

Holden, Robert, *Shift Happens*, Hay House, 2010

Jeffers, Susan, *End the Struggle and Dance with Life*, Hodder Mobius, 2005

Jeffers, Susan, *Feel the Fear and Do it Anyway*, Vermilion, 2007

Loyd, Alexander, and Ben Johnson, *The Healing Code*, Hodder & Stoughton, 2011

Mohr, Barbel, *The 21 Golden Rules for Cosmic Ordering*, Hay House, 2011

Myss, Caroline, *Why People Don't Heal and How They Can*, Bantam Books, 1998

Scovel-Shinn, Florence, *The Game of Life and How to Play it*, Vermilion, 2005

Metaphysical causes of disease

Dethlefsen, Thorwald and Rudiger Dahlke, *The Healing Power of Illness*, Vega Books, 2004

Hay, Louise L., *Heal Your Body*, Hay House, 2004

Hay, Louise L., *You Can Heal Your Life*, Hay House, 2004

Linn, Denise, *Unlock the Secret Messages of Your Body*, Hay House, 2010

Shapiro, Debbie, *Healing Mind, Healing Body: Explaining How the Mind and Body Work Together*, Collins and Brown, 2007

Shapiro, Debbie, *Your Body Speaks Your Mind*, Piatkus, 2007

Physical body

Atkinson, Dr Mark, *The Mind Body Bible*, Piatkus, 2007
Bloom, William, *The Endorphin Effect*, Piatkus, 2001
Holford, Patrick, *New Optimum Nutrition Bible*, Piatkus 2004
Holford, Patrick, *The 10 Secrets of 100% Healthy People*, Piatkus 2010
Waugh, Anne, and Alison Grant, *Ross and Wilson Anatomy and Physiology in Health and Illness*, Churchill Livingstone, 2006

Emotional body

Goleman, Daniel, *Emotional Intelligence*, Bloomsbury, 1996
Hamilton, David R., *Why Kindness is Good for You*, Hay House, 2011
Hicks, Esther and Jerry, *The Astonishing Power of Emotions*, Hay House, 2008
Hicks, Esther and Jerry, *Getting into the Vortex*, Hay House, 2010
Lynch, Paul and Valerie, *Emotional Healing in Minutes*, Thorsons, 2001
McKenna, Paul, *I Can Make You Happy*, Bantam Press, 2011
Neill, Michael, *Feel Happy Now*, Hay House, 2007
Pert, Candace B., *Molecules of Emotion*, Pocket Books, 1999

Mental body

Carnegie, Dale, *How to Stop Worrying and Start Living*, Pocket Books, 2004
Dyer, Wayne W., *Change Your Thoughts, Change Your Life*, Hay House, 2007
Dyer, Wayne W., *You'll See It When You Believe It*, Arrow, 1990
Hamilton, David R., *The Contagious Power of Thinking*, Hay House, 2011
Hamilton, David R., *How Your Mind Can Heal Your Body*, Hay House, 2008
Hamilton, David R., *It's the Thought that Counts*, Hay House, 2005
Leahy, Dr Robert I., *The Worry Cure*, Piatkus, 2006

Spiritual body

Armstrong, Karen, *Twelve Steps to a Compassionate Life*, The Bodley Head, 2011
Hicks, Esther and Jerry, *Ask and it is Given*, Hay House, 2005
Hicks, Esther and Jerry, *Getting into the Vortex*, Hay House, 2010
Myss, Caroline, *Anatomy of the Spirit*, Bantam Books, 1997
Myss, Caroline, *Sacred Contracts*, Bantam Books, 2002
Ruiz, Don Miguel, *The Four Agreements*, Amber-Allen Publishing Inc., 1997
Tolle, Eckhart, *A New Earth: Awakening to Your Life's Purpose*, Penguin Books Ltd, 2006

Tolle, Eckhart, *The Power of Now: A Guide to Spiritual Enlightenment*,
  Hodder Mobius, 2001
Walsch, Neale Donald, *Conversations with God*, Books 1, 2 and 3,
  Hodder & Stoughton, 1996, 1997, 1998

Visualisation and guided meditation

For CDs from Penelope Quest: website: www.reiki-quest.co.uk;
email: info@reiki-quest.co.uk

For tapes/CDs from Gill Edwards: website: www.livingmagically.co.uk;
email: info@livingmagically.co.uk

For CDs from William Bloom: website: www.williambloom.com

For CDs from Esther and Jerry Hicks: website:
www.abraham-hicks.com

Index

Note: page numbers in **bold** refer to illustrations, page numbers in *italics* refer to information contained in tables.

Also available by Penelope Quest, published by Piatkus:

THE BASICS OF REIKI

The Basics of Reiki offers a clear and accessible introduction to Reiki for people who want to find out more about this holistic healing method and the benefits it can offer. In this helpful and easy-to-follow book, you will discover:

- The origins and development of Reiki as a healing system
- What to expect when receiving a Reiki treatment
- How Reiki treats both the symptoms and the causes of illness, easing physical pain and helping to clear emotional blockages
- How easily you can be attuned to Reiki, and what to expect at each level of training
- How to use Reiki for self-healing and for healing other people, animals, plants and the environment
- Practical exercises and visualisations to encourage relaxation and develop insight and energy awareness

978-0-7499-2774-5

Also available by Penelope Quest, published by Piatkus:

SELF-HEALING WITH REIKI

Many people attending a Reiki workshop are taught the basics of self-treatment, but few discover Reiki's real potential for self-healing. It is an amazing tool for healing mind, body, emotions and spirit to create wholeness and harmony, personal peace and a sense of purpose.

Self-healing with Reiki is packed with innovative yet easy-to-use techniques and is aimed at everyone who has worked with Reiki at any level. This book includes:

- The four essential steps to self-healing – acknowledgement, acceptance, awareness and action
- New ways of using Reiki to heal the whole person, from the subtle energies of the aura to the physical body, for a healthier and more balanced life
- A 'whole life' approach to self-healing, including psychological, emotional, social and environmental issues
- Unique methods of using Reiki more creatively for spiritual development and self-understanding
- Techniques from both Eastern and Western Reiki traditions
- Plus exclusive special meditations and easy-to-follow diagrams

978-0-7499-2972-5

Also available by Penelope Quest, published by Piatkus:

THE REIKI MANUAL
(with Kathy Roberts)

The Reiki Manual provides guidance and much-needed support
for students, practitioners and teachers who want to ensure best
practice of this ancient healing art. It can be used as preparation
for, or during Reiki workshops, and also by people who have
already taken Reiki courses and want more information, or wish
to update their skills and work professionally, or simply treat
themselves, family and friends informally.

The first few sections cover all the essential theory and practice
for the first two levels of Reiki. The information is given in an
accessible, structured and interactive way, including a wealth of
helpful illustrations to increase understanding, knowledge and
experience, along with revision questions to consolidate your
learning. The final two sections of the manual contain reference
material specifically for students who want to become professional
practitioners, as well as information about how to become a Reiki
Master, and a teaching guide for Masters who wish to expand the
scope of the training they can offer to their students.

The Reiki Manual can also be used as the foundation for additional
courses or workshops on topics such as health and safety and
managing a successful practice.

978-0-7499-4251-9